The Thyroid Encyclopedia

AN EVERYDAY THYROID DISEASE REFERENCE BOOK

"A little bit of everything about Thyroid Disease"

By Kylie Wolfig

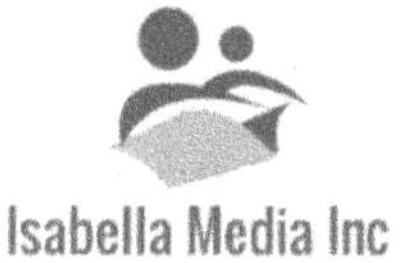

The Thyroid Encyclopedia by Kylie Wolfig
An Everyday Thyroid Disease Reference Book
Published by Isabella Media Inc 270 Bellevue Ave #1002,
Newport RI 02840
www.IsabellaMedia.com

ISBN-13: 978-1-7330416-0-7

For permissions contact: requests@isabellamedia.com

Disclaimer:

This publication is strictly for educational purposes. The methods described in these pages are the author's personal thoughts and experiences. They are not intended to be a definitive set of instructions or treatments for your health.

It is not intended for advice, self-diagnosis, treatment or a substitute for the medical advice of physicians. The reader should regularly consult a physician in matters relating to his / her health and particularly with respect to any symptoms that may require diagnosis or medical attention.

The author shares her own experiences and makes no claims as to its effectiveness on others, nor guarantees the accuracy of any healing properties claimed and disclaims all liability for any use or misuse of the information in this book.

Although the author and publisher have made every effort to ensure that the information in this book was correct at the time of press, the author and publisher do not assume and hereby disclaim any liability to any party for any loss, damage, or disruption caused by errors or omissions, whether such errors or omissions result from negligence, accident, or any other cause.

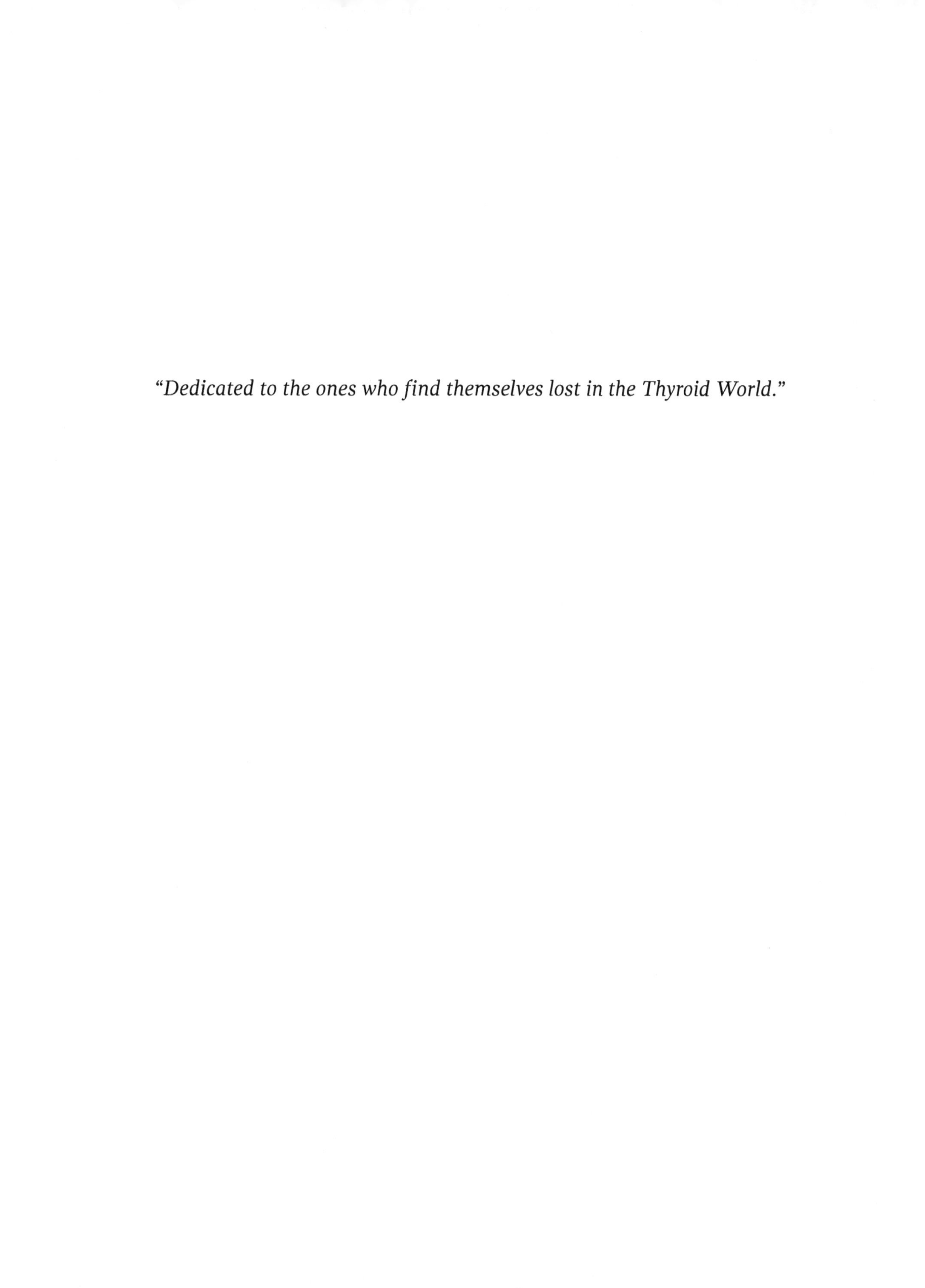

"Dedicated to the ones who find themselves lost in the Thyroid World."

Contents

Acknowledgements

To my Publisher: thank you for understanding the need for such a book and being so easy to work with and patient with me as I found my voice.

My love and gratitude will forever go out to Helen Redford. From the beginning you supported all of my visions, and with Michaels Wings, you helped me with the biggest dream so far.

Dr Gladys Ato, for your mentorship, laughter, support and encouragement to hit "submit" even when the timing seemed all wrong and so many other things were a jumble in my world. I will forever be in your debt.

To Mum, Dad, Stacy and Jonathon I thank you for always being a sounding board and understanding my sometimes lengthy absences from family Skype sessions. I am grateful I can text at anytime and one of you will always answer.

To Jakob, I thank you for understanding that mothers are people too, and for choosing to be patient with me no matter how many movie plots I forgot when my brain just didn't have room to remember them.

And to my husband Oliver, the man who had seen my dream long before I remembered it, I thank you. For always being the voice of reason, the devil's advocate and the idea's man, I thank you. But most of all, for saving me from myself by encouraging me to let go of the brakes, dance all night, and find the joy... for those things I could never ever thank you enough.

Introduction

When I was in Grade 9 my science teacher wrote in my end of year report card "The day I can turn science into poetry is the day Kylie will understand it." Admittedly, I did write poetry in science class, and actual science held no real appeal or relevance for me. But somewhere deep inside it was the start of me believing I was not cut out for higher learning, particularly not in the field of maths or science.

When I was diagnosed with thyroid disease, it was a whole new world of strange science language that I didn't understand. Oddly enough, I didn't see the importance of looking up those words or learning about this disease that I had been told I now have for the rest of my life.

Maybe it was my age (I was only 21) or maybe it was my belief that I would never understand anyway that stopped me from becoming familiar with thyroid disease, either way it led me to a couple of decades of "just getting by" and an ever growing list of symptoms.

Imagine my surprise when at the age of 39 I found myself enrolled in a Bridging course, which, if successful would see me studying Naturopathy, Nutrition and Western Herbal Medicine.

Sitting at the family computer that very first night I opened a rather large textbook. As I began reading the first paragraph, I stopped and let my eyes settle back at the beginning again. I read it 3 more times only to get a horrible sinking feeling that there were about 10 words in that first paragraph I could not even pronounce let alone understand.

But I couldn't turn back. It was a one-way only street I had put myself on by telling the whole world and then some that I was studying to be a Naturopath!

So, thanking the gods that I now live in the era of google (unlike when I sat in Year 9 science) I looked up each and every word. Some words found me having to look up more words until I had gone down a rabbit hole so deep I struggled to remember what word I had started with.

During my 4 years at college and the years since then, I have kept notebooks filled with all kinds of snippets of information about thyroid disease. Everything I learned in college I immediately linked it to how it affected the thyroid. It was my why, it was the whole reason I was there, so it became my anchor.

When I launched Thyroid School in 2015, I quickly found myself answering questions day in and day out.

Since there is only so much my thyroid brain will actually hold at any given time, I would refer to all of my notebooks and binders, for details when writing answers.

It wasn't until my 3rd book Thyroid Habits, where I found myself looking up specifics I knew I had written that I suddenly understood that my books were simply my own reference system.

I made a mental note that it would be so awesome to have a huge book that contained all of my notes and snippets in one place, in alphabetical order to make it quick and easy to refer to when answering questions on the Facebook Page.

The Thyroid Encyclopedia was born in that moment and I decided this book would be the reference book we all needed to interpret all of those other thyroid books and articles. It is not a book you buy instead of another thyroid book, it is the one you keep handy while you are reading the other one.

This book is the one you write notes in the margins, highlight and underline words, dog ear your most often read entries and open at random pages to learn more.

It has been a beast of a book to write, and each time I came close to giving up in overwhelm, I would remind myself I was simply gathering all of my notes in an organised way to make life easier and more streamlined.

And that is what I hope it is for you. A streamlined, organised compilation of snippets, descriptions, explanations and ideas, to make your life easy, and encourage you to learn the thyroid language and find hope in the new Thyroid World you have found yourself in.

Love & Hugs

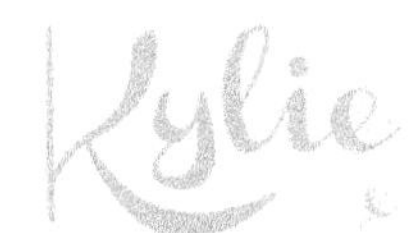

Acknowledge

Stop where you are right now. I want you to acknowledge that the reason you are in the predicament you are in is most likely because of your lifestyle choices.

Yes, you may have a genetic weakness and thyroid issues run in your family, but all defective genes do not get turned on until the body is overloaded with the things that flick the switch.

Although I most likely had a genetic weakness in my thyroid from the day I was conceived, I can't ignore that it was my lifestyle that actually turned that switch on.

I was living on Hamilton Island, off the coast of Queensland Australia. The Great Barrier Reef was my backyard and I was living the kind of life that most would envy (what a shame instagram wasn't around in those days).

Slowly though I was adding habits to my life that would eventually make my thyroid stop working.

You see I began to get fit by swimming in the chlorinated staff pool everyday, which one would say is healthy, however chlorine blocks iodine to the thyroid.

I was also drinking about 10 cans of diet cola every day. This excessive amount of aspartame also contributed to my thyroid going on strike.

I ate fish every single day because I was the supervisor of a fish and seafood take-out (Harpoon Harry's if you have ever been there). While we would all think that fish has iodine and that is fine, fish also contains mercury and anything in excess is as bad as deficiency.

So while I was looking extremely thin and active, all of these lifestyle choices were beginning to add up.

The final nail was stress.

After meeting a man from Perth on the Island I moved to the other side of Australia to be with him. Within the first couple of months I knew I had made a mistake. His life was not what I wanted for my life but I was too proud to speak up. But my body and my thyroid knew what I was feeling and within another couple of months after that the incredible fatigue set in and the weight began to pile on.

The weight piled on so fast that literally one day I could zip up my jeans and the next day I couldn't. I slept whenever I wasn't working and the thought of going out and socialising made me feel sick.

Add to that the stress of my boyfriend thinking I was hiding away binge eating, which actually led to me hiding when I did eat, even if it was healthy! One particular day after walking up to the corner shop for milk he kissed me passionately out the front of the house. I smiled and asked him what that was for. He laughed and said he was checking to see if I had eaten any chocolate while I was up there. I was heartbroken and felt so small I wanted to curl up and disappear.

It was quite some time before I was actually diagnosed, but back then, as it is now, it's an invisible illness that nobody understands unless they are in the trenches with it.

From somebody who knows the heartache and the helplessness, trust me when I gently take your hand and tell you... first you must acknowledge your part in it. Then we can move forward together.

A

A Vitamin

Vitamin A is a fat soluble vitamin required right at the beginning of the thyroid pathway. Fat soluble means it needs some kind of fat to actually absorb it and use it.

The pituitary gland needs Vitamin A to make TSH and if you do not have enough the Pituitary Gland is forced to increase the making of TSH, which can look like we have a lowered thyroid function.

Vitamin A deficiency also reduces the thyroids uptake of iodine which is vital in the making of thyroid hormone.

Deficiency symptoms of Vitamin A include:

- ☐ Acne
- ☐ Allergies
- ☐ Bone loss
- ☐ Diabetes Type 1
- ☐ Dry hair
- ☐ Dry Skin
- ☐ Weak / ridged fingernails
- ☐ Night blindness
- ☐ Lowered immunity
- ☐ Sinus issues
- ☐ Tinnitus

Factors that contribute to Vitamin A deficiency:

- ☐ Alcohol
- ☐ Diabetes

- ☐ Diarrhoea
- ☐ Gall bladder dysfunction
- ☐ Pancreas dysfunction
- ☐ Smoking
- ☐ Stress

Food Sources of Vitamin A include:

- ☐ Apricots
- ☐ Barley Grass
- ☐ Carrots
- ☐ Egg Yolk
- ☐ Fish liver oils
- ☐ Green leafy vegetables
- ☐ Sweet Potatoes

Daily Requirements of Vitamin A:

- ☐ Adults - 5000 - 9000 IU
- ☐ Pregnancy - <5000 IU
- ☐ Toxic Dose - >75000 IU

Abhyanga Massage

This is a traditional full body oil massage performed daily to boost health in Ayurvedic Medicine.

I experienced this for the first time in India, at an Ayurvedic Hospital and found it to be the most stimulating and yet relaxing massage I had ever experienced. It also changed my body shape dramatically in just days, due to its ability to loosen toxins, encouraging them to be eliminated from the body via the digestive tract.

This is a treatment that can and should be done daily at home, on ourselves, with practice. Using sesame oil, it not only aids detoxification but also helps to relieve stress and increase circulation.

Abraham Hicks

The name given to the group consciousness or entity that is channelled by Esther Hicks in The Law of Attraction.

Whether you believe in this kind of thing or not, the teachings of Abraham on Joy, Abundance and living our best life is inspirational.

Abraham encourages us to search for the "better feeling" within us and gives us plenty of practical exercises to help us.

There are an abundance of videos of Esther and Abraham in action on YouTube.

Acanthosis

A skin condition where the folds and creases become darker and thicker in appearance and texture.

Mostly affecting places like the groin, neck, armpits it is more common when obesity, insulin resistance and hormonal disorders are in play, particularly an underachieve thyroid and adrenal fatigue.

It can be treated by losing weight, balancing hormones (neither of which is easy I know) and surgery, if the issue is caused by cancer, which is rare.

Acetaminophen

Acetaminophen is an analgesic used for mild to average pain and fever. Available over the counter it is also sold under the names of Tylenol and Paracetamol. Studies suggest it is one of the leading causes of liver failure.

Seventy percent of the thyroid hormone T4 is converted into its active form of T3 in the Sulfation Pathway in the liver. This is the same pathway Acetaminophen is processed through, so for those of us with lots of aches, pains, migraines and the like, this could be a common way to seek relief that may be causing bigger, underlying problems.

If you take a lot of these types of pain medications it may be a great starting point to count the number you take and start physically reducing that number each day.

Other natural options for pain relief include Turmeric, California Poppy, and Cat's Claw, but it's important to work with an herbalist who can tailor to your individual needs.

Acetyl-L-Carnitine

Primarily used in supplement form for weight loss, acetyl-L-carnitine boosts energy, cognition and memory BUT it is also a thyroid antagonist, so this is one for the hyperthyroid people as it will worsen hypothyroid symptoms.

Food sources to avoid or consume depending on your thyroid issues are:

- ☐ avocado
- ☐ beef
- ☐ chicken
- ☐ fish
- ☐ milk
- ☐ liver
- ☐ Any supplements containing carnitine or Acetyl-L-Carnitine

Achlorhydria

The fancy medical name for an absence of hydrochloric acid in the gut.

We actually need this acid in our thyroid pathway as it helps us to absorb iron and break down amino acids.

For good gut acid levels we need:

- ☐ Iron (we need iron to make gut acid, and then need gut acid to absorb iron... amazing hey?)
- ☐ Vitamin B12 (clams, egg yolk, meat, salmon, liver)
- ☐ Zinc (beef, peppers, oysters, pumpkin seeds)
- ☐ Histidine (found in bananas, chicken, cottage cheese, egg, fish, meat, legumes)
- ☐ Betaine (found in echinacea, astragalus, broccoli, spinach, beetroot, wheat)
- ☐ Pepsin (made in the stomach)

Want to test your stomach acid levels?

- ☐ Mix ¼ teaspoon baking soda in 250ml of water
- ☐ Drink first thing in the morning before anything else.
- ☐ Set a timer to see how long it takes until you burp.
- ☐ If it takes longer than 5 mins or not at all then you are low.

Acidosis

Our body is constantly battling to be in a state of balance between acid and alkaline. Too far either way and health issues can arise.

Acidosis is when the body has become extremely acid including the blood, tissues and organs.

We only have a small pH range between 6.8 and 7.8 in which we are healthy so our body does everything it can to keep things in balance.

One of the ways it does this is "robbing from Peter to pay Paul" so to speak. If our blood becomes too acidic, our body takes its biggest supply of alkaline matter available and leaches it into the bloodstream. What's our biggest source? Calcium from our bones!

High acidity in thyroid disease:

- Increases thyroid inflammation
- Lowers release of T4 & T3
- Raises TSH levels

In one clinical trial subjects were induced into a state of acidosis and then given an alkaliser. T3 levels increased to normal range after alkalising.

Acne

Acne can be an issue for many thyroid people as often it is hormone derived.

Particularly in the case of hypothyroidism, when there is not enough thyroid hormone being produced the body struggles to make steroids from cholesterol, in particular progesterone.

The other issue we have is our impaired ability to convert beta-carotene into Vitamin A.

We need both progesterone and Vitamin A to prevent acne.

Clearly the first step here is to stabilise the thyroid so that we are converting these ingredients, and then if that fails it is worth seeing a specialist about supplementing with straight Vitamin A and progesterone.

Here are a few other things that may help: Vitamin A

- Nutrients: Vitamin A, Vitamin B2, Vitamin B B5, Vitamin B12, Biotin, Zinc
- Internal Herbs for Acne: Andrographis, Blue Flag, Burdock, Calendula, Chaste Tree, Golden Seal, Oregon Grape
- Topical Herbs for Acne: calendula, Oregon Grape, Licorice, Poke Root
- Clean up the diet making sure you are not eating too many processed and fatty foods.

Acrylamides

Acrylamide's are the chemical bi-product formed in carbohydrates cooked above 120 degrees Celsius. It is generally the golden brown colouring on our toast, cookies and other baked or fried foods.

This bi-product has been associated with causing tumours in the thyroid, causing nerve damage and cancer in some animals in very high doses. It is not known what the safety cut off is for humans however most ingested exposure come from French Fries. Still want that fry?

Acute Suppurative Thyroiditis

Accounting for less than 1% of thyroid sufferer's, this uncommon form of thyroid disease is caused by a bacterial infection.

Most commonly it comes from an infection in the sinus cavity of Streptococcus agalactiae.

Symptoms include:

- ☐ Enlarged thyroid gland
- ☐ Rapid onset of pain in either side of the neck
- ☐ Red marks on the neck
- ☐ Painful swallowing
- ☐ Swollen lymph glands
- ☐ Fever
- ☐ General feeling of cold and flu symptoms

While it's easy to ignore the general cold and flu symptoms, any time there is sudden onset of pain in the thyroid area and red markings should send us to the doctor to check it out no matter what our healing preferences are.

Acupuncture

A tool used in Ancient Chinese Medicine, acupuncture is the practice of using extremely fine needles to stimulate certain points in the body.

The Chinese work on meridians that flow through our body, and each meridian has many many points that reflect a system, an organ or tissue. Stimulating that point is a way to stimulate the corresponding internal tissue.

The main point for both overactive and underactive thyroid issues is at Kidney 27. I know that sounds foreign but it is the point below the collarbone and next to the breastbone on both sides. It is a small depression, and I find it is usually quite tender to touch (maybe it's not tender when your thyroid is functioning correctly?).

When looking for an acupuncturist, try to find an old-school little old Chinese man. I have been to a few different practitioners, and it is the older ones that were trained for many years in Chinese hospitals and seem to have more of an intuitive knowledge because of their experience.

Adaptogen

Something which helps the body accommodate to any kind of stress or change. A balancer of symptoms, will lower too much and increase too little.

Eg: Withania, Brahmi, Astragalus, Rhodiola, Gotu Kola

Addiction

Have you heard the saying "... she has an addictive personality". I'm not entirely sure this isn't a real thing, but I do know addictions can be caused by everything from a nutrient imbalance to emotional trauma.

Whatever the cause the starting point is to first recognise we have an addiction to something (without justifying it) and then see what options are out there to help us overcome the addiction and heal the root cause. If we don't dig down to the root cause, that is when we just end up replacing one addiction for another. Eg. give up smoking, start eating more.

There are herbs that can help with addictions of various kinds including: California Poppy, Kava, Korean Ginseng, Passionflower, Siberian Ginseng, Skullcap, St John's Wort, Valerian and Withania.

Nutrients that can help with addictions (and in some cases may be the root cause) include: Tyrosine, dl-phenylalanine, tryptophan, acetyl-l-carnitine, NAD, magnesium, adenosine, and valine.

Addison's Disease

An autoimmune disorder of the Adrenal Glands, in which they don't produce enough hormones due to the destruction of the adrenal cortex.

Symptoms include dizziness, fainting, fatigue, loss of appetite, low blood pressure, low blood sugar, nausea, vomiting, excess urination, craving of salty foods, muscle weakness and pain, weight loss, low libido, and abdominal pain.

Addison's Disease can only be diagnosed medically and is treated with steroids. If left untreated it can be fatal, and is not something ordinarily that can be treated with herbs.

Adipose Tissue

The correct medical term for fat.

It is now considered an organ in its own right due to its content of estrogen.

Adrenal Glands

We have two small glands that sit above our kidneys (one on each). Their role is as our bodies pharmacy and they produce steroid hormones to help with injury, infection and stress.

The hormones they produce are Adrenaline, Nor-adrenaline and cortisol.

The adrenals work in balance with the Thyroid Gland. If one is up the other is down kind of like a see saw. The aim is to get them in balance, like when you were a kid, remember when you and your mate used to shimmy up and down along the length of the seesaw until you were both in the air? We want that for our thyroid and adrenal mates too.

There are basic rules with our adrenals to keep them from going into "fight or flight" which in turn stresses our body and releases cortisol unnecessarily.

- ☐ Eat regularly, including within an hour of rising
- ☐ Include protein (plant or animal) in your meals
- ☐ Don't make coffee your first drink of the day
- ☐ Include good quality pink salt in your diet

There are some herbs that are called Adrenal Adaptogens, because they help to balance the adrenals no matter where they are at. They include: Panax Ginseng, Siberian Ginseng, Ashwagandha (Withania), Holy Basil Leaf Extract, Rhodiola

For Adrenal Exhaustion the following is helpful: Glycyrrhiza glabra (licorice), B Vitamins, Dehydroepiandrosterone (DHEA), andPregnenolone

When trying to address any kind of adrenal stress at all (and really who isn't?) the following nutrients will help: Vitamin B5, Vitamin C, Potassium, Magnesium, Copper (be careful if you have allergies) and tyrosine.

Finally, when it comes to knowing if your adrenals or your thyroid should be the main focus, then it is a simple matter of running a Basal Temperature Test for a full month instead of 5 days. If the graph looks like a roller coaster, then it is your adrenals that is in most need of a hand, if it looks more normal then stick with thyroid as the focus.

Aggression

Although it is a symptom of many disorders such as bipolar, ADHD and schizophrenia, aggression can also be caused by excess heavy metals and toxins.

High copper and cadmium excess has shown up on hair mineral analysis done on extremely aggressive inmates in a high security prison.

Removing all excess sources of these heavy metals and adjusting the diet may help.

Nutrients to include in the diet if aggression is an issue include:

- Phenylalanine
- Tryptophan
- Selenium
- Vitamin B12
- DHA/EPA

Air Hunger

Air Hunger is the odd but unsettling feeling of not being able to breathe in enough air no matter how large a breath is taken (assuming asthma or other lung diseases have been ruled out)

It is commonly reported in thyroid disease but is not life threatening.

Often, finding something to distract you or take your mind off it makes it go away. It is when concentrating on it that can lead to a type of panic that makes the issue worse.

Alanine

A non essential amino acid that the body uses for our metabolic pathways, lean muscle mass, exercise and athletic performance.

Alanine helps our body with:

- Metabolising tryptophan (mental health)
- Metabolising Vitamin B6 (mental health)

- ☐ Regulating glucose
- ☐ Energy for muscles
- ☐ Strengthens the immune system (produces antibodies)

Alcohol

I will preface this entry with a warning that this is not about how you can drink alcohol now! This is simply a reason why so many of us can't drink alcohol and what message it is sending us.

For many years (a good 20 at least) I couldn't drink alcohol without feeling sick within the hour.

Where most people would have a fun night out then suffer the consequences in the morning, I would be heaving over a toilet bowl before the night was in full swing.

I wasn't always like that, it just started in my early 20's around the same time my thyroid disease came along... coincidence??

Fast forward 20 years, and after studying naturopathy and applying many of the learnings, including a lot of work on my liver and a night out with friends revealed my ability to now drink alcohol and not get sick!

Because liver health is one of the major things I incorporate in my life every single day, I can now drink alcohol if I want to, enjoy it and move on.

Do I drink everyday? Of course not! But now if I want to have a cocktail at a party, I know exactly what is going on and that I will need to up my liver health game after the party in return. Let's have a look at what alcohol actually does to our body and why I don't take my sudden new found ability to drink lightly:

- ☐ Leaches out Vitamin A (Thyroid pathway)
- ☐ Leaches out Vitamin B1 (Thyroid health)
- ☐ Leaches out Vitamin B2 (Thyroid pathway)
- ☐ Leaches out Vitamin B3 (Mental health & fatigue)
- ☐ Leaches out Vitamin B5 (Nervous system, muscles, hair & immune system)
- ☐ Leaches out Vitamin B6 (Depression, fatigue, fluid retention, insomnia)
- ☐ Leaches out Folate (MTHFR, cognitive function, muscle weakness, restless legs)
- ☐ Leaches out Vitamin B12 (Cognitive function, Anemia, mental disturbances, restlessness, weakness)
- ☐ Leaches out Vitamin D (Bone health, immune health, Glucose intolerance, nervousness)

- ☐ Leaches out Vitamin E (Thyroid Pathway, Antioxidant, fluid retention, muscle wasting, Liver disease, immune health, cholesterol)
- ☐ Leaches out Magnesium (Fatigue, Fluid retention, chronic pain, unstable blood sugar, insomnia, anxiety, depression, concentration)
- ☐ Leaches out Selenium (Thyroid Pathway, autoimmune, Depression, Arthritis)
- ☐ Flushes out Zinc (healing, thyroid health, mental health)

Clearly in some way or another alcohol finds a way to chase out pretty much all the nutrients in our body that we need.

Just to be clear, my liver improvement wasn't instant either. It happened over a couple of years, so don't think you can do one or two things, pop a multivitamin this week and go out partying this weekend ok? But this is what did and still do to improve my liver:

- ☐ Coffee Enemas
- ☐ Lemon Water
- ☐ Green Juicing
- ☐ Hippocrates Soup & lots of Vegetables
- ☐ St Mary's Thistle & Globe Artichoke

Alcohol Ablation

Used for removal of thyroid cystic nodules, the procedure involves using a needle to drain fluid from the nodule and then inject a small amount of ethanol which stops the blood supply to any dangerous, cancerous cells in the attached lymph nodes.

Aldosterone

A hormone produced by the adrenal glands.

The job of this hormone is to tell the kidneys how much sodium to release into the blood and how much potassium to release in the urine.

Excess aldosterone causes low levels of potassium and high blood pressure.

Low levels of aldosterone are a sign of Addisons' Disease, a rare adrenal disease which is fatal if untreated.

Alkaline Diet

Our entire bodies focus is actually to keep our blood in the correct pH. This is referred to as homeostasis.

Once we become to acid then it has to find a way to alkalise our blood to get back to homeostasis. In most cases it does this by pulling calcium from our bones which is our bodies biggest source of alkalising minerals.

And before you think "...calcium? oh I will drink some milk" it is actually acidifying to us as it was not designed for our body, plus milk is heated and treated so much prior to drinking which makes it worse.

So how do we alkalise?

- ☐ Eating your greens
- ☐ Eating your greens
- ☐ Eating fruit
- ☐ Eating your greens
- ☐ Eating vegetables
- ☐ Eating your greens

Oh and did I say eat your greens????

And believe it or not, lemons are ALKALISING in the body. True - don't believe me, research it lol.

Allergies

Food Allergies

Anything that we are allergic or intolerant to causes inflammation of some degree in our body. It doesn't have to be a full blown allergy such as celiac disease, it can simply be an intolerance to something as simple as lettuce (27% of people at any one time are intolerant to it)!

A reminder that Thyroid Disease is an inflammatory disease so anywhere we can reduce the inflammation so that our body can focus on healing then we should.

A big clue will be those foods we don't eat often cause we "don't feel quite right" after eating it. It could be we are intolerant to it and it's causing some inflammation.

Trying an elimination diet can be helpful in figuring out what may be causing you an issue. Having an allergy test or food intolerance test can be problematic because they can change in as little as 6 months.

Environmental Allergies

Having hay fever and sinusitis is miserable. Taking a tablet everyday to combat it is also pretty hard on our liver.

When we get a lot of allergies we get a build up of histamines in our body (which is why we take antihistamines such as clarytine).

Common causes of a build up of histamines include:

- ☐ Medications including heart, antidepressants, antipsychotics, gut medications
- ☐ Diuretics, muscle relaxants, malaria drugs
- ☐ Aspirin, NSAIDS, Voltaren
- ☐ Alcohol, extreme stress, liver disease
- ☐ Deficiencies in Vitamin B6, Vitamin C, Copper or Zinc

Allopathic Medicine

The collective term for western medicine. Use this terminology when you want to sound fancy.

Aloe Vera

An evergreen succulent, the aloe vera plant is hard and spiky on the outside yet soft and gooey on the inside. And so easy to grow that everyone should have it in their garden or a pot.

Uses I have found in research for Aloe vera include:

- ☐ Improve digestion, soothe reflux
- ☐ Anti-inflammatory
- ☐ Soothe sunburn and burns
- ☐ Blocks plaque when used as a mouthwash
- ☐ Lowers blood sugar
- ☐ Natural laxative
- ☐ Antimicrobial
- ☐ Protects the skin from sun damage
- ☐ Protects the skin from damage after radiation therapy
- ☐ Improves cognition and lowers depression
- ☐ Make up remover

And a final tidbit, I read that Jennifer Anniston stays so young by cutting open an Aloe leaf every day and rubbing it all over her face. You can decide if it's true or not. I actually had a go and it is very tightening on the skin, so maybe there is some validity.

I guess I would only find out if I did it everyday, and sadly after the first time I forgot to do it again!

Alopecia

As it is an autoimmune disease, thyroid people are susceptible to alopecia.

This disease usually has a sudden onset and is characterised by small patches of hair falling out all over the scalp.

There is no known cure for it, however working on the immune system and stopping the overall attack may help both the thyroid and alopecia at the same time.

Some deficiencies that can be involved include:

- Biotin deficiency
- Vitamin A Deficiency (common in thyroid disease)
- Zinc deficiency
- Protein deficiency

Alpha-Lipoic-Acid

Alpha-Lipoic Acid is classed as an antioxidant and a fatty acid.

- Involved in metabolism and energy production
- Reduces inflammation
- Chelates heavy metals (will cross the blood-brain barrier to chelate metals in the brain)
- Protects against Arsenic, cadmium, mercury, lead
- Increases glutathione levels
- Can reduce liver fibrosis in Hepatitis
- Promotes liver regeneration

Dietary sources of Alpha-Lipoic Acid include:

- Red meat, organ meat
- Spinach, brussels sprouts, carrots, beets
- Potatoes, yams, tomatoes
- Rice Bran

Side effects from taking supplement form (over 2,400mg) include:

- Skin rashes
- Muscle cramps
- Headaches
- Pins and needles

ALT

Alanine Aminotransferase (ALT) is an enzyme in the blood that is generally found in small amounts. The test is run at the same time your doctor orders a full liver panel.

High ALT results show that the liver has suffered damage with common causes being hepatitis, alcohol abuse, kidney damage, heart failure, autoimmune disorders including celiac disease and non-alcoholic fatty liver disease.

This test is the one that told me many years ago that my liver was damaged due to Non-Alcoholic Fatty Liver Disease (NAFLD), so the damage was simply being done by the excess weight I had carried for so many years.

It is a great idea to track your liver results over time to keep an eye on this level.

Alterative

An agent used to improve elimination of metabolic waste to facilitate the restoration of normal bodily functions.

It provides gradual beneficial change over time in the body.

Examples include: Alfalfa, Burdock, Chickweed, Comfrey

Aluminium

Considered one of our toxic metals, in excess it exhibits symptoms such as:

- Mood swings
- Brain irritation
- Depleted calcium in joints
- Interferes with normal immune function
- Grumpiness
- Associated with Dementia and Alzheimers.

For thyroid people, it is important to also know that high parathyroid activity will make the body absorb even more aluminium which results in lowered thyroid function.

In the year 2000 childhood vaccinations, which originally contained mercury as the irritant that causes the immune system to notice the pathogens, were swapped out for aluminium due to concerns about the toxicity of mercury.

As with all heavy or toxic metals, they have opposing nutrients in the body, that stop them taking up residence. In the case of Aluminium it is Silica, so as long as we have a lot of silica in our diet and body it should counteract any aluminium. The problem here is that our depleted soils no longer have much silica in them, so we are not getting enough in our natural diet.

Add to that, we seem to be getting aluminium from so many sources now that it is hard to avoid. Some sources include bakeware, soft drinks and cola tins, underarm deodorant, baking soda, and some bakery products.

American Thyroid Association

Founded in 1923, ATA is a support group and information base for thyroid sufferer's in America. They have a mass amount of information, papers and articles on their site and they run conventions regularly.

Thyroid.org

Amines

Although amines are referred to as a group of foods, it actually is a term for a natural byproduct of bacteria that is produced during fermentation, storage or breakdown of certain foods. These chemicals have a cumulative action, meaning they continue to build up in the body

The main culprit in this group are called histamines and are responsible for many allergies but there are many others.

As you can see from the following list, there are so many foods involved here that it is easy to see how it could be a hidden cause of migraines, nasal congestion, sinusitis, fatigue, hives, and digestive problems.

Fruits high in Amines:

- ☐ Avocado
- ☐ Banana

- ☐ Berries
- ☐ Custard Apple
- ☐ Cherries
- ☐ Citrus
- ☐ Dates
- ☐ Figs
- ☐ Mango
- ☐ Papaya
- ☐ Kiwifruit
- ☐ Passionfruit
- ☐ Pineapple
- ☐ Plums
- ☐ Dried Fruits

Vegetables high in Amines:

- ☐ Broccoli & broccolini
- ☐ Cauliflower
- ☐ Radicchio
- ☐ Rocket
- ☐ Tomatoes
- ☐ Sauerkraut
- ☐ Pickled vegetables
- ☐ Vegetable juice & vegetable stock
- ☐ Vegetable soups
- ☐ Truffles
- ☐ Spinach, Chinese spinach, choy sum
- ☐ Mushrooms
- ☐ Seaweed

Dairy high in Amines:

- ☐ Cheese, cheese slices, soft cheese
- ☐ Soy cheese
- ☐ Fruit flavoured yoghurt
- ☐ Chocolate milk

Animal Products high in Amines:

- ☐ Chicken Skin
- ☐ Pork, Turkey, Prawns, aged Beef
- ☐ Fish Fingers & Frozen Fish
- ☐ Canned salmon, tuna & sardines
- ☐ Bacon, Ham, Salami
- ☐ Chicken nuggets, meat pies, sausages
- ☐ Offal, liver, fritz
- ☐ Fish and meat pastes

Legumes, Nuts & seeds high in Amines:

- ☐ Almonds, brazil nuts, chestnuts, coconut, hazelnuts, macadamia nuts, peanuts, pecans, pine nuts, pistachio nuts, walnuts
- ☐ Linseeds, flaxseed, pumpkin seeds, sesame seeds, sunflower seeds, black nigella seeds, mustard seeds
- ☐ Nut flours, falafel, humus, nut pastes, tahini, broad beans

Baking Aids & condiments high in Amines:

- ☐ Gravy, sauces, stock cubes, stock liquid, stock powder
- ☐ Coconut milk & Cream
- ☐ Tomato paste, sauce & puree
- ☐ Vinegar (excluding Malt vinegar)
- ☐ Mustard, curry powder, chicken salt
- ☐ Fish sauce, oyster sauce, soy sauce, miso
- ☐ Tamari, tempeh
- ☐ Coconut oil, Olive oil, peanut oil, copha, almond oil, avocado oil, sesame oil, walnut oil, flavoured oils, salad dressings
- ☐ Applesauce, fruit jams, fruit conserves
- ☐ Lemon Butter, chocolate spread, yeast spread
- ☐ Maple flavoured syrup, chocolate syrup

Snacks high in Amines:

- ☐ Chocolate
- ☐ Flavoured Corn chips, flavoured rice crackers
- ☐ Cough lollies, throat lozenges, Butter Menthols
- ☐ Cakes, Cookies, granola bars
- ☐ Pastries with chocolate, fruit, nuts, jelly and coconut

Amino Acids

These are organic compounds that make up the building blocks of protein.

There are two kinds of Amino Acids - essential and non-essential.

The essential amino acids are named because our bodies cannot make these on its own, they must come from a food source. Non-essential amino acids our body has the ability to make from other ingredients.

Essential amino acids are:

- Isoleucine
- Leucine
- Lysine
- Methionine (needed for methylation)
- Phenylalanine (precursor to Tyrosine)
- Threonine
- Tryptophan (mental health)
- Valine

Non Essential Amino Acids are:

- Alanine
- Arginine
- Asparagine
- Aspartic Acid
- Cystine
- Glutamic Acid
- Glutamine (joint health)
- Glycine
- Proline
- Serine
- Tyrosine (a major ingredient in thyroid hormone)

Analgesic

An agent used to relieve pain either orally or topically.

Examples Include: Arnica (topically), California Poppy, Devil's Claw, Kava, Peppermint (topically), Willow Bark

Anaphrodisiac

An agent used to lessen sexual function and desire.

Example: Hops.... that explains beer right?

Androgens

A collective name for the group of steroids produced by the testes, ovaries and adrenal glands, that stimulate male characteristics such as a deep voice and excess facial hair.

Often females can suffer from an excess of androgens. This can be tested through your doctor and is generally tested via blood or saliva.

Herbs to help reduce excess androgens include: Chaste Tree, Licorice, and Paeonia.

Andrographis

An herb used to help improve the liver, Immune system, and parasites.

Avoid in the first Trimester of Pregnancy.

Use with caution if on immunosuppressive drugs.

Anger

The liver is known as the "Seat of Anger" so if you or someone you know struggles with anger issues, liver health might be a great place to start.

Angina

Chest pain occurring when the heart is deficient in oxygen.

The underlying cause is Coronary Heart Disease and can be both stable (after activity or emotion) or unstable (sudden and without cause).

Angina is NOT a heart attack, but is a sign that you are at high risk of one if changes are not made.

Nutrients to help reduce symptoms include: a plant based diet, low salt, reduce processed foods, reduce alcohol and smoking.

Herbs to help reduce angina symptoms include: coleus, Dan Shen, Ginger, Hawthorn, Lime Flowers, Olive Leaf, and Turmeric.

Angiogenesis Inhibitors

Angiogenesis is the formation of new blood vessels. Inhibitors are something that stops the creating of those new blood vessels.

Why do we want that? New blood vessels help support the growth of tumours, cancer and fat deposits. If they don't have a blood supply, they can't be there.

Dietary sources of naturally occurring Angiogenic foods include:

- Strawberries and blackberries
- Oranges, grapefruit, lemons
- Apples, pineapple, cherries, red grapes
- Bok choy, kale, mushrooms, artichokes, pumpkin, tomato, avocado
- Green tea, red wine, dark chocolate
- Olive oil, grape seed oil
- Licorice, cinnamon, turmeric, nutmeg, parsley, garlic

Anodyne

Similar to an analgesic, this is an agent used to soothe or ease pain.

Examples include: California Poppy, Arnica, Devil's Claw, Kava, Willow Bark

ANS

The shortening for the Autonomic Nervous System. The system in the body that acts "automatically" by regulating functions such as the heart, breathing, arousal, and urination.

Antacid

An agent used to neutralise acid in the stomach. This could mean herbal as well as medicinal.

Example includes: Meadowsweet

Anthelmintic

An agent used to expel or destroy parasitic worms in the gastro-intestinal tract.

Examples Include: Black Walnut, Cloves, Feverfew, Garlic, Myrrh, Wormwood

Anti-arthritic

An agent used to relieve and heal arthritic conditions.

Examples Include: Cat's Claw, Turmeric, Boswelia

Antibacterial

A substance that destroys or arrests the growth of microorganisms.

Examples include: Barberry, Garlic, GoldenSeal, Green Tea, Myrrh, Oregano, Pau d'Arco, Pelargonium, Thyme

Antibiotics

Although most of us know that antibiotics wreak havoc on our gut health, requiring a good round of probiotics afterwards to improve the flora again, not many know that a particular type of antibiotic can also wreak havoc on the thyroid.

There is a type of commonly prescribed antibiotics called Fluoroquinolones and the problem is that they are based on fluoride.

Fluoride is a known neurotoxin and it also blocks iodine from the thyroid. The side effects are alarming, so they should only be used in the absolute worst bacterial cases after exhausting all other options.

Next time your doctor writes you a script, be sure it isn't one of these, and if it is, ask them to write a script for one that isn't based on fluoride.

Antibodies

Fighters that come out to attack and neutralise any pathogens (bad guys) that don't belong in the body such as bacteria or viruses.

When we are tested for Autoimmune disease, it is the number of antibodies that are tested because that then tells us that our thyroid has sent out its fighters for protection against something.

To be diagnosed with autoimmune thyroid disease the following antibody blood tests need to be ordered by a physician. You may need to ask them to do it though!

- ☐ TPO Ab - Anti-thyroperoxidase - will be found in both Hashimoto thyroiditis and Graves Disease and also in preterm labour
- ☐ TGAb - this detects an attack on thyroglobulin, a protein involved in T3 transport to the cells. These antibodies can show up in Thyroid cancer.

- TSHR Ab - Thyroid Stimulating Hormone Receptor antibodies - These antibodies can indicate Grave's Disease.

Anticarcinogenic

An agent that reduces the frequency or occurrence of spontaneous or induced cancers.

Examples Include: Green Tea, Licorice

Anticarrhal

An agent which reduces catarrh or excessive mucus secretion.

Examples Include: Elder Flower, eyebright, Golden Seal, Horseradish, Mullein, Ribwort

Anticoagulant

An agent which slows or prevents clotting of blood.

Examples Include: Dan Shen, Garlic, Turmeric, Ginger, Gingko, Vitamin E

Antidepressant

An agent that prevents or relieves depression. This could be a pharmaceutical based agent or a natural one.

Examples of natural anti-depressants include: Lavender, St John's Wort, Schisandra and the combination of turmeric & black pepper.

Many people who are on antidepressants start taking St John's Wort, but it must be monitored as you will likely need less of the anti-depressant. The other thing to note with this herb is that it takes about 4 weeks to have an effect as it is accumulative.

Antigen Presenting Cell

APC is a cell created when a macrophage cell (an immune system cell that eats intruders, parasites, bacteria etc) attaches to an intruder.

The APC then raises the alarm which lets the immune system know it needs to come and help.

Antihistamine

An agent that reduces or inhibits Histamines, a response in allergies.

Examples Include: Astragalus, Nettle Leaf, Spirulina

Anti-inflammatory

An agent that works to contain the inflammatory process. Pharmaceutical ones are NSAIDS such as Nurofen plus there are many natural options.

Topical Examples of anti-inflammatory herbs include: Arnica, Calendula, chamomile, Licorice, Myrrh, Yarrow

Gut Examples of anti-inflammatory herbs include: Bilberry, Calendula, Chamomile, Fenugreek, Licorice, Meadowsweet, Yarrow

Musculoskeletal Examples of anti-inflammatory herbs include: Boswelia, Cat's claw, Celery Seed, Ginger, Rosehips, Turmeric, Withania

Immune System Examples of anti-inflammatory herbs include: Baical Skullcap, Bupleurum, Feverfew, Gotu Kola, Rehmannia, Sarsaparilla

Let's also remember that exercise is an amazing natural anti-inflammatory!

Antilithic

An agent used to prevent the formation of calculi (stones) or gravel in the urinary system or gallbladder.

Examples Include: Corn Silk, Gravel Root, Hydrangea

Antimitotic

An agent which inhibits the division of cells (a process called mitosis). It is used for cancer cells that grow as they divide.

Antioxidant

An agent that prevents oxidation, a process believed to be the initiating factor in the development of many disease conditions such as cancer and heart disease.

Examples Include: Bacon, Cat's Claw, Elder Berry, Garlic, Gingko, Green Tea, Hawthorn, Oregano, Rhodiola, Rosemary, Sage, Thyme, St Mary's Thistle, Turmeric

Antipruritic

An agent that stops itching.

Topical Examples Include: Kava, Peppermint

Antiseptic

An agent used to prevent, resist and counteract infection.

Examples include: Iodine, Calendula, Boswelia, Aloe Vera, and Eucalyptus.

Antispasmodic

An agent used to reduce or prevent excessive involuntary muscular contractions or spasms.

Examples Include: Cayenne, chamomile, Cinnamon, Coleus, Cramp Bark, Fennel, Hops, Kava, Lavender, Lemon Balm, Lime Flowers, Passionflower, Peppermint, Rosemary, Shatavari, Thyme, Valerian, Yarrow

Antisudorific

An agent which stops or prevents sweating.

Examples include: Valerian root, chamomile, sage

Antithyroid Drugs

Drugs used to decrease or stop the output of thyroid hormone in the treatment of Graves' Disease and hyperthyroidism.

Because hyperthyroidism and Graves is extremely dangerous to the heart, if these drugs cannot stabilise the disease within 2 years, surgery is recommended by doctors.

These include:

- Carbimazole - inhibits the making of hormone
- Methimazole - inhibits the making of hormone
- Propylthiouracil - inhibits the making of thyroid hormone
- Iodine - inhibits the release of thyroid hormone
- Radioactive Iodine - kills the thyroid

It is a valuable piece of information here to know that many years ago fluoride was also used to treat hyperthyroidism.

Antithyroid

Drugs used to decrease or stop the output of thyroid hormone in the treatment of Graves' Disease and hyperthyroidism.

Because hyperthyroidism and Graves is extremely dangerous to the heart, if these drugs cannot stabilise the disease within 2 years, surgery is recommended by doctors.

These include:

- ☐ Carbimazole - inhibits the making of hormone
- ☐ Methimazole - inhibits the making of hormone
- ☐ Propylthiouracil - inhibits the making of thyroid hormone
- ☐ Iodine - inhibits the release of thyroid hormone
- ☐ Radioactive Iodine - kills the thyroid

It is a valuable piece of information here to know that many years ago fluoride was also used to treat hyperthyroidism.

Antitussive

An agent which relieves or reduces coughing.

Examples Include: Bupleurum, Licorice, Peppermint, Schisandra, Wild Cherry, Bromelain

Antiviral

An agent which kills or inhibits viral action.

Examples Include: Elder Berry, Propolis, St John's Wort, Thyme

Topical Examples: Calendula, Celandine, Green Tea, Lemon Balm

Anxiety

This is a big topic today and a very common issue in thyroid people. As we have many T3 receptors (remember they are the homes for our active hormone) in our brains, if we don't have any hormone getting to them, mental health symptoms will arise very quickly. In fact it is often the first sign of thyroid disease that we don't recognise.

There are several types of anxiety, they include:

- Generalised Anxiety Disorder - constant, excessive worry about general every-day things.
- Social Anxiety Disorder - a phobia about being in social situations, generally a fear of embarrassment, rejection or feeling like they don't belong.
- Panic Disorder - regular panic attacks couples with severe physical symptoms like shortness of breath and dizziness.

If anxiety is an issue, making sure your thyroid pathway is optimal is the first step. If the receptors in your brain are not getting any thyroid hormone it doesn't matter what else you try.

Other things to try:

- Meditation
- Breathing techniques
- Get regular exercise
- Cut down on caffeine & alcohol
- Quit Smoking
- Cut out processed foods and junk foods
- Try an elimination diet (I found that dairy was the cause of my panic attacks years ago)
- Eat fresh whole foods
- Herbs to help reduce anxiety include: Bacopa, California poppy, Corydalis, Damiana, Hawthorn, Hops, Kava, Lavender, Lemon Balm, Lime flowers, Passionflower, St John's Wort, Valerian, Zizyphus
- Micronutrients to help include: Vitamin B3, Vitamin B6 and zinc

It is important to not try and cope with this on your own. Seek help from whomever you need to for support around this.

Anxiolytic

An agent that reduces anxiety.

Examples Include: Bacon, California Poppy, Green Oats, Kava, Lavender, Mexican Valerian, Passionflower, Valerian, Zizyphus

Aphrodisiac

An agent used to stimulate sexual interest.

Examples Include: Shatavari, Tribulus Leaf, Damiana, Oysters, Figs, chocolate, strawberries

Apple Cider Vinegar

A fermented vinegar made from apples sugar and yeast, Apple Cider Vinegar is considered a miracle liquid by many, and is said to be able to cure everything from warts to reflux. I know several people who use it to improve digestion with great success and drink a tablespoon in water with every meal.

The Gerson Institute uses a dressing of ACV, FlaxSeed Oil and Raw Honey for their salad dressings, and it's really yummy.

Let's look at a small list of what it is said to do:

- ☐ Improves allergies
- ☐ Improves sinus infections
- ☐ Alkalises the body
- ☐ Anti-viral
- ☐ Anti-fungal
- ☐ Anti-bacterial
- ☐ Reduces toxicity in the body
- ☐ Soothes insect bites
- ☐ Soothes skin allergies
- ☐ Helps with weight loss
- ☐ Relieves acid reflux
- ☐ Regulates blood sugar levels
- ☐ Lowers Cholesterol
- ☐ Reduces Blood Pressure
- ☐ Improves Gut Health
- ☐ Reduces varicose veins (topically)
- ☐ Treats warts (topically)

- □ A Natural deodorant (topically)
- □ As a rinse, improves Hair health

Be careful though if:

- □ you have diabetes, it can alter insulin levels
- □ you already have low potassium as it can lower potassium levels
- □ you have weak tooth enamel as it can damage it further, best to use a straw
- □ you have excess gut acid

When purchasing Apple cider vinegar, ensure you have a brand that is organic and still contains the "mother" which will be evident in the bottle. Look for floating bits that make it look like it is old and fermented! Yep really!

Aquaretic

An agent that makes us pee more by increasing kidney function but without the loss of electrolytes such as potassium that you may get from taking diuretics.

Arginine

This is a non-essential amino acid, however, when we are in sickness or disease, it becomes an essential amino acid.

Arginine is a neurotransmitter and helps our body with:

- □ Relaxing blood vessels (better circulation)
- □ Methylation
- □ Modulates the immune system
- □ Wound healing
- □ Involved in making insulin
- □ Involved in making collagen
- □ Sperm motility
- □ Increases natural killer cells
- □ Stimulates the release of Human Growth Hormone
- □ Helps block tumour formation

Sources of Arginine include:

- □ Almonds, cashews, peanuts, pecans

- ☐ Carob, chocolate
- ☐ Seafood
- ☐ Dairy products, soy protein
- ☐ Beans, peas
- ☐ Garlic, ginseng

Armour Medication

Also called Natural Desiccated Thyroid, Armour is made from the thyroid gland of a pig. It contains both T3 and T4 and is measured in grains instead of mcg.

It is only available on script and some people swear by it for feeling better.

One thing to keep in mind is that because it is actual pig thyroid hormone that is being ingested, sometimes sufferers with autoimmune disease finds that it makes the issue worse as it is more "thyroid" for the immune system to attack. In my case personally, I became depressed while taking it, and that disappeared as soon as I stopped taking it.

Work closely with your doctor and monitor symptoms for 6 months before deciding if it is a right fit for you.

Arsenic

Most people think of old fashioned murder mysteries when they think of arsenic. But it is actually a common issue in the groundwater of many countries such as Mexico, India, and the US where there are naturally higher occurring amounts of arsenic in the ground.

Arsenic has the ability to block Selenium, Vitamin E and Boron in the body which can have a direct affect on the thyroid pathway, cause sensory issues, anaemia, jaundice and hyperpigmentation.

Unusual sources of arsenic include:

- ☐ Fish, shrimp, shellfish, clams, oysters and seafood
- ☐ Rice
- ☐ Tobacco and cigarettes
- ☐ Living near industrial areas that use arsenic in their processes
- ☐ Drinking water
- ☐ Pesticides and weed killers
- ☐ Copper smelters

Arthritis

A painful condition that inflames and damages joints, arthritis can affect all ages, and autoimmune Rheumatoid Arthritis is a common addition to many thyroid sufferers.

Unfortunately the general way to treat this condition is through NSAIDS which presents its own problems, so anything that can reduce the pain and inflammation naturally is going to be beneficial to our thyroid health.

Natural options to try include:

- Using anti-inflammatory herbs such as Turmeric
- Eating an anti-inflammatory diet
- Removing nightshades
- Removing grains
- Acupuncture
- Omega 3 fatty acids

Asparagine

Asparagine is a non essential Amino Acid which means we can make it in our own body from other ingredients if needed.

Asparagine is needed for the following:

- Maintain nervous system control
- Increase oxidative metabolism
- Contributes to Collagen assembly
- Involved in antibody production (immune system)
- Precursor to RNA & DNA (Disease growth)
- Precursor to ATP (energy)
- Involved in brain function
- Involved in Nervous System control

The main sources of asparagine are asparagus, eggs, fish and meat.

Asparagus

That lovely green stalk of health that makes our pee smell weird!!!

1 cup (about 180g) of Asparagus contains:

- ☐ 67% of DRI in Folate (MTHFR, Liver)
- ☐ 20% of DRI in Selenium (thyroid pathway)
- ☐ 14% of DRI in Manganese (thyroid pathway)
- ☐ 14% of DRI in Phosphorus (bones, liver health)
- ☐ 14% of DRI in Fibre (hormone clearance, gut health)
- ☐ 12% of DRI in Potassium (thyroid, fluid, fatigue)
- ☐ 10% of DRI in Zinc (thyroid, healing, mental health)
- ☐ 9% of DRI in Iron (thyroid pathway)
- ☐ 9% of DRI in Protein (thyroid pathway)
- ☐ 6% of DRI in Magnesium (stress, sugar)
- ☐ 4% of DRI in Calcium (bones)
- ☐ 2% of DRI in Omega 3s (mental health, joints)
- ☐ 24% of DRI in Vitamin B1 (thyroid, hair, hyperthyroidism)
- ☐ 19% of DRI in Vitamin B2 (thyroid pathway)
- ☐ 12% of DRI in Vitamin B3 (mental health)
- ☐ 8% of DRI in Vitamin B6 (mental health)
- ☐ 18% of DRI in Vitamin C (thyroid pathway, adrenals)
- ☐ 10% of DRI in Vitamin A (thyroid pathway)
- ☐ 18% of DRI in Vitamin E (thyroid pathway, antioxidant)
- ☐ 101% of DRI in Vitamin K (blood, bones)

As awesome as Asparagus is, it also contains:

- ☐ 33% of DRI in Copper (so if you have allergies, hayfever etc it is possible you may already be too high in this)
- ☐ 1% of DRI in Fluoride. (not a massive amount, but good to know)

So apart from the fluoride, and possibly the copper for some people, the asparagus is an absolute powerhouse of nutrients that we need.

Aspartame

Made up of phenylalanine, methanol and aspartic acid, aspartame is used as an artificial sweetener in many food products and beverages.

Just prior to my thyroid taking a holiday, I was drinking about 10 cans of diet cola a day (which isn't going to help anyone) but in my defence, I was 20 and living on an island in the Great Barrier Reef where my biggest concern was how I looked. Plus I didn't know any better!

Now, this was not the only thing that contributed to my thyroid downfall but it was a biggy!

Let's look at what Aspartame does in the body:

- It breaks down into formaldehyde in the body
- ***Inhibits Tyrosine getting to the thyroid***
- Headaches, dizziness, vertigo, memory loss
- Heart palpitations
- General weakness, numbness and muscle spasms
- Depression
- Behavioural issues
- Nausea

Studies are now showing that long-term use of artificial sweeteners actually impair weight loss! As in, long term use actually makes you fatter! What's the point then??

We really should not be using artificial sweetener of any kind if we have any hope of returning to good thyroid health. But we are all grown ups so if we choose to do so, at least we know what we are doing after this read!

Aspirin

Aspirin is made from Willow Bark and is high in Salicylates.

It works by stopping chemical signals getting through which helps reduce fever and pain. It is also used to reduce blood clots and reduce the risk of heart attacks and strokes.

Natural pain relievers that can be used as an alternative include ginger, turmeric, valerian root, boswellia, magnesium, cats claw and ACTUAL white willow bark.

If you are using it for blood clotting and heart attack risk, please be smart and talk to your doctor before changing anything.

Astragalus

An herb that increases white blood cells and Natural Killer Cells (NKC). It is classed as an adaptogen herb, which balances issues by reducing them if too high or increasing them if too low.

Astragalus is considered an immune system booster and disease fighter and will also assist with chronic infections, night sweats, fatigue, fibromyalgia, mild congestive cardiac failure.

To be used cautiously with immunosuppressive drugs

Astringent

An agent that contracts tissue, skin and mucous membranes making them firmer and reducing their discharges. An astringent can also be used to reduce bleeding, inflammation and diarrhoea.

Astringent foods are helpful in fluid retention, which thyroid disease goes hand in hand with.

Examples Include: Apples, Beans, Bearberry, Chickweed, Cinnamon, Cos Lettuce, Cranberry, Eyebright, Green Tea, Hawthorn, Horsetail, Lentils, Meadowsweet, Myrrh, Pears, Potatoes, Raspberry Leaf, Rosehip, Sage, Wild cherry and Witch Hazel Leaf.

Atherosclerosis

This is a disease where plaque forms inside your arteries and can cause heart disease, cardiovascular disease, heart attacks and strokes.

Risk factors include: a family history, lack of exercise, high blood pressure, smoking, diabetes,

Signs and symptoms of atherosclerosis include angina, shortness of breath, fatigue, confusion, muscle weakness and chest pain.

I have also found in my research that if you are the kind of person who builds up a lot of plaque in your teeth, then you are also the kind of person who will build up plaque in your arteries.

Herbs to use include: Garlic, Ginkgo, Globe Artichoke, Grape Seed, Green Tea, Hawthorn, Polygonum *cuspidatum*, and Turmeric.

Foods to help include: asparagus, avocado, broccoli, watermelon, fatty fish, and spinach.

Atkins Diet

A Low Carb diet developed by Dr Robert Atkins in the 1970's that emphasised consumption of meat and fat similar to the modern Paleo Diet.

Atkins works on the premise of turning the body from glucose (carbohydrate) burning into fat burning for health and wellbeing.

Although it is said that the weight loss from this type of diet is due to the fat burning, others believe it is because you are eating far less calories on this diet because appetite is reduced.

The types of food eaten in this protocol include Beef, pork, chicken, lamb, bacon, fatty fish, seafood, eggs, full fat dairy, nuts, seeds, coconut oil, avocado, extra virgin olive oil and low carb veg such as spinach, broccoli, and asparagus.

The Atkins diet, unlike Paleo is divided into 4 phases

- Phase 1 - Induction - under 20g carbs per day for 2 weeks to kick start weight loss
- Phase 2 - Balancing - some carbs are added back to your diet
- Phase 3 - Fine tuning - As you approach your goal weight, the number of carbs eaten daily is tweaked until the weight loss slows down
- Phase 4 - Maintenance - Once you arrive at phase 4 you know how many carbs you can eat a day without putting weight back on again.

Autoimmune Disease

A disorder of the body's immune system causing it to attack itself or various organs in the belief it is attacking a virus, toxin or other pathogen.

In most cases it is looking for the virus or toxin hidden within our organs, and they become collateral damage as the immune system tries to kill off the invaders. It is never about the body just randomly turning on itself I believe.

There are over 100 Autoimmune Diseases studied, including Hashimoto's (hypothyroidism), Graves Disease (hyperthyroidism), Rheumatoid Arthritis (joints), Type 1 Diabetes (pancreas), Lupus (immune system), Addison's Disease (Adrenal Glands), Celiac Disease (gut & gluten) and Multiple Sclerosis (nerve endings).

After the body experiences one autoimmune disease, the likelihood of developing more greatly increases, due to the high alert the immune system is always operating in.

An estimated 90% of all thyroid disease is caused by autoimmune disease, even if it has not been diagnosed as such. Often, doctors do not run the tests to diagnose thyroid disorders as an autoimmune disease because in most cases there is nothing extra they can do about it, unless it is Graves Disease.

As a patient though, if we know we have an autoimmune disease we can go about finding ways to calm it down, to stop it attacking other organs and tissues.

Autoimmune Paleo Diet

Developed by Mickey Trescott, the Autoimmune Paleo Diet takes the basic Paleo diet and removes further food triggers that may contribute to immune dysfunction such as eggs, nuts, seeds and the nightshade family of foods (tomatoes, potatoes, eggplant etc).

Many thyroid sufferer's swear by her protocol, feeling well and losing weight on it. It is fairly restrictive, but if you are motivated and love the paleo way of life, but still feel like you could go further then this might be for you.

Avocado

I remember the first time I tried avocado. I was about 13 and I was at a ceramics class with my mother on a Saturday morning and one of the other ladies had it. Back then, it was a rather pricey item to have, but she let me try some.

I thought it was awful and didn't understand why someone would pay so much for something so yucky!!!

I can safely say now that Avocado is definitely one of those foods that is an acquired taste. Right up there with Olives I think. The more you have them, the more you want them.

So let's have a look at why the experts think Avocado is so good for us:

1 cup (150g) of Avocado gives us:

- ☐ 40% of our DRI in Fibre (hormone clearance, gut health)
- ☐ 35% of our DRI in Copper (careful if you have allergies)
- ☐ 30% of our DRI in Folate (MTHFR, liver)
- ☐ 23% of our DRI in Vitamin B6 (mental health)
- ☐ 21% of our DRI in Potassium (fluid, fatigue, thyroid)
- ☐ 21% of our DRI in Vitamin E (thyroid pathway)
- ☐ 20% of our DRI in Vitamin C (thyroid pathway)
- ☐ 6% of our DRI in Protein (thyroid pathway)
- ☐ 15% of our DRI in Vitamin B2 (thyroid pathway)
- ☐ 16% of our DRI in Vitamin B3 (mental health)
- ☐ 2% of our DRI in Calcium (bones)
- ☐ 2% of our DRI in Iodine (thyroid pathway)

- ☐ 11% of our DRI in Magnesium (stress, sugar)
- ☐ 11% of our DRI in Manganese (thyroid pathway)
- ☐ 9% of our DRI in Zinc (thyroid, immunity, mental health, wound healing)
- ☐ 1% of our DRI in Selenium (thyroid pathway)

My fave way to eat it is on GF toast with lemon pepper.

Ayurveda

A traditional eastern system of medicine originating in India.

Meaning Science of Life (Ayur = Life, Veda = Science) it is classed as the sister science of Yoga and Vedic Astrology.

Ayurvedic practitioners concentrate on gut health to help heal the body and focus on balancing the three doshas in our body to attain good health.

When the three doshas - Kapha, Pitta & Vata are out of balance, disease can grow in the body. We are born being more dominant in one or two of these doshas, which makes it very easy to get out of balance if our lifestyle and diet are not ideal.

Kapha is the dominant dosha when talking about hypothyroidism

Vata is the dominant dosha when talking about hyperthyroidism

Pitta comes into play often with both of them as it is involved with inflammation.

I attended an Ayurvedic Hospital in India last year where the doctors told me I was Kapha / Pitta dominant. To correct this a lot of Vata remedies were used to increase that dosha to bring them all into alignment.

Gut health is a major priority within this form of medicine, and it is believed that once the gut it right, everything will be right.

One of the best books to explain this way of living and eating in detail is Deepak Chopra's "Perfect Health". It was actually recommended by the doctors at the hospital and it is a book I refer to often.

B

Bravery

To feel better with Thyroid Disease, no matter what your presentation or manifestation it takes bravery.

Often the things that actually make us feel better and start to reverse some of our symptoms and issues are against mainstream medical science.

I personally am not for or against allopathic medicine. We need it for sure. But when it comes to a chronic disease that in many cases has been brought on by lifestyle choices, then we have to be brave enough to take ownership of that and learn what it will take to turn our own health around.

We must learn it for ourselves because we each have a completely unique presentation of this disease. We each breathe different air, eat different foods, have different gut flora, think different thoughts, react to stress differently, so it makes sense that we would all have a slightly different manifestation.

But it is because of this that only we can figure out what is going to make us feel better.

Are you brave enough to:

- ☐ Speak up if you don't understand your doctor?
- ☐ Find another doctor if you don't have a good relationship with your current one?
- ☐ Eat differently to your family if necessary?
- ☐ Learn new strategies such as meditation?
- ☐ Accept that people who don't have thyroid disease will NEVER understand how you feel?
- ☐ To try new and different modalities that may not be mainstream?

I ask you again... are you brave enough?

B Cells

Immune cells that make antibodies (Wanted Posters) against antigens (Bad Guys).

This then allows the body to remember the antigen (Bad Guy) next time it comes to visit.

B1 Vitamin

Also called Thiamin, Vitamin B1 is required for:

- ☐ Carbohydrate metabolism
- ☐ Sugar metabolism
- ☐ Protein metabolism
- ☐ Energy Production
- ☐ Hydrochloric acid release

Deficiency Symptoms of Vitamin B1 include:

- ☐ Appetite Loss
- ☐ Backache
- ☐ Brain Fog
- ☐ Chronic Fatigue syndrome
- ☐ Constipation
- ☐ Fatigue
- ☐ Fluid Retention
- ☐ Hair Loss
- ☐ Slow reflexes
- ☐ Depression
- ☐ Memory loss
- ☐ Moodiness
- ☐ Muscle weakness
- ☐ Nervous Exhaustion
- ☐ Shortness of breath
- ☐ Sleep disturbance
- ☐ Restless Legs

Factors that contribute to Vitamin B1 deficiency:

- ☐ Alcohol
- ☐ Coffee

- ☐ Diuretics
- ☐ Diarrhoea
- ☐ Excess Copper levels
- ☐ Excess Aluminium
- ☐ Excessive Exercise
- ☐ Excessive amounts of highly refined foods
- ☐ Folate deficiency
- ☐ Hyperthyroidism
- ☐ Liver Disease
- ☐ Pregnancy
- ☐ Stress
- ☐ Sulphites
- ☐ Surgery

Food sources of Vitamin B1 include:

- ☐ Asparagus
- ☐ Beef
- ☐ Brewers Yeast
- ☐ Legumes
- ☐ Nuts
- ☐ Pork
- ☐ Whole Grains

Daily Requirements of Vitamin B1:
Adults - 1-5 mg
Toxic Dose - > 125mg / kg

B2 Vitamin

Also called Riboflavin, Vitamin B2 is required for:

- ☐ Activates Vitamin B6 and Folate
- ☐ Eye & Mouth tissue health
- ☐ Reduces edema
- ☐ Myelin Sheath maintenance
- ☐ Mucous Membrane health
- ☐ Thyroid Pathway

Deficiency Symptoms of Vitamin B1 include:

- ☐ Alopecia / Hair Loss
- ☐ Anemia
- ☐ Bloodshot eyes & Blurred vision
- ☐ Cracks on the lips and corners of the mouth
- ☐ Cataracts & Eye Fatigue
- ☐ Conjunctivitis
- ☐ Dermatitis
- ☐ Sensitivity to cold
- ☐ Inflammation
- ☐ Sore tongue & sore throat
- ☐ Oily facial skin
- ☐ General Weakness

Factors that contribute to Vitamin B2 deficiency:

- ☐ Alcohol intake
- ☐ Coffee intake
- ☐ Diabetes
- ☐ Heart Disease
- ☐ Lactose Intolerance
- ☐ Malabsorption
- ☐ Oral Contraceptive Pill
- ☐ Smoking
- ☐ Stress
- ☐ Sugar & Refined Foods
- ☐ Surgery
- ☐ Thyroid Disease
- ☐ High Cadmium, Boron & Copper Levels

Food sources of Vitamin B2 include:

- ☐ Almonds
- ☐ Asparagus
- ☐ Avocados
- ☐ Barley Grass
- ☐ Beans
- ☐ Broccoli

- ☐ Eggs
- ☐ Organ Meats
- ☐ Sprouts
- ☐ Wholegrain Cereals
- ☐ Yeast

Daily Requirements of Vitamin B2:

- ☐ Adult RDA - 1.5 - 2.0mg

B3 Vitamin

Also called Niacin, Vitamin B3 is required for:

- ☐ Energy Production
- ☐ Neuroprotective (brain protector)
- ☐ Hormone production
- ☐ Stimulates Tyrosine hydroxylase
- ☐ Fat metabolism (lowers cholesterol)
- ☐ Protein metabolism
- ☐ Carbohydrate metabolism
- ☐ DNA repair
- ☐ Gastric Acid secretion
- ☐ Bile secretion

Deficiency Symptoms of Vitamin B3 include:

- ☐ Anxiety, Depression, Confusion
- ☐ Fatigue, Headaches, Insomnia
- ☐ Sore tongue and mouth
- ☐ Canker sores in mouth
- ☐ Scaly Dermatitis
- ☐ Muscle fatigue and weakness
- ☐ Nausea, Diarrhoea, Vomiting
- ☐ Indigestion
- ☐ Anorexia

Factors that contribute to Vitamin B3 deficiency:

- ☐ Alcohol & coffee intake
- ☐ Diarrhoea & fever

- Diabetes
- High Cholesterol
- Smoking
- Ulcerative colitis
- High Aluminium Levels

Food sources of Vitamin B3 include:

- Almonds, Peanuts, Sunflower Seeds
- Chicken, Meat, Eggs
- Mackerel, Salmon, Sardines
- Legumes
- Yeast

Daily Requirements of Vitamin B3:

- Adult RDA - 15-20 mg

B5 Vitamin

Also called Pantothenic Acid, Vitamin B5 is required for:

- Antibody production
- Stress resistance
- Decrease lactic acid build up
- Improves Immune system
- Fat metabolism
- Protein metabolism
- Steroid hormone production
- Reduces Arthritis Pain
- Maintains uric acid levels

Deficiency Symptoms of Vitamin B5 include:

- Depression, fatigue, nervousness
- Irritability, Insomnia, sleep disturbances
- Arthritis
- Low Blood Pressure
- Anemia
- Fatigue
- Muscle spasms & Cramps

- ☐ Poor coordination
- ☐ Low immunity (many infections)
- ☐ Hair loss
- ☐ Dermatitis
- ☐ Tender heels & burning feet

Factors that contribute to Vitamin B5 deficiency:

- ☐ Alcohol, coffee intake
- ☐ Pregnancy
- ☐ Stress
- ☐ Copper Excess
- ☐ Mercury exposure
- ☐ Fluid Retention

Food sources of Vitamin B5 include:

- ☐ Avocado, Green veg, mushrooms, sweet potato
- ☐ Beans, lentils & whole grains
- ☐ Baker's Yeast
- ☐ Egg yolks
- ☐ Oranges

Daily Requirements of Vitamin B5:

- ☐ Adult RDA - 5-10 mg

B6 Vitamin

Also called Pyridoxine, Vitamin B6 is required for:

- ☐ Progesterone Production
- ☐ Carbohydrate metabolism
- ☐ Fat metabolism
- ☐ Protein metabolism
- ☐ Nervous system function
- ☐ Serotonin, dopamine synthesis
- ☐ Histamine synthesis
- ☐ Oxygenation of cell tissues
- ☐ Required for Vitamin B3 synthesis

Deficiency Symptoms of Vitamin B6 include:

- ☐ Acne, facial oiliness
- ☐ Anemia & anorexia
- ☐ Depression & confusion
- ☐ Kidney stones
- ☐ Poor coordination
- ☐ Low blood sugar
- ☐ Poor immunity
- ☐ Sleep walking
- ☐ Weakness & fatigue

Factors that contribute to Vitamin B6 deficiency:

- ☐ Diabetes
- ☐ Coffee, Tea, Alcohol consumption
- ☐ Pregnancy
- ☐ Celiac Disease
- ☐ Copper Excess
- ☐ Low Zinc and Vitamin B2

Food sources of Vitamin B6 include:

- ☐ Avocado, Bananas, carrots
- ☐ Brewer's Yeast
- ☐ Chicken & egg yolks
- ☐ Mackerel, salmon, tuna
- ☐ Oatmeal, legumes, lentils
- ☐ Peanuts, walnuts, sunflower seeds

Daily Requirements of Vitamin B6:

- ☐ Adult RDA - 1.6-2.6 mg

B9 Vitamin

Also called Folate, Vitamin B9 is required for:

- ☐ Purine metabolism (meats, beer & seafoods)
- ☐ DNA Repair

- ☐ Metabolism of Tyrosine (required in Thyroid Pathway)
- ☐ Methylation pathway of the liver
- ☐ Synthesis of serotonin
- ☐ Reduces chromosome mutation

Deficiency Symptoms of Vitamin B9 include:

- ☐ Anemia
- ☐ Skin irritations, cracked lips, red tongue
- ☐ Rheumatoid arthritis, osteoporosis
- ☐ Restless legs & weak muscles
- ☐ Constipation
- ☐ Mental sluggishness, Irritability
- ☐ Depression, Apathy
- ☐ Poor sleep & memory

Factors that contribute to Vitamin B9 deficiency:

- ☐ Alcohol
- ☐ Antibiotics & Gastric Surgery
- ☐ Celiac Disease
- ☐ Pregnancy & Oral Contraceptive Pill
- ☐ Diarrhoea
- ☐ Copper excess
- ☐ Antacid use
- ☐ Potassium sparing diuretics

Food sources of Vitamin B9 include:

- ☐ Beans & Lentils
- ☐ Eggs, Organ meats
- ☐ Green leafy vegetables
- ☐ Yeast

Daily Requirements of Vitamin B9:

- ☐ Adult RDA - 400 ug

B12 Vitamin

Also called Cobalamin, Vitamin B12 is required for:

- ☐ Bone marrow maintenance
- ☐ Fat metabolism
- ☐ Protein metabolism
- ☐ Growth maintenance
- ☐ Methylation

Deficiency Symptoms of Vitamin B12 include:

- ☐ Bursitis
- ☐ Restlessness & weakness
- ☐ Mood swings, Irritability, depression
- ☐ Dizziness, poor memory
- ☐ Anemia
- ☐ Brown areas over joints
- ☐ Sore, pale smooth tongue
- ☐ Nausea & Diarrhoea
- ☐ Paranoia, Schizophrenia, Psychosis
- ☐ Temper outbursts, violence, negative thinking
- ☐ Dementia, Nightmares

Factors that contribute to Vitamin B12 deficiency:

- ☐ Diabetes, Celiac Disease
- ☐ Ulcerative colitis & Crohn's disease
- ☐ Gastric Surgery
- ☐ Helicobacter
- ☐ Alcohol & Smoking
- ☐ Bacterial gut overgrowth
- ☐ High copper, lead and mercury levels

Food sources of Vitamin B12 include:

- ☐ Brain, kidney & liver
- ☐ Egg yolk & meat
- ☐ Clams, herring, oysters, salmon, sardines

Different kinds of Cobalamin are:

- ☐ Methylcobalamin - already activated for issues like MTHFR
- ☐ Cyanocobalamin - Synthetic version of B12
- ☐ Adenosylcobalamin - used in cases of myelin sheath issues, nerve & spinal cord degeneration, and energy metabolism.
- ☐ Hydroxocobalamin - Potent detoxifier of cyanide. Particularly amazing for smokers.

Daily Requirements of Vitamin B12:

- ☐ Adult RDA - 2-50ug

Bacopa monnieri

Also called Brahmi, this well known brain and cognition herb, helps to improve memory, concentration and mental performance.

Studies have been done that prove its effectiveness, and some have pointed to Bacopa's ability to regrow brain neurons, particularly after a physical trauma.

Bacopa is also a thyroid stimulant, so is useful in hypothyroidism, particularly if trying to reduce medication needs.

It is also helpful for Alzheimer's, Insomnia and Anxiety.

It may cause oesophageal reflux.

Bacterial Thyroiditis

See Acute Suppurative Thyroiditis

Balms

I love my balms and have enjoyed making them and selling them. But my vision has always been to teach people to do things for themselves.

So with that in mind here are my recipes!

Balancing Balm

- ☐ 300 ml Coconut Oil
- ☐ 50g Beeswax
- ☐ 150 ml Macadamia Oil
- ☐ 25 ml Thyroid Oil Mix (see essential oils)

Melt the coconut oil and beeswax, then add the macadamia oil. Remove from the heat and stir in the thyroid essential oil mix. Pour into tins or glass containers.

To use, rub over neck on a daily basis.

This is also lovely to use as a perfume which both benefits your thyroid and removes the toxins of traditional perfume. Win Win!

Clarity Balm

- ☐ 300 ml Coconut Oil
- ☐ 50 g Beeswax
- ☐ 150 ml Macadamia Oil
- ☐ 10 ml Lavender essential oil
- ☐ 10 ml Bergamot essential oil
- ☐ 10 ml Peppermint essential oil

Melt the coconut oil and beeswax, then add the macadamia oil. Remove from the heat and stir in the essential oils. Pour into tins or glass containers.

To use, rub into your wrists, behind your ears and the back of your neck when you are feeling overwhelmed, stressed or have a headache.

Heel Balm

- ☐ 300 ml Coconut oil
- ☐ 50g Beeswax
- ☐ 150 ml Calendula Oil
- ☐ 150 ml Macadamia Oil
- ☐ 100g Jarrah Medicinal Honey or Manuka Medicinal Honey
- ☐ 15ml Lavender essential Oil

Melt the coconut oil and beeswax, then add the calendula and honey stirring until the honey is dissolved. Remove from the heat and stir in the lavender oil. Pour into tins or glass containers that has a really wide diameter.

To use, take the lid off and rub directly onto your heels using the pot as your applicator. This avoids getting it on your hands (quite sticky). Then cover your feet with dark socks for an hour or two.

Banana

Nature's ultimate fast food! Comes in its own packaging and everything.

What's not to love about Bananas? We can add them to smoothies, oats, fruit salad, pancakes, cakes (put down the cake) the list is endless. Plus they are full of things we thyroid people need in our day.

1 medium banana gives us:

- ☐ 3% of DV in Protein (thyroid pathway)
- ☐ 12% of DV in Dietary Fibre (hormone clearance, gut health)
- ☐ 2% of DV in Vitamin A (thyroid pathway, skin)
- ☐ 17% of DV in Vitamin C (thyroid pathway, adrenals)
- ☐ 1% of DV in Vitamin E (thyroid pathway, antioxidant)
- ☐ 5% of DV in Vitamin B2 (thyroid pathway)
- ☐ 4% of DV in Vitamin B3 (mental health)
- ☐ 22% of DV in Vitamin B6 (mental health, progesterone)
- ☐ 6% of DV in Folate (MTHFR, liver)
- ☐ 4% of DV in Vitamin B5 (Food conversion, energy)
- ☐ 1% of DV in Calcium (bones)
- ☐ 2% of DV in Iron (thyroid pathway, fatigue, gut acid)
- ☐ 8% of DV in Magnesium (stress, sugar)
- ☐ 3% of DV in Phosphorus (bones, liver)
- ☐ 12% of DV in Potassium (thyroid, fatigue, fluid)
- ☐ 1% of DV in Zinc (thyroid, immunity, wound healing, mental health)
- ☐ 5% of DV in Copper (skin, collagen, nerves, bones)
- ☐ 16% of DV in manganese (thyroid pathway)
- ☐ 2% of DV in Selenium (thyroid pathway)
- ☐ Glycemic Load of 10

All of that from one medium banana?! Surely we can squeeze one in every day right?

Barnes, Broda Dr

An American doctor who specializes in endocrine dysfunction in the 70's. He published several books and papers on thyroid disease, particularly hypothyroidism stating that it was under diagnosed.

It was this belief that led him to believe Basal Temperature Testing was the only true way to know what the function of the thyroid was like.

His work has been compiled into a book called Hypothyroidism: The Unsuspected Illness

Basal Temperature Testing

The original Gold Standard of testing the thyroid developed by Dr Broda Barnes.

As the thyroid is the body's temperature regulator, Dr Barnes developed the method of taking the temperature every morning to ascertain if the thyroid was running efficiently.

If the temperature is too high, it indicates the thyroid is running too fast (hyperthyroidism) and if the temperature is too low, it indicates the thyroid is running too slow (hypothyroidism).

This test is simple to perform and all you need is a thermometer on the bedside table.

Every morning when you wake up, before you cuddle anyone or go to the bathroom, put the thermometer in your mouth. A digital one that records your temperature till the next time you turn it on is awesome for early mornings!

Do this 5 mornings in a row and check your average temperature.

- Normal - 36.5 - 37.2 / 97.0 - 97.7
- Low - below 36.5 / 97.0
- High - above 37.2 / 97.7 (excluding fevers and illness)

If you are one of those people that always say, the doctor says my test is fine but I don't feel fine, doing this will tell you just how fine you are!

If you are menstruating then do this on days 1-5 of your cycle (while bleeding) and if you are male or after menopause then you can do this at any time.

Base Chakra

Also called the root chakra, the first of the seven chakras is located between the anus and the genitals.

This is the chakra we use when grounding ourselves, which puts us in the same vibration as the earth, and it is also the one we use to get rid of negative emotions. If we are not in touch with the earth and "grounded" we cannot let go of the negative emotions.

- ☐ Colour - Red
- ☐ Key Issues - Sexuality, obsession
- ☐ System - Reproductive
- ☐ Endocrine Gland - Gonads and ovaries
- ☐ Crystals - carnelian and emerald
- ☐ Aromatherapy - Cedarwood, Patchouli and Myrrh

Basil

If you have eaten any kind of Italian food in your life, you have eaten basil. The fragrance of this herb is intoxicating and just makes you want to exhale. I love it... clearly!

Since we only tend to eat in small amounts (unless you are eating pesto) it is hard to show just how packed with nutrients it is. So I am going to show you how much is in 100g of Basil instead of say a sprinkling. I have included it because it is an herb that would be great to have many times a week, so if you think of these amounts as what you would gain over that time, we are on the same page!

100g of Basil contains:

- ☐ 6% of DV in Protein (thyroid pathway)
- ☐ 6% of Dietary Fibre (hormonal clearance, gut health)
- ☐ 106% of DV in Vitamin A (thyroid pathway, skin)
- ☐ 30% of DV in Vitamin C (thyroid pathway, adrenals)
- ☐ 4% of DV in Vitamin E (thyroid pathway, antioxidant)
- ☐ 518% of DV in Vitamin K (blood, bones)
- ☐ 2% of DV in Vitamin B1 (thyroid, hair, hyperthyroid)
- ☐ 4% of DV in Vitamin B2 (thyroid pathway)
- ☐ 5% of DV in Vitamin B3 (mental health)
- ☐ 8% of DV in Vitamin B6 (mental health, progesterone)
- ☐ 17% of DV in Folate (MTHFR, liver)
- ☐ 2% of DV in Vitamin B5 (food conversion, energy)
- ☐ 18% of DV in Calcium (bones)
- ☐ 18% of DV in Iron (thyroid pathway, fatigue, gut acid)
- ☐ 16% of DV in Magnesium (stress, sugar)
- ☐ 6% of DV in Phosphorus (liver, bones)
- ☐ 8% of DV in Potassium (fluid, fatigue, thyroid)

- ☐ 5% of DV in Zinc (mental health, wound healing, thyroid, immunity)
- ☐ 19% of DV in Copper (skin, nerves, bones, collagen)
- ☐ 57% of DV in Manganese (thyroid pathway)
- ☐ Glycemic Load of 1

All of this adds up to basil being amazing for:

- ☐ Lowering inflammation
- ☐ Lowering Stress
- ☐ Lowering pain
- ☐ Boosts the immune system
- ☐ Antioxidant
- ☐ Protects our blood vessels and cardiovascular health
- ☐ Protects our DNA

Growing basil is pretty easy too, even on the window sill where you can easily grab a few leaves for your meals.

Basmati Rice

Of all the rice available on the market, basmati rice is the one of most interest to thyroid people, particularly if there is excess weight and fluid retention at play.

This rice is considered in Chinese Medicine to help reduce "damp" in the body and in doing so help reduce weight. Thyroid disease (particularly hypothyroidism) used to be called Edema or Myxedema, meaning excess fluid, so any way that we can release this is going to be a good thing.

1 cup of basmati rice contains:

- ☐ 17% DV in Vitamin B1 (thyroid, hair, hyperthyroid)
- ☐ 12% DV in Vitamin B3 (mental health)
- ☐ 7% DV in Vitamin B6 (mental health, progesterone)
- ☐ 23% DV in Folate (MTHFR, liver)
- ☐ 2% DV in Calcium (bones)
- ☐ 11% DV in Iron (thyroid pathway, gut acid, fatigue)
- ☐ 5% DV in Magnesium (stress, sugar)
- ☐ 7% DV in Phosphorus (liver, bones)
- ☐ 5% DV in Zinc (thyroid, immunity, mental health, wound healing)

- □ 37% DV in Manganese (thyroid pathway)
- □ 17% DV in Selenium (thyroid pathway)
- □ 8% DV in Protein (thyroid Pathway)
- □ 3% DV in fibre (hormone clearance, gut health)

It should be noted that all rice now seems to contain arsenic and 1 cup of basmati rice also contains 64.9mcg of fluoride (all rice contains fluoride) so if goitre or low iodine is an issue then eating in excess would not be recommended.

I have added this in simply because if we are going to eat rice, this is probably the one we should choose (it's the one I eat, if I am going to eat it).

Beans

See Legumes

Bearberry

I don't have UTI's very often but I am never without this liquid herb (which I mix with a few others) just in case!

I literally may only get one every few years, but it is a saviour when I do.

Bearberry is a urinary antiseptic, astringent and also has anti-inflammatory properties.

It works by melting the little hooks on the bacteria that attach to the uterine wall and cause so much pain and discomfort when we have a UTI, and it works like a dream.

It is not for use in pregnancy, lactation, kidney disease, and children under 12.

Beautiful on Raw

Beautiful on Raw is the online presence and brain child of Tonya Zavesta, a beautiful woman who defies her 60 years and shares her devotion to turning back the clock by eating raw foods and practising hot yoga.

Tonya has written many books, developed body and hair products and shares many recipes and lifestyle advice on her website and across her social media pages.

I particularly love her hair care range which is so natural you could eat it but also doesn't feel like many of the other natural shampoos out there. It leaves my hair feeling beautiful and soft, plus after using her hair stimulating serum, my hairdresser noticed many new soft hairs growing in.

Beef

When eating any animal foods, it is best for our hormonal situation if we can get organic grass fed. Although this is a pricier option, it is better to only eat it occasionally and get what is not going to interrupt our hormones .

Commercially raised beef is fed on grains, and are treated with antibiotics and hormones. Although this may not cause an issue with non-thyroid people, anyone with hormonal issues need to avoid extra hormones.

There are so many different cuts of beef and fat contents, so I have put the details for grass fed, which will be completely different to commercially raised beef.

100g grass fed beef strip steaks contain:

- 46% of DV in Protein (thyroid pathway)
- 1% of DV in Vitamin E (thyroid pathway, antioxidant)
- 1% of DV in Vitamin K (bones, blood)
- 3% of DV in Vitamin B1 (thyroid, hair, hyperthyroid)
- 7% of DV in Vitamin B2 (thyroid pathway)
- 34% of DV in Vitamin B3 (mental health)
- 7% of DV in Vitamin B5 (food conversion, energy production)
- 33% of DV in Vitamin B6 (mental health, progesterone)
- 3% of DV in Folate (MTHFR, liver)
- 21% of DV in Vitamin B12 (Energy, gut health)
- 1% 0f DV in Calcium (bones)
- 10% of DV in Iron (thyroid pathway, gut acid, fatigue)
- 6% of DV in Magnesium (stress, sugar)
- 21% of DV in Phosphorus (liver, bones)
- 10% of DV in Potassium (fluid, fatigue, thyroid)
- 24% of DV in Zinc (immunity, thyroid, wound healing, mental health)
- 30% of DV in Selenium (thyroid pathway)

I don't eat meat often, simply because I don't crave it, but when I do, I enjoy it and get the best quality I can.

Beets

Beets or Beetroot are a powerhouse of nutrients. I would almost call the Beet Greens (the leaves on top) a thyroid superfood, and the root (the beet) is so great for our liver.

If you can get the leaves, then make them part of your regular salads or stir fries.

Beet Greens

Let's start with the amazing little green leaves with gorgeous red veins running through them.

These are an amazing source of nutrients for Thyroid People.

1 cup of Beet Greens contains:

- ☐ 220% of DV in Vitamin A (thyroid pathway, skin)
- ☐ 60% of DV in Vitamin C (thyroid health, adrenals)
- ☐ 13% of DV in Vitamin E (thyroid pathway, antioxidant)
- ☐ 871% of DV in Vitamin K (not a typo!) (bones, blood)
- ☐ 11% of DV in Vitamin B1 (thyroid, hair, hyperthyroid)
- ☐ 24% of DV in Vitamin B2 (thyroid pathway)
- ☐ 4% of DV in Vitamin B3 (mental health)
- ☐ 5% of DV in Vitamin B5 (food conversion, energy)
- ☐ 10% of DV in Vitamin B6 (mental health, progesterone)
- ☐ 5% of DV in Folate (MTHFR, Liver)
- ☐ 16% of DV in Calcium (bones)
- ☐ 15% of DV in Iron (thyroid pathway, fatigue, gut acid)
- ☐ 24% of DV in Magnesium (stress , sugar)
- ☐ 6% of DV in Phosphorus (liver, bones)
- ☐ 37% of DV in Potassium (thyroid, fatigue, fluid)
- ☐ 14% of sodium (electrolytes, adrenals)
- ☐ 5% of DV in Zinc (immunity, thyroid, mental health, wound healing)
- ☐ 18% of DV in Copper (skin, collagen, nerves, bones)
- ☐ 37% of DV in Manganese (thyroid pathway)
- ☐ 2% of DV in Selenium (thyroid Pathway)
- ☐ 17% of DV in Dietary Fibre (hormonal clearance, gut health)
- ☐ 7% of DV in Protein (thyroid pathway)
- ☐ Glycemic Load of 4
- ☐ Contains Trace amounts of ALL amino Acids

How amazing are those numbers? I haven't had any in a while but typing this up, I'm going to get some for dinner!

Beets

I live Down Under, and here some people consider it un-Australian to not have beetroot (as we call them) on our burger!!

Beets are fantastic for the liver! And since 70% of our thyroid hormone is converted in our liver, anything we can do to help it along is a good thing.

1 cup of this amazing root vegetable will bestow upon our bodies the following:

- ☐ 1% of DV in Vitamin A (thyroid pathway, skin)
- ☐ 11% of DV in Vitamin C (thyroid pathway, adrenals
- ☐ 3% of DV in Vitamin B1 (thyroid, hair, hyperthyroidism)
- ☐ 3% of DV in Vitamin B2 (thyroid pathway)
- ☐ 2% of DV in Vitamin B3 (mental health)
- ☐ 5% of DV in Vitamin B6 (mental health, progesterone)
- ☐ 37% of DV in Folate (MTHFR, Liver)
- ☐ 2% of DV in Calcium (bones)
- ☐ 6% of DV in Iron (thyroid pathway, fatigue, gut acid)
- ☐ 8% of DV in Magnesium (stress, sugar)
- ☐ 5% of DV in Phosphorus (liver, bones)
- ☐ 13% of DV in Potassium (thyroid, fatigue, fluid)
- ☐ 4% of DV in Sodium (electrolytes, adrenals)
- ☐ 3% of DV in Zinc (thyroid, immunity, mental health, wound healing)
- ☐ 5% of DV in Copper (skin, collagen, nerves, bones)
- ☐ 22% of DV in Manganese (thyroid pathway)
- ☐ 1% of DV in Selenium (thyroid pathway)
- ☐ 15% of DV in Dietary Fibre (hormonal clearance, gut health)
- ☐ 4% of DV in Protein (thyroid pathway)
- ☐ Trace amounts of all amino acids
- ☐ Glycemic load of 5

I buy my beetroot fresh and bake it in the oven. I then peel the skin off and slice it or dice it depending on what I want to do with it. If I am organised I will do many at once and then pop them in a glass jar in the freezer. Then I always have some on hand without using a tin which is usually loaded with sugar.

Belief Systems

I have had many clients sit in front of me since becoming a naturopath and sometimes I find that all seems lost to them. Like nothing can make them feel better and they are doomed to suffer thyroid symptoms for the rest of their perceived miserable lives.

It is with these particular clients that I ask about their belief systems.

In all cases so far, these people had no belief systems. By that I mean, they did not subscribe to a religion, a deity, or any thought process around past lives, reincarnation, the universe ... whatever you want to call it.

So their actual belief systems were this:

I am born, I have a crappy diseased life, then I die.

Very often they don't realise they have this type of belief system, or lack of, until I state it to them.

I am not suggesting we all need a deity to bow down to, however if we have some kind of belief around why we are put on this planet, then it can sometimes make it easier to walk the path we have been given, and change that path if we want to. What's your belief system?

Benign Thyroid Nodules

Benign means not dangerous. These types of nodules may be caused by cysts or simply overgrowth of thyroid tissue. 95% of thyroid nodules are benign and are diagnosed via ultrasound. However a fine needle aspiration biopsy will be used as further diagnosis if your specialist wants to confirm if they are benign or malignant.

As a side note, I have many people that follow Thyroid School who have reversed their nodules using a good diet and essential oils rubbed on their neck daily.

Bentonite Clay

A clay that is used for its ability to absorb toxins.

Often used for mould ingestion, heavy metals and chemicals, it is also used in face masks and bath treatments.

Bergamot

From the citrus family, bergamot is the featured flavour in Earl Grey Tea and the fragrant oil is considered to be a relaxant, reducing tension, stress and anxiety.

Betaine

Betaine is a naturally occurring Amino Acid made from Choline and Glycine. It is a "methyl donor" which is the key here!

One of our liver pathways is the Methylation pathway and this is the one under the spotlight for everyone that is out getting a gene test for the MTHFR gene mutation. For those of us taking supplements for this, or eating more folate-rich foods for it, then Betaine is needed just as much as folate and Vitamin B12 (they are all methyl donors).

Betaine helps us with:

- ☐ Improved mental health
- ☐ Fat metabolism
- ☐ Convert homocysteine in the blood
- ☐ Improves cardiovascular disease
- ☐ Improves heart disease
- ☐ Improves muscle mass
- ☐ Lowers body fat
- ☐ Improves muscle strength
- ☐ Improves the flow of bile
- ☐ Improves Tyrosine pathway (mental & thyroid health)

So how do we get this handy amino acid?? Well besides our body making it we can up our consumption of beetroot and spinach!! There are also two herbs you can take called Astragalus and Echinacea.

Beta Blocker

A drug used to manage irregular heart rhythms. Often used after a heart attack to prevent another one.

Side effects include:

- ☐ Slow heartbeat
- ☐ Fatigue, weakness, weight gain
- ☐ Nausea, dizziness
- ☐ Cold and swelling of hands and feet

Beta Blockers don't really affect thyroid function although they do ease symptoms such as fast heat rate in hyperthyroid people.

Like anything, when starting a medication, always track your thyroid symptoms and temperature test to see if it is affecting your thyroid function.

Beta-carotene

A member of the carotenoid family, beta carotene is required for:

- Making Vitamin A
- Is an antioxidant
- Increases number of Natural Killer Cells
- Decreases plaque formation
- Protects skin from sunburn
- Decreases damage to DNA
- Protects the lining of the nose, mouth, throat, lungs

Deficiency Symptoms of beta-carotene include cancer, cataracts, and inflammation of the stomach lining (atrophic gastritis)

Factors that contribute to a beta-carotene deficiency include:

- ageing
- cystic fibrosis
- smoking
- pesticides

Food sources of beta-carotene include:

- carrots (particularly juiced)*
- broccoli, red peppers, spinach, sweet potatoes, tomatoes, papaya

*When you eat raw carrot you get 1% of the beta carotene. When you juice a carrot you get 100% of the beta carotene

Daily Requirements of Vitamin B1:

- Adults - 5-8mg

Bija Mantras

You know when you watch someone meditating and they are singing or chanting the word “OMMMMMM”??

Well Om is a Bija Mantra!

That is just the easiest way to describe what a Bija Mantra is and each chakra has a different one that connects us to our inner selves.

- Base Chakra - Om (note of B)
- Sacral Chakra - Vam (Note of D)
- Solar Plexus Chakra - Ram (note of E)
- Heart Chakra - Yam (note of F)
- Throat Chakra - Ham (note of G)
- Brow Chakra - Om (note of A)
- Crown Chakra - Om (Note of B)

Keep in mind when chanting all of these notes (assuming you can hold the tone cause I sure can’t) they are all pronounced in the posh way.

For example the Throat Chakra is pronounce Harm as are the rest of them.

So when do we chant these? I use the throat one often because I want to stimulate my thyroid. If you know a lot about Chakra’s though, you will know when you want to chant away.

Bile

The fluid produced by the liver and stored in the gallbladder to enable us to digest and absorb fats and fat soluble vitamins.

Slower emptying of the bile ducts is common in hypothyroidism but they can also become obstructed (not as common) presenting with symptoms such as:

- Weight loss
- Fever
- Fatigue
- Light brown urine
- Jaundice skin (yellow)
- Low appetite
- Greasy looking stools
- Pain on the right side of the trunk

Bioflavonoids

A group of plant compounds that include Hesperidin, Quercetin and Rutin, bioflavonoids are required for:

- ☐ antioxidant ability
- ☐ anti inflammatory ability
- ☐ antiviral ability
- ☐ anti allergic ability
- ☐ anti ageing
- ☐ inhibitor of cancer growth
- ☐ reduction of blood sugar
- ☐ strengthening of capillaries
- ☐ Immune stimulation
- ☐ free radical scavengers

Deficiency Symptoms of bioflavonoids include:

- ☐ bruising
- ☐ inflammation
- ☐ autoimmune disease
- ☐ purple/blue spots on the skin

Factors that contribute to bioflavonoid deficiency include:

- ☐ allergies
- ☐ asthma
- ☐ high blood pressure
- ☐ burns
- ☐ fragile capillaries
- ☐ cataracts
- ☐ depression
- ☐ inflammation
- ☐ mastectomy patients
- ☐ rheumatoid arthritis

Food sources of bioflavonoids include:

- ☐ apricots, cherries, rosehips, berries
- ☐ apples, lemons, citrus
- ☐ garlic, olives, onions, red wine

Bio-identical hormones

Hormones derived from yams or soy that are identical in molecular structure to hormones made in our body.

There is no clear answer as to its safety or effectiveness over synthetic hormones as there are still side effects.

Side effects may include:

- ☐ weight gain, fatigue, mood swings
- ☐ acne, facial hair, breast tenderness, spotting, cramping
- ☐ bloating, indigestion, headaches, blurred vision

Biotin

This vitamin I have been taking everyday for a while now as it helps with so many thyroid type symptoms.

Also called Vitamin B7, Biotin is a water soluble vitamin synthesised in our gut and is required for:

- ☐ Energy conversion from food
- ☐ Hair, skin, nail health
- ☐ Sugar metabolism
- ☐ Fat metabolism
- ☐ Liver function
- ☐ Reducing plaque in blood vessels

Deficiency Symptoms of Biotin include:

- ☐ Alopecia, hair thinning, grey hair
- ☐ Anemia, fatigue
- ☐ Depression, hallucinations
- ☐ scaly and seborrheic dermatitis

Factors that contribute to Biotin deficiency:

- ☐ Ageing, pregnancy, lactation, athletes
- ☐ Alcohol, coffee, raw egg white consumption
- ☐ Gastric sleeve or bypass surgery
- ☐ Anticonvulsant medication

Food sources of Biotin include:

- ☐ Bean sprouts, bulgar wheat, oats
- ☐ Cashews, peanuts, soy beans
- ☐ Egg yolks, milk
- ☐ Kidney, liver

Daily Requirements of Biotin is:

- ☐ Adults: 30-100ug

Birth Defects

When a thyroid woman falls pregnant, first of all that's a huge thing to be celebrated because it is more difficult for us, but the second most important piece of information is that thyroxine levels must be extremely closely monitored throughout the pregnancy. Like, every 6 weeks if possible.

Lack of thyroid hormone (actively in hypothyroidism) can cause birth defects in the baby, so while it will be hard not to stress about this, it is something that needs to be aware of.

While I'm hesitant to tell you the possible side effects I feel I need to if it means you will be proactive about getting regular checkups and also making sure that your levels are stable before you get pregnant.

Here's the dreaded list:

- ☐ Increased risk of heart defects
- ☐ Increased risk of brain abnormalities
- ☐ Increased risk of kidney defects
- ☐ Increased risk of cleft lip and palate
- ☐ Increased risk of extra fingers
- ☐ Increased risk of developmental delays
- ☐ Increased risk of intellectual problems
- ☐ Increased risk of preterm birth
- ☐ Increased risk of low birth weight
- ☐ Increased risk of congenital thyroid disease

Please don't be put off by this list. I managed to give birth to a perfectly healthy child, even though my thyroid was only checked once through my pregnancy (I just didn't know enough 19 years ago!).

This is just a reminder to keep on top of your own thyroid health so that it does not impact your future babies health.

Bisphenol A

A chemical that acts as an estrogen mimic found in hard plastics, that interfere with our normal hormone balance.

Many food and drink containers are made with this, along with it being in the plastic lining of many tinned food items, although, due to consumers becoming more educated, its presence has been slightly reduced, particularly in water bottles.

Bitter Tonic

An agent that has a bitter taste but also promotes digestive function and improves appetite.

Examples Include: Barberry, Dandelion Root, Gentian, Globe Artichoke, Golden Seal, Hops, Olive Leaf, Polygonum multiform, Wormwood, Yarrow

Bitter Melon

Also called Bitter Gourd and Balsam-pear, this is an amazing fruit type vegetable that is incredible for our gut health and so much more.

They are bitter as their name suggests, but I ate it many times in India last year and when it is mixed in with a curry or other veggies it is really tasty!

1 average bitter melon contains:

- □ 2% of DV in Protein (thyroid pathway)
- □ 14% of DV in Dietary Fibre (hormonal clearance, gut health)
- □ 12% of DV in Vitamin A (thyroid pathway, skin)
- □ 174% of DV in Vitamin C (thyroid pathway, antioxidant, adrenals)
- □ 3% of DV in Vitamin B1 (thyroid, hair, hyperthyroidism)
- □ 3% of DV in Vitamin B2 (thyroid pathway)
- □ 2% of DV in Vitamin B3 (mental health)
- □ 3% of DV in Vitamin B5 (food conversion, energy)
- □ 3% of DV in Vitamin B6 (mental health, progesterone)
- □ 22% of DV in Folate (MTHFR, liver)
- □ 2% of DV in calcium (bones)

- ☐ 3% of DV in iron (energy, thyroid, gut acid)
- ☐ 5% of DV in magnesium (stress, sugar)
- ☐ 4% of DV in phosphorus (liver, bones)
- ☐ 10% of DV in Potassium (thyroid, fatigue, fluid)
- ☐ 7% of DV in Zinc (thyroid, mental health, immunity, wound healing)
- ☐ 6% of DV in Manganese (thyroid pathway)
- ☐ Glycemic Load of 1

This all adds up to these benefits:

- ☐ Improved immune function
- ☐ Reduced inflammation
- ☐ Blood sugar regulation
- ☐ Boosts fat metabolism
- ☐ Improve insulin sensitivity

Black Pepper

When I attended an Ayurvedic Hospital in the south of India last year, a common ingredient in all of the food was black pepper. I don't tolerate hot spicy food too much, so it was never an extreme amount of it, but it was present in small amounts in all of the food I was served.

With an extremely high level of potassium and other boosting micronutrients such as Vitamin A, Vitamin K and Zinc, it aids thyroid health by:

- ☐ Improving digestion by increasing the level of hydrochloric acid in the stomach (low levels are often a problem with people low in iron)
- ☐ Increasing weight loss due to the breaking down of fat cells by the outer layer of the peppercorn
- ☐ Helping lessen skin issues such as vitiligo
- ☐ Clearing sinus passages by breaking up mucus and phlegm
- ☐ improves memory and cognitive function
- ☐ reduces the risk of cancer
- ☐ reduces cardiovascular disease
- ☐ relieves peptic ulcers
- ☐ helps in liver malfunction
- ☐ improves bio-availability of the food it is served with

- promotes sweating and urination which then lowers fluid retention
- is antibacterial and antitumor

It should be noted that black pepper can be an irritant in large quantities and may cause allergic reactions in some people.

Black Tea

The strongest of the tea leaves from the camellia sinensis plant it is more oxidised than green tea, white tea or oolong tea and is sold under the labels of Black Tea and English Breakfast Tea.

Black tea naturally contains high levels of caffeine and fluoride, which it makes it a less than ideal beverage for a thyroid person.

Caffeine blocks iron absorption, plus is overstimulating to the adrenal glands. Many drink tea thinking it is only a very small amount of caffeine compared to coffee, but (depending on how they are both made) it can be almost half the amount. So if you are having 4 or 5 cups of tea a day thinking it is a better choice, you are consuming the same amount of caffeine as a 2 cups of coffee.

Add to that the naturally occurring fluoride content and you have a lovely cup of "blocking iodine getting to the thyroid" nobody wants that now do they?

Like anything, balance is the key. If you are having multiple cups of anything a day, then you need to look at what it is very closely. It is always the little things we do everyday that make the biggest difference to how we feel.

Bladderwrack

An herb specifically for hypothyroidism which also helps with excess weight caused by low thyroid function.

Bladderwrack is a seaweed and therefore extremely high in iodine, selenium and many other nutrients required by the Thyroid Pathway.

It is NOT for use with hyperthyroidism and goiter related thyroid issues.

Use cautiously and under supervision in pregnancy and lactation.

Bloating

Bloating is both uncomfortable and makes us feel less than attractive in our clothes.

There are many reasons for bloating, so it is up to you to find the reason specific to you. Most often it is a food intolerance of some kind. They include:

- ☐ food intolerance or allergies (celiac)
- ☐ constipation, Irritable Bowel Syndrome
- ☐ bad gut health / bacteria
- ☐ hormonal fluctuations (endometriosis, ovarian cysts)
- ☐ medications
- ☐ weight gain
- ☐ stress

Ways to improve bloating, will firstly be to clean up your diet and remove all the nasties, then follow with an elimination diet (FODMAPS) to see if you can find an offending food item. Adding fibre slowly will also help to alleviate the issue.

Also avoid chewing gum, drinking sodas or any fizzy drinks.

Peppermint oil, leaves or tea are great for relieving both bloating and intestinal discomfort.

Some helpful herbs include: Cloves, Gentian, Ginger, Globe Artichoke, St Mary's Thistle, and Wormwood

Blood Flow

An herb specifically for hypothyroidism which also helps with excess weight caused by low thyroid function.

Bladderwrack is a seaweed and therefore extremely high in iodine, selenium and many other nutrients required by the Thyroid Pathway.

It is NOT for use with hyperthyroidism and goiter related thyroid issues.

Use cautiously and under supervision in pregnancy and lactation.

Blood Pressure

The measurement of how hard or fast our blood is circulating in our body resulting in either high or low blood pressure.

A measurement is given in two numbers for example 120/80.

The first number (systolic) represents the pressure in our arteries while the heart is pumping and the second number (diastolic) represents the pressure when the heart relaxes.

- ☐ low - less than 90 / less than 60
- ☐ optimal - less than 120 / less than 80
- ☐ normal - 120 to 129 / 80 to 84
- ☐ high/normal - 130 to 139 / 85 to 89
- ☐ high - above 140/90

Low blood pressure causes:

- ☐ parathyroid issues
- ☐ adrenal issues
- ☐ low blood sugar
- ☐ dehydration
- ☐ heart problems
- ☐ pregnancy
- ☐ septicaemia (septic blood infection)
- ☐ anaphylaxis (severe allergic reaction)
- ☐ low B12 and B9
- ☐ medications (diuretics, alpha blockers, beta blockers, antidepressants, drugs for erectile dysfunction)

High blood pressure causes:

- ☐ thyroid disease
- ☐ birth defects
- ☐ medications (OCP, decongestants, pain relief, cocaine, amphetamines)
- ☐ Obstructive sleep apnea
- ☐ kidney disease
- ☐ adrenal gland tumour
- ☐ family history
- ☐ being overweight
- ☐ sedentary lifestyle
- ☐ smoking
- ☐ salt intake
- ☐ low potassium
- ☐ stress
- ☐ chronic disease

If you don't have your blood pressure checked regularly, ask your doctor to do it each year when you are having a full check up (like you should be if you have thyroid disease, wink wink).

Blood Sugar

Blood sugar refers to the measurement of levels of sugar in our blood at any particular time.

- ☐ normal - 4.0 to 5.4 mml/L
- ☐ up to 2 hours after eating - <7.8mmol/L

Anything outside of this range is considered high.

At a conference I attended once, the diabetes educator said that most of the damage done is from the "postprandial response" so that is the time directly after eating.

Now if it takes 2 hours for our blood sugar to return to normal after our meal, and we are in the habit of snacking or eating every couple of hours, our bodies stay permanently in the state of heightened blood sugar which is when the damage occurs.

Blood Tests

The first thing I always say about blood tests is that they are yours. You own them!

Whenever your doctor is writing a slip for you to have blood taken, always ask that you can have a copy sent to you. Then keep them in a file where you can compare them as time goes by, depending on what different things you have tried.

The tests you want for thyroid disease are:

- ☐ TSH - Thyroid Stimulating Hormone
- ☐ FT4 - Free T4 (inactive hormone)
- ☐ FT3 - Free T3 (active hormone)
- ☐ RT3 - Reverse T3 (T3 blocker)
- ☐ Antibodies - Autoimmune disease

In some cases you may need to pay for a couple of these tests as they won't be covered, but all of these together will give you a good picture of what is going wrong or right in your thyroid pathway.

Here in Australia, to do this we need to ask the doctor to write on the path form that the patient gets a copy. Once we are at the path lab then we need to tell them again there that the doctor has written on the form that we can have a copy, and then they will stamp it.

I have found over the years that this is the way to absolutely ensure I get a copy in the mail.

We want our own copies because the ranges are HUGE in the grand scheme of things and often we are simply told "you are in range" and to continue on the same dosage.

However, we may be really close to the outer edge of that range which tells us that either we are not paying attention to our diet or lifestyle or something else is not quite right.

Things that can change our results could be holidays, stress, family tragedies, visitors or even a cold or flu. I know my TSH always went up during exam time, even if I had changed nothing else.

When I receive my results in the mail, I always write beside them what dosage I was on at the time.

This is really helpful if you change doctors, are travelling, need to see a specialist or even engage a naturopath. It also helps you remember that you are in control of your own health.

Blood Type Diets

Developed by Dr Peter D'Adamo and presented in his book "Eat Right 4 your Type", this way of eating found its way into the households of many, and also became the go-to protocol for many nutritionists and naturopaths in the late nineties and into the naughties.

It centres around eating certain foods that are helpful to your blood type. Here is an example of the top foods that are recommended for each type:

- ☐ Type O - Red meat, oily cold water fish, spinach, kale, seaweed
- ☐ Type A - Pineapple, broccoli, onions, cultured soy products, olive oil
- ☐ Type B - Red meat, broccoli, cultured dairy products, onions, pineapple
- ☐ Type AB - Tofu, cultured dairy products, broccoli, walnuts, cauliflower

Conversely, the foods that most need to be avoided according to this diet are:

- ☐ Type O - wheat, corn, kidney beans, navy beans, white potatoes
- ☐ Type A - Red meat, milk, lima beans, white potatoes, oranges
- ☐ Type B - chicken, corn, peanuts, lentils, buckwheat
- ☐ Type AB - chicken, corn, buckwheat, lima beans, kidney beans

I never personally got into this diet (although some people swear by it) because as a B type, I am supposed to eat cultured dairy products yet my body disagrees with them badly.

But if it appeals to you and these lists make sense to you then maybe it's worth a trial?

Blueberries

These amazing little morsels of joy are packed with thyroid goodness and very easy to get these days.

1 cup of blueberries contain:

- ☐ 2% of DV in protein (thyroid pathway)
- ☐ 14% of DV in Dietary Fibre (hormonal clearance, gut health)
- ☐ 2% of DV in Vitamin A (skin, thyroid pathway)
- ☐ 24% of DV in Vitamin C (thyroid pathway, adrenals)
- ☐ 4% of DV in Vitamin E (thyroid pathway, antioxidant)
- ☐ 36% of DV in Vitamin K (blood, bones)
- ☐ 4% of DV in Vitamin B1 (thyroid, hair, hyperthyroidism)
- ☐ 4% of DV in Vitamin B2 (thyroid pathway)
- ☐ 3% of DV in Vitamin B3 (mental health)
- ☐ 2% of DV in Vitamin B5 (food conversion, energy production)
- ☐ 4% of DV in Vitamin B6 (mental health, progesterone)
- ☐ 2% of DV in Folate (MTHFR, liver)
- ☐ 2% of DV in Iron (thyroid pathway, fatigue, gut acid)
- ☐ 2% of DV in magnesium (stress, sugar)
- ☐ 2% of DV in Phosphorus (liver, bones)
- ☐ 3% of DV in Potassium (thyroid, fatigue, fluid)
- ☐ 2% of DV in Zinc (thyroid, mental health, immunity, wound healing)
- ☐ 25% of DV in Manganese (thyroid pathway)
- ☐ Glycemic Load of 6

The Medical Medium says that wild blueberries are particularly helpful for removing toxic metals, to halt a shrinking thyroid and reduce nodule growth.

Blue Cohosh

An herb that is considered spasmolytic (calms spasms), uterine and ovarian tonic, emmenagogue (promotes menstrual flow), and an oxytocic (contracts uterus).

It helps with:

- Ovarian pain
- Uterine prolapse
- Endometriosis
- Period cramping
- Assists labour in late pregnancy (with specialised help from a herbalist)

Blue Flag

An herb (the rhizome) that is considered a depurative (detoxifier), mild laxative, lymphatic and cholagogue (releases bile) and is used for:

- Dermatitis, eczema, acne, psoriasis, rosacea
- Liver deficiencies causing nausea, headaches and constipation
- Enlarged lymph glands
- Weight loss

Body Mass Index

This is a tool to categorise your weight into an area of perceived illness or health.

It is determined by maths, are you ready?

Your weight divided by (Your height in metres) times 2

If you like maths as much as I do, the easy way is to google "BMI calculator" and voila! Many will pop up to save your brain.

Unfortunately our BMI can be misleading and does not take into account many factors like muscle mass.

Depending on your score, you are placed into a classification of health.

- <18.5 - underweight
- 18.5 - 24.9 - Healthy weight
- 25.0 - 29.9 - Overweight
- 30.0 - 34.9 - Obese Class 1

- 35.0 - 39.9 - Obese Class 2
- >40.0 - Morbid Obesity

Body Temperature

As the thyroid is the body temperature regulator, it is extremely common for us to be affected by temperature in general.

Often we go on holidays, or move to a different location and don't feel as great as we could and that may be down to the temperature of the destination.

Generally (not always) hypothyroid people prefer warmer temperatures because they are always cold. And hyperthyroid people prefer the cooler temperatures because they are always hot.

If you move or holiday in a location that is the opposite of what you are used to, it is possible your thyroid medication will need adjusting.

Bone Broth

Bone Broth has always been a healing remedy and used for convalescence and rebuilding the body after childbirth in many cultures, even some vegans use it when necessary.

Bone Broth is amazing for:

- Gut health
- Joint health
- Immune system health
- Skin, hair and nail health
- Detoxification
- Boosts metabolism

Many years ago I was at an international natural health conference and one particular Doctor was taking questions about gut health. He was asked the quickest way to heal the gut in his opinion.

His reply was "... hands down bone broth"

The GAPS protocol for gut healing uses bone broth 5 times a day both on its own and sometimes with a few veggies thrown in. Either way, learning how to make it and keeping it on hand in the fridge or freezer is better for our health than the stock we purchase full of preservatives and numbers.

A broth can be made from various bones such as chicken, fish or beef, boiled for extremely long periods of time (up to 24 hours) with other herbs and vegetables. I use a slow cooker in the garage to keep the ongoing smell out of the house.

To make a Chicken Broth:

- 1 whole chicken
- 2 chicken feet
- 1 tbsp sea salt
- 6 peppercorns
- 2 bay leaves
- 1 onion
- ¼ cup apple cider vinegar
- Place all ingredients in a large stock pot or slow cooker with enough filtered water to cover the chicken
- Bring to the boil and then lower heat to simmer for 24 hours
- Strain the broth, and pour into glass jars for later use

I have in the past, kept a pot heated on the stove with a carrot and zucchini grated into it for a little texture plus some thyme for a little flavour kick, but you could add any veg you like if you are not a fan of it straight up.

Boron

Boron is required for:

- Insulin secretion
- Antibody production
- Bone development & maintenance
- Parathyroid hormone function
- Activates Vitamin D

Deficiency Symptoms of Boron include:

- Osteoarthritis, Rheumatoid arthritis, osteoporosis
- Low antibody levels, autoimmune disorders
- Fatigue, Lethargy

- ☐ Poor concentration, poor attention span, poor memory
- ☐ Lowered testosterone levels

Factors that contribute to Boron deficiency:

- ☐ Low magnesium
- ☐ Low Methionine
- ☐ Low Vitamin D
- ☐ Fluoride
- ☐ Blocked by Copper & Arsenic

Food sources of Boron include:

- ☐ Almonds, hazelnuts, peanuts
- ☐ Pears, Apples, dates, raisins, prunes
- ☐ Tomatoes

Daily Requirements of Boron:

- ☐ Adult RDA - 2 - 3 mg

Boswellia

Not so much an herb, but a resin, Boswellia is anti-inflammatory, anti-arthritic, and antitumor.

It is particularly useful for Rheumatoid Arthritis, osteoarthritis, Crohns' Disease, ulcerative colitis,.

Useful also in lupus, gout, urticaria, multiple sclerosis & hay fever.

No major safety issues.

Bowel Movements

As a naturopath I have spent many many hours talking poop with fellow naturopaths. We love talking about it! Seriously we do!

Our poop can tell us so much about what is going on in our body from its color, size, shape, if it floats (possible malabsorption) or leaves skid marks (too much fat in the diet), the odour (possible bacterial infection).

The main issues with thyroid disease are generally constipation in hypothyroidism and diarrhoea in hyperthyroidism.

If you are not sure where yours are at, google the Bristol Stool Chart and it will show you pictures of what is considered normal and what is not.

It is also good to know the colours and understand that if any colour change lasts longer than 2 weeks it must be checked out by the doctor.

- Black - iron supplements, liquorice, stout, or possible gastric bleeding
- White - liver or gallbladder issues, anti-diarrhoea medications
- Green - Consumption of lots of green veg, or too much bile
- Red - possible gastric bleeding, haemorrhoids, drinking beet juice
- Orange - drinking carrot juice, eating excessive orange vegetables, antibiotics or blocked bile ducts
- Yellow - excess fatty diet

Bowen Therapy

A modality that involves a therapist using small flicking movements at specific points in the body to release the fascia (lining) of the muscles.

This is said to reduce many types of musculoskeletal pain, and I have to say, for me it worked! After 2 decades of back pain, I went to a Bowen therapist and after about 3 treatments, it was gone. Poof! Just like that.

Bovine Adrenal Gland

This is the medical term for an adrenal supplement that has been made from the adrenal gland of a cow.

It is up to you if you have issues with this idea or a vegan.

Bradycardia

This is the medical term for a slow heart beat.

In adults, a resting heart beat of less than 60 beats per minute would fall under the category of bradycardia, which may indicate not enough oxygenated blood is pumping around the body.

As heart rate is modulated by thyroid hormone it is common to have a low heart beat when hypothyroid as everything slows down.

This is something that should always be monitored by your practitioner.

Brain Damage

A Head trauma can initiate a thyroid problem.

Because the Thyroid Pathway begins in the brain with the hypothalamus, and the pituitary gland, any trauma to the brain can then initiate a breakdown in that pathway.

Brain Fog

Brain fog is a really common thyroid symptom where we literally feel like we are living in a fog. Everything is slow to react and our cognitive function is just not there.

This is a scary symptom which often leads us down the road of Dr. Google and thinking the worst.

For the most part, our brain fog is simply due to the fact that there are a higher concentration of T3 receptors in our brain which need thyroid hormone.

If our thyroid pathway is not functioning correctly then our receptors are not getting hormone and our brain will suffer not just with brain fog but with memory, anxiety, depression, indecision and the list goes on.

The lesson here, is that there is not a lot you can do directly for the brain (except maybe the herb brahmi which also increases T4 levels) except for cleaning up your thyroid pathway in general, which will have the indirect effect of helping with all of the brain issues.

Brain Food

With our foggy brains, forgetful memory and confusion, our thyroid brains need all the help they can get don't you agree?

There are some major nutrients we need for brain health which include:

- ☐ Pretty much all the B Vitamins
- ☐ Omega 3's
- ☐ Zinc

Also if we can add the following herbs we are onto a winner:

- ☐ Brahmi
- ☐ Gingko
- ☐ Rosemary

The foods that best fit these criteria are:

- Avocados (like we needed a reason) full of healthy fats, folate and B vitamins.
- Fatty Fish (salmon, Mackerel etc) High in Omega 3's and zinc - just make sure they are wild caught.
- Turmeric. Nature's anti-inflammatory! So that also means inflammation in our head.
- Blueberries (wild if possible) - the anthocyanins in them do all kinds of amazing things in our brain.
- Pumpkin Seeds - so full of zinc, B vitamins and tryptophan (the precursor to serotonin) these are a great addition to our meals and snacks
- Macadamia Nuts. (ok, all nuts) but mostly macadamias because they have a much higher Omega 3 : Omega 6 Ratio.
- Tomato's - full of lycopene which helps against free radicals that attack the brain.

Just as a side note, I want to talk about the herb Brahmi! It is BRILLIANT for brain stuff.

I have been giving it to my teenager for several months now, and a week or so ago he ran out.

I hadn't ordered more bottles yet, and he came to me last night and asked where his brain tablets were at.

I was shocked he asked for them and said so. He told me "Oh they make such a difference, and I have exams at the moment can you get some more"

So that is coming from a 17 year old boy!!

Brassica Family

Brassica family of vegetables are all types of cruciferous vegetables. It's confusing but Brassicas, Cruciferous and Goitrogenic vegetables are pretty much all the same veggies.

They include broccoli, Brussels sprouts, cabbage, cauliflower, kale, collards, arugula, turnips, collards and bok choy.

It is said that this family of veg loses its goitrogen ability once it is cooked, and that you would have to eat a LOT of them everyday to cause an effect however many years ago I tested this theory and began eating it again after staying clear for decades.

Within about 2 months of eating just a small amount 3-4 times a week, my hair began to fall out which I had not experienced before.

After stopping my consumption, it returned to normal within about 2 weeks.

With anything you want to try, always keep a diary of symptoms and judge for yourself if it works for you.

Brazil Nuts

Brazil Nuts are Nature's Selenium Pill and since Selenium appears multiple times in the Thyroid Pathway we need to make sure we are getting enough of it.

Here is what I love about food instead of supplements. A study has shown that just 2 Brazil Nuts per day over a 12 week period can increase blood levels of selenomethionine levels by 64% as opposed to a selenium pill which raised it by 61%. How cool is that?

Unless you are allergic to nuts, then brazil nuts would be my go-to for getting enough selenium for our thyroid pathway.

Let's look at what else 2 of these little power houses have inside them:

- ☐ 2% of the DV of Vitamin E (Thyroid Pathway)
- ☐ 4% of the DV of Vitamin B1 (thyroid health)
- ☐ 2% of the DV of Protein (thyroid pathway)
- ☐ 2% of the DV of Calcium (bones)
- ☐ 2% of the DV in Iron (fatigue, thyroid, gut acid)
- ☐ 10% of the DV in Magnesium (Stress & Sugar)
- ☐ 8% of the DV in Phosphorus (Liver)
- ☐ 2% of the DV in Potassium (thyroid health)
- ☐ 2% of the DV in Zinc (healing & metabolism)
- ☐ 8% of the DV in Copper (nerves, bones, skin, collagen)
- ☐ 6% of the DV in Manganese (thyroid pathway)
- ☐ 274% of the DV in Selenium (Thyroid Pathway)

All of this adds up to the following health benefits:

- ☐ Anti-inflammatory
- ☐ Boosts the immune system
- ☐ Regulates thyroid function
- ☐ Lifts mood and decreases depression, anxiety and fatigue
- ☐ Pure anti-cancer Food
- ☐ Boosts testosterone

- ☐ Excellent deplaquer
- ☐ Lowers Heart Disease

WARNING: if you are already taking selenium supplements, 2 kernels a day would replace it. Like anything, too much of something can be as bad as not enough, so you don't want toxic doses in your body!!

Bread

Although bread is just one of the most amazing, time management helping food item put on this planet, it is really not helpful to us at all.

If you have read the section on gluten you will understand the risks, and before you can say "but Kylie... mine is Gluten Free" generally the GF varieties are jam packed with additives and sugar and other things that make it as close to resembling our normal bread as possible.

So, let's take a breath, and where we can let's replace our addiction for bread and the easy solution it offers us when we are in a hurry and start to replace it with something else.

Some ideas when time is short:

- ☐ Replace the bread with Romaine Lettuce Leaves
- ☐ If you are ok with eggs, google vegan Cloud Bread... you will thank me later!
- ☐ Thinly sliced, baked sweet potato
- ☐ Flatbread made from chickpeas or buckwheat
- ☐ Vegetable waffles (homemade) with grated veg of choice pressed into a waffle maker. These can be made ahead of time and stored in the freezer
- ☐ Try my Jar Food idea and skip the sandwiches all together

Breakfast

For so many years I couldn't stomach the idea of breakfast. Like so many others, it consisted of a sweet milky coffee on my way out the door to work. Then around 10.30 I would finally feel my hunger and go looking for something to eat at the nearest cafe or have another coffee if I couldn't leave my office.

The problem with this is that coffee puts our adrenals into fight or flight. So immediately in the morning our adrenals are pumping out cortisol. Add to that, the calcium in the milk interferes with the thyroid medication I had just taken and it really adds up to a thyroid adrenal disaster! Every morning!

Generally not wanting breakfast is a sign of a sluggish liver, which is extremely common in thyroid people.

Although it is hard to force yourself to eat when you don't want to, a small amount of protein within an hour of rising will calm your adrenals which in turn will stop the surge of cortisol that contributes to too many thyroid issues.

Getting the timing right is crucial though. As soon as you wake up then thyroid medication gets taken, then about 50 mins later (to allow for food interfering with the medication) have a protein rich (plant or animal) breakfast, preferably though with no dairy still to avoid the calcium so close to the medication.

Eventually as you clean up your liver, you will find that eating first thing will be less of an issue.

Breast Cancer

Although opinions and research seems to be mixed on the topic of thyroid and breast cancer, one study suggest that a patient with hyperthyroidism (overactive) is at an increased risk of breast cancer.

However, since many hypothyroid patients carry extra fat, which translates to excess estrogen, it is not uncommon to find the two linked.

Some breast cancers are estrogen based and need estrogen to thrive and grow. This type of breast cancer is treated with hormone therapy, amongst other things.

I came across some research some time ago that suggests there is a direct correlation between root canals and breast cancer. So while that is not thyroid related I thought it was worth mentioning.

Breast Discharge

Assuming you are not lactating to feed your child, if you have any discharge coming from your nipples it is unusual. The medical term for this is galactorrhea due to the overproduction of prolactin.

Potential causes are:

- Pituitary disorder - The pituitary gland is part of our thyroid pathway and is responsible for making our TSH so if that is not in range and you have leaking nipples then a closer look at the pituitary gland is needed.

- Excessive Breast and nipple stimulation - not much to say here except lucky you!
- Some medications - particularly some types of birth control, antidepressants, blood pressure, antipsychotics, marijuana, cocaine, opioids
- Some herbs - fenugreek (often used to increase breast milk in nursing moms), fennel and anise
- Male testosterone deficiency - let's not forget men may experience this too
- Possible emotional response - there have been cases reported where women have had all other physical causes ruled out when they experienced discharge when being near a newborn. It was decided that this was down to an extreme emotional response to being around an infant.

Breast feeding

After having my son in 2000 I struggled to breastfeed. It actually took about 4 days for even my colostrum to come in and then for the 3 weeks following that, I battled constantly to supply enough milk for him which was heartbreaking.

It was not as well known back then the effect of thyroid disease on milk supply so I had no idea it was a symptom, instead I assumed it was just me. I now know that thyroid hormones are involved in the making of breast milk, so if our hormone is low, then milk supply will be also.

What to do:

- Have ***extremely regular*** blood tests after bub is born to keep an eye on levels.
- Herbs that help increase levels are fennel, fenugreek, goat's rue, shatavari and vervain
- Herbs that stop milk supply include sage and peppermint, so be careful you are not drinking too much peppermint tea!

And finally if you struggle to breastfeed regardless of your levels being ok then don't feel bad about it. It's hard enough being a new mum without feeling like your child is going to suffer because you can't feed him. The stress of those thoughts alone will worsen your thyroid issues.

Breathing

See Air Hunger

Bromelain

This is a substance derived from the Pineapple and it has incredible health benefits, in case we needed a reason to eat it.

Bromelain is:

- □ Anti-inflammatory
- □ Anti-tumour
- □ Helps wound healing
- □ Breaks down plaque in the arteries
- □ Improves circulation
- □ Is an immune modulator
- □ Reduces fluid retention
- □ Reduces Blood pressure
- □ Reduces cholesterol
- □ Reduces coughing

It does though have interactions with some drugs. It promotes the action of warfarin and increases the absorption of antibiotics so it is wise to not go crazy with pineapple juice or diet if taking these.

Bromelain is unstable to heat, so it is important to recognise that these benefits would only come about having pineapple fresh, not canned or ready juiced from the grocer which will have been heat treated.

Bronchodilator

An agent which increases the diameter or width of the respiratory airways making it easier to breathe.

Examples include: Coleus, Reishi mushroom, Licorice.

Bronchospasmolytic

An agent which calms bronchial airways.

Examples Include: Black haw, Coleus, Elecampane, Grindelia, Inula racemosa

Brow Chakra

Also called the Third Eye Chakra it is located between the Brows.

The Chakra of psychic ability it is also about stepping into the bigger picture and looking beyond what is right in front of us. It is about us trusting our inner wisdom and balancing knowledge from our higher selves with the disbelieving lower selves.

- Colour - Deep blue
- Key Issues - Trust and Balance
- Location - Between the brows
- System - Endocrine & Nervous
- Endocrine Gland - Pineal & Pituitary
- Imbalances - Thyroid Disease, Sleep disorders, Serotonin disruption
- Crystals - Diamonds, Emeralds, Sapphire, Lapis Lazuli
- Aromatherapy - Frankincense, Basil,

Brownstein, David MD

Dr Brownstein is an expert in his field and is the author of "Iodine, Why You Need It, Why You Can't Live Without It".

It is a fantastic book which covers Autoimmune Disease, cancer, detoxification, fatigue and thyroid disease.

Bruising

Bruising is generally the result of tissue damage under the skin after we knock ourselves in some way.

If there is no obvious reason for bruises then other reasons may include:

- Low iron
- Low Vitamin C
- Less Collagen or thinner skin
- Some medications and supplements including Omega 3 and flaxseed oil
- Heavy weight lifting (can burst vessels)

- Autoimmune Disorders (Rheumatoid Arthritis), fibromyalgia, hyperthyroidism, hypothyroidism
- Diabetes
- Blood Cancers

Herbs to help heal existing bruises include: Arnica (topically), Butcher's Broom, Grape Seed, Horsechestnut

Herbs for people prone to easy bruising include: Bilberry, Butcher's Broom, Grape Seed, Horsechestnut

Buckwheat

Buckwheat is actually a pseudo grain. It looks and tastes like a grain however it is actually a seed from the rhubarb family which makes it gluten free and grain free.

It's really nice and nutty tasting and helps bulk out a salad if you are avoiding grains.

1 cup of buckwheat boasts:

- 11% of DV in Protein (thyroid pathway)
- 18% of DV in Fibre (hormone clearance, gut health)
- 6% of DV in Vitamin B1 (thyroid, hair, hyperthyroid)
- 5% of DV in Vitamin B2 (thyroid pathway)
- 10% of DV in Vitamin B3 (mental health)
- 8% of DV in Vitamin B6 (mental health, progesterone)
- 6% of DV in Folate (MTHFR conversion, liver)
- 1% of DV in Vitamin E (thyroid pathway)
- 4% of DV in Vitamin K (blood, bones)
- 1% of DV in Calcium (bones)
- 28% of DV in Copper (skin, nerves, collagen, bone)
- 7% of DV in Iron (thyroid pathway, gut acid)
- 21% of DV in Magnesium (stress, sugar)
- 34% of DV in Manganese (thyroid pathway)
- 17% of DV in Phosphorus (liver, bones)
- 4% of DV in Potassium (thyroid, fluid, fatigue)
- 7% of DV in Selenium (thyroid pathway)
- 9% of DV in Zinc (thyroid, healing, immunity, mental health)
- 1% of DV in Omega 3s (mental health, joints)

This all add up to blood sugar regulation, prevention of gallstones, lowering of heart disease and breast cancer prevention.

Bugleweed

An herb for supporting hyperthyroidism. It is antithyroid and acts as a mild sedative to help calm the associated symptoms of hyperthyroidism.

NOT to be used in hypothyroidism, pregnancy or lactation.

Bulging Eyes

A symptom of Graves Disease, the official name for the phenomenon is Exophthalmic eyes and is related to high levels of inflammation.

Bupleurum

The root of this herb is anti-inflammatory, liver protective, and encourages elimination through the skin.

Helpful in autoimmune diseases that involve the liver or kidneys it also helps to improve liver damage and poor liver function.

Also useful in the common cold when a chronic cough will not go away.

May cause reflux.

Burdock

The root of this herb has diuretic properties to help release fluid and is a depurative which is a soothing agent.

It is useful in the support of fluid related conditions such as gout, rheumatism, rheumatoid arthritis, and also skin conditions such as dermatitis, acne, eczema and psoriasis

Bursitis

Bursitis is an inflammation of the bursa sacs that act as cushions in our joints. And boy is it painful!

The first time I experienced this, I thought I had sciatica or something because it was so painful. I couldn't straighten my hip without crying in pain. Admittedly I had been sitting in bed for a few hours in a strange position typing on my laptop!

After a trip to my chiropractor the next day, still feeling sorry for myself he explained it was Bursitis and was a red flag that I was letting inflammation get out of hand in my body. I need those reminders sometimes, no matter how painful, and really that's all pain is - our body talking to us.

Bursitis develops over time and generally through repetitive activities, so for example painful knees when kneeling is part of your job can be a sign of inflamed bursa sacs in the knees.

Apart from reducing inflammation in general, there is not much else you can do. Mine went away, after addressing that and only comes back now if I have not been keeping an eye on inflammation.

- ☐ Turmeric for inflammation
- ☐ Vitamin B12 - a deficiency seems to be related to bursitis
- ☐ Essential oils Thyme, Rose, Fennel, Bergamot, Clove, Eucalyptus
- ☐ Anti-inflammatory foods: pineapple, papaya, leafy greens, omega 3s

Butcher's Broom

The root and rhizome of this herb is helpful for the health of our veins (venotonic) and to reduce fluid retention (angioedema). As a bonus for thyroid disease it is anti-inflammatory.

It is useful with venous insufficiency where our fluids settle due to gravity and don't circulate as well as it should.

also used for Varicose veins, haemorrhoids, Lymphedema, Deep vein thrombosis, restless leg syndrome, leg cramps, spider veins, and bruising.

It may cause reflux.

C

Change

There is a saying... Nothing ever changes if nothing ever changes.

There are two ways to look at this.

- ☐ In most cases something changed for us to get thyroid disease
- ☐ In most cases we have to change something to reverse our thyroid disease

It doesn't matter what we change to start the process. You may just get up one morning and decide to shave your legs or beard and do your hair or put on a tie even though it is not date night!

This simple change can spark an avalanche of positive steps in improving your thyroid health.

If you are not ready to change your mindset or beliefs (I know they are tough to budge) then start with the physical things that are easy and in your control.

Easy Changes:

- ☐ Have a lemon water instead of a coffee
- ☐ Use organic shampoo instead of commercial
- ☐ Replace perfume for essential oils
- ☐ Swap plastic food storage containers for glass
- ☐ Drink filtered, distilled water instead of tap water
- ☐ Swap 1 takeaway a week for home cooked

Just start somewhere. Doing one little thing that you know improves your thyroid and your health will have a ripple affect into other areas of your life.

I promise.

C Vitamin

Also called Ascorbic Acid, Vitamin C is required for:

- ☐ Antihistamine production
- ☐ Major antioxidant
- ☐ Bone & teeth health
- ☐ Collagen production
- ☐ Heavy metal excretion
- ☐ Sperm motility
- ☐ Connective tissue strength
- ☐ Regulates fat metabolism
- ☐ Wound Healing

Deficiency Symptoms of Vitamin C include:

- ☐ Iron deficiency, asthma
- ☐ Depression, malaise, listlessness
- ☐ High cholesterol, High Blood Pressure
- ☐ Fluid Retention
- ☐ Painful joints, weak joints, weak muscles
- ☐ Bruising, Bleeding gums, rough skin
- ☐ Lowered immunity, increased infections
- ☐ Poor healing

Factors that contribute to Vitamin C deficiency:

- ☐ Thyrotoxicosis
- ☐ Allergies
- ☐ Antibiotics & Oral Contraceptive Pill
- ☐ Smoking
- ☐ Cancer, infections, chronic inflammatory conditions
- ☐ Pregnancy & lactation
- ☐ Stress
- ☐ Surgery & Scar Tissue
- ☐ Heavy metal excess
- ☐ Arthritis, Diabetes, AIDS

Food sources of Vitamin C include:

- Citrus fruit & berries
- Guava, pineapple, rosehips, papaya
- Broccoli, Peppers, Potatoes
- Parsley, sweet potato, tomatoes

Daily Requirements of Vitamin C:

- Adult RDA - 75-125 mg

Cadmium

Cadmium is a neurotoxin that loves to disrupt and destroy hormones. It causes damage to our mitochondria (energy centres) and depletes the body of selenium, a vital mineral for the thyroid pathway to work.

There are some studies that show a correlation between hyperthyroidism and high levels of cadmium and mercury.

It can also be associated with:

- Bone Disease
- Kidney Disease
- High Cholesterol
- High Blood Pressure
- Emphysema
- Headaches
- Reproductive Disorders
- Aggression
- Self Destruction
- Blocks zinc, magnesium, selenium, copper, melatonin, SAMe, and sulphur

And before you say you don't come into contact with this toxic metal, let me assure you that you do! Cadmium sources include:

- Cigarette smoke
- Traffic - is released whenever people apply the car brakes
- Is used in some fertilisers and is therefore in soils and produce
- Industrial areas emissions

- ☐ In PVC Pipes
- ☐ Pigment in some paints

Zinc is Cadmium's arch enemy so where we have plenty of zinc stores, there will be no room for cadmium to hang around and since cadmium seems to play a role with many hormonal disruptions getting plenty of Zinc is the key.

Caffeine

Caffeine is a wonderful thing. Gives us a giddy up when we need it and for most of us tastes sublime and smells even better!

But there are a few issues with caffeine that need to be kept in mind before deciding if we are going to consume it, how much, and how often.

- ☐ Caffeine lowers absorption of thyroid medication if consumed within an hour of each other
- ☐ Caffeine is a stimulant, so hyperthyroid people who are already wired and tired may want to rethink this
- ☐ Makes TH2 Dominant autoimmune people worse
- ☐ Inhibits the absorption and encourages the excretion of calcium, magnesium, potassium and iron
- ☐ It can cause anxiety, insomnia, digestive issues
- ☐ Impairs insulin production

Now caffeine is not just in coffee we also find it in:

- ☐ Black tea, oolong tea, green tea, rooibos tea, herbal tea infusions
- ☐ Chocolate, hot chocolate, decaf coffee (yes it does contain a small amount)
- ☐ Weight loss supplements, protein bars
- ☐ Guarana, energy drinks, some sodas, vitamin waters
- ☐ Some medications
- ☐ Any foods that contain coffee or chocolate - ice cream, cake, cookies, yogurt, candy bars, breakfast cereals ... and the list goes on

Calcitonin

A hormone secreted by the thyroid to help regulate calcium and phosphate levels in the blood.

Its job is to keep parathyroid hormone in check by monitoring the levels and then increasing their secretion through urine if there is too much present.

Calcium

Calcium is required for:

- ☐ Activates insulin
- ☐ Activates calcitonin and thyroid hormone release
- ☐ Blood clotting
- ☐ Bone & tooth formation
- ☐ Outer Cell membrane
- ☐ Muscle contraction
- ☐ Regulate heartbeat

Deficiency Symptoms of Calcium include:

- ☐ Brittle nails, eczema
- ☐ Heart palpitations, irregular heart beat
- ☐ High Blood pressure
- ☐ Muscle spasms & cramps
- ☐ Soft bones & teeth
- ☐ Depression, agitation, insomnia
- ☐ Cognitive impairment, hyperactivity

Factors that contribute to Calcium deficiency:

- ☐ Hypothyroidism
- ☐ High Phosphate intake
- ☐ High protein intake
- ☐ Lack of exercise
- ☐ Lack of magnesium
- ☐ Pregnancy
- ☐ Blocked by lead
- ☐ Water softeners
- ☐ Rhubarb, spinach, chard, grains & cereals decrease absorption of calcium

Food sources of Calcium include:

- ☐ Almonds, buckwheat

- Molasses
- Egg yolk, sardines
- Leafy green vegetables, turnips, broccoli

Daily Requirements of Calcium:

- Adult RDA 800-1400mg
- Elevated calcium = parathyroid dominance

Calendula

This beautiful bright orange flower is used extensively in skin balms and is an excellent topical treatment for wounds, ulcers, bed sores, minor burns, haemorrhoids and insect bites. This is due to its anti-inflammatory, antimicrobial, antiviral and antifungal properties.

Internally it is used for enlarged lymph glands as it has a lymphatic action.

Californian Poppy

I have a quick story about California Poppy. Several years ago I had just ordered a bottle of this for a client's Sciatica.

After sitting at my desk for about 10 hours working on a book, I got up and realised I couldn't walk without incredible back and hip pain.

After being grumpy with myself for spending so long sitting, I remembered the bottle of Poppy. I quickly poured myself the highest therapeutic safe dose, and threw it down (disgusting). I then proceeded to walk to the back of the house to say goodnight to my son.

We had a little chat and then I headed to the front of the house and as I was about to climb into bed it hit me...

I WAS NO LONGER IN PAIN...

Yes it was that quick!

California Poppy has a mild sedative action is an anxiolytic, meaning it calms anxiety and is also an analgesic (pain reliever) and hypnotic.

So it is fantastic for any pain caused by nerve issues such as neuralgia, sciatica and toothache but also very useful for insomnia emotional stress and panic attacks.

Although I don't use it very often it is one of the bottles of herbs I always have on hand.

Cancer

This is not a big long entry about how to conquer it or reverse it or stop it in its tracks. I don't have enough experience around it to speak to these things, although I do think anything is possible.

These are the things I do know and want to share:

- Cancer has only two fuel sources - sugar and glutamate
- 20-50% of all human cancer is associated with dietary factors
- Cancer is literally something eating away at you - what do you need to forgive yourself or someone else for?
- The Gerson Therapy is a nutrition based program for reversing cancer in Mexico and is amazing with melanoma particularly
- Cancer cannot live with oxygen - oxygenate the cells
- Aromatherapy cancer fighters are - myrrh, frankincense, lavender
- Red food dye increases the risk of thyroid cancer

I am lucky enough to have not experienced this myself so I cannot imagine how I would navigate it if I did, but honestly I think my first step would be The Gerson Therapy, even if I needed the chemo or whatever else.

In the meantime I will try and reduce sugar and glutamate (think MSG here) and make sure my body is not a cancer friendly host.

Candida

Although candida is a normal bacteria in our body (I'm sure I read somewhere that it is the bacteria that breaks down our bodies when we die), candida overgrowth seems to have been the headline on every woman's health site for decades now.

The connection I want to tell you about is that candida overgrowth symptoms can be eerily similar to hypothyroid symptoms which leads me to suggest, if you have tried everything in your power to reduce your thyroid symptoms, perhaps it's not your thyroid?

I saw a test once that said if you spit into a glass of water first thing in the morning and the spit starts to form tendrils reaching down, then you have a candida overgrowth. I have never done any forms of medical testing to follow that up, but it is interesting. Testing usually involves a Candida antigen blood test and possibly IgG, IgA and IgM if the doctor thinks it is food allergy related.

Getting rid of it is simple but yet the hardest thing on earth. It is a yeast, and it feeds off sugar. So removing sugar, perhaps heading in the direction of a paleo type diet for awhile may improve the situation.

Herbs to help reduce gut candida include: Andrographis, Aniseed, Barberry, Echinacea, Garlic, Golden Seal, Grape Seed, Green Tea, Oregano, pau d'Arco, and St Mary's Thistle

Herbs to help vaginal candida: Andrographis, Echinacea, Chaste Tree, and pau d'Arco.

Cannabis Oil

I don't know a lot about cannabis oil, nor have I tried it, however many people on Thyroid School have reported that using it reduces their aches and pains (particularly those that also have arthritis and fibromyalgia) and swear by it.

There have been no official trials on CBD oil and thyroid people that I have found so far, although I did find some science sites that said we have cannabinoid receptors on our thyroid gland which means using CBD may influence the health of the thyroid, but if that is a good or bad influence is still unknown.

One study (on rats) found that the receptors may be a target for nodules or lesions so it is unclear if this is a good option for thyroid people long term at this time.

Canola

A vegetable oil from the rapeseed plant that is high in mono and polyunsaturated fats.

There is a lot of information for both the good and the bad of consuming canola including it being a GMO, is said to be rancid by the time we purchase it, is said to contain trans fats due to it being highly processed and heated.

Regardless of those points, I don't use any polyunsaturated oils, and you can read about why under PUFAs.

Carbamazepine

An anti-seizure medication that also decreases thyroid hormones. Sold under the brand name Tegretol.

Carbimazole

Carbimazole (also called Neo-Mercazole) is an antithyroid drug used for the treatment of hyperthyroidism. Most people are not kept on it for more than a couple of years, because doctors don't like hyperthyroidism and its dangerous complications to be long term.

The least sciency explanation I can think of what carbimazole does is that it reduces the production of thyroid hormones by blocking the joining of Tyrosine with Iodine which forms T4 & T3 (The T stands for Tyrosine and the 3/4 are the number of molecules of Iodine).

So not only is it used to try and control hyperthyroidism, but it is also used prior to thyroid removal and radio-iodine treatment.

when I went researching I found under the category called "Undesirable effects" the following line up of side effects:

- ☐ Nausea
- ☐ HeadachesRash on hands and feet
- ☐ Facial Swelling
- ☐ Mouth Ulcers
- ☐ Hoarseness
- ☐ Difficulty breathing
- ☐ Blood in Urine
- ☐ Arthralgia (joint pain)
- ☐ Mild gastrointestinal disturbance
- ☐ Fever
- ☐ Malaise
- ☐ Bruising
- ☐ Skin Rashes
- ☐ Pruritus (severe itching)
- ☐ Insulin autoimmune syndrome
- ☐ Angioedema (swelling under the skin)
- ☐ Loss of sense of taste
- ☐ Salivary gland swelling
- ☐ Polyneuropathy (peripheral nerve damage)
- ☐ Abnormal liver function tests

- □ Hepatitis
- □ Haemolytic anaemia
- □ Cholestatic hepatitis
- □ Jaundice
- □ Cutaneous vasculitis
- □ Multi-system hypersensitivity
- □ Urticaria
- □ Hair Loss
- □ Myopathy (muscle disease)
- □ Generalised lymphadenopathy

This is not to alarm you if this is your medication. This is about knowing what you are doing, knowing your body and knowing when to speak up if something is wrong.

If you have any of these symptoms you need to tell your Doctor! Even the ones that don't seem related because they sound like a thyroid issue - it could actually be a medication issue!

Carbohydrates

Some are scared by them, some use them for emotional eating, and yet others lose weight eating them as the main part of their diet.

It is always individual. Here are some things to keep in mind:

- □ Dr John McDougall centres his whole health regime around high carb (mostly potatoes) and no fat with great results.
- □ An excess in any carbohydrates (particularly refined such as bread, pasta) will cause high blood sugar followed by insulin which is a fat storing hormone
- □ There is evidence to suggest that a strict ketogenic diet (no carbs) will reduce blood levels of thyroxine
- □ Very low carb diets may inhibit thyroid conversion

I guess like anything, maybe it's not the potato we eat, but the stuff we put on it.

Cardiovascular disease

Cardiovascular Disease (CVD) is an umbrella term for diseases of the heart and blood vessels, including heart attacks, stroke, high blood pressure, atherosclerosis and angina.

Experts are saying there are three main drivers of CVD:

- Oxidation
- Inflammation
- Immune dysfunction

Thyroid disease plays a part in heart function and particularly hypothyroidism can be a high risk factor for CVD. Since the heart generally pumps slower in hypo patients, blood pressure needs to rise to get it around the body effectively.

So a couple of things to keep in mind here.

- Gut health - you can't fix your vascular system if your gut health is not good.
- Food related CVD is from post prandial reactions, meaning your body is always in digesting mode. Keep meals 3 times a day making sure there is 5 hours between eating so the body has a chance to rest.

Remember this is not a death sentence, this is a reminder of the job we have at hand to keep our body in the best working order we know how to.

Cardioprotective

An agent which has a beneficial action on the heart.

Examples Include: Astragalus, Coleus, Dan Shen, Hawthorn, Korean Ginseng, Tienchi Ginseng

Carminative

An agent that has a calming, tranquillising, sedating affect either physically or mentally

Examples Include: aniseed, Cayenne, Chamomile, Cinnamon, Cloves, Dill, Fennel, Ginger, Juniper, Lavender, Lemon Balm, Peppermint, Rosemary

Carnitine

See Acetyl - L-carnitine

Carpal Tunnel Syndrome

A condition where the median nerve is squashed as it goes through the carpal tunnel in the wrist.

It shows up by exhibiting numbness, tingling and sudden shooting spasms (they hurt, let me tell you) and is caused by repetitive movements such as writing a book.

In the case of thyroid disease, inflammation of the synovial membrane around the tendons can cause the problem also.

Treatments include resting, corticosteroid injections, wearing splints to stop the repetitive movement, physiotherapy exercises, diuretics to reduce fluid in the wrist and surgery.

Herbs and nutrients that may help include:

- ☐ Vitamin B6
- ☐ Manganese
- ☐ Butcher's Broom
- ☐ Grape Seed
- ☐ Horsechestnut
- ☐ St John's Wort

Carrot Juice

Carrot juice was my first major juice addiction. It tastes like the nectar of the gods to me. On the rare occasion I am feeling off, then some fresh organic carrot juice followed by a coffee enema (yes, I know some of you won't cope with that) and I am good as gold. In fact, I can't even remember the last time I was sick with this dual action weapon at my side.

I started drinking carrot juice after reading some of Dr Norman Walker's books on juicing and health and before you say, "Well Kylie, why not just eat the carrot" I will tell you that in a carrot we can obtain about 1% of the beta-carotene inside. In a juiced carrot, we can get 100% of the beta-carotene.

Whcn it comes to gaining instant nutrients, juicing is our best friend.

Let's look at the humble carrot up close! According to the science people, 1 cup of raw sliced carrots contains:

- ☐ 113% of DRI of Vitamin A (thyroid pathway)
- ☐ 20% of DRI of Biotin
- ☐ 18% of DRI in Vitamin K (Blood & Bone Health)
- ☐ 14% of DRI in Fibre (hormone clearance)
- ☐ 14% of DRI in Molybdenum

- ☐ 11% of DRI in Potassium (thyroid health & fatigue)
- ☐ 10% of DRI in Vitamin B6
- ☐ 10% of DRI in Vitamin C (adrenals)
- ☐ 9% of DRI in Manganese (thyroid health)
- ☐ 8% of DRI in Vitamin B3 (mental health)
- ☐ 7% of DRI in Vitamin B1
- ☐ 6% of DRI in Phosphorus (liver health)
- ☐ 6% of DRI in Folate (liver & MTHFR)
- ☐ 5% of DRI in Vitamin E (thyroid pathway
- ☐ 5% of DRI in Vitamin B2 (thyroid Pathway)
- ☐ 4% of DRI in Calcium (bones & thyroid pathway)
- ☐ 2% of DRI in Iron (fatigue & thyroid pathway)
- ☐ 3% of DRI in Zinc (healing)
- ☐ 1% of DRI in Chromium (sugar balance)
- ☐ Extremely high in antioxidants and carotenoids
- ☐ Helps to improve the Cardiovascular system
- ☐ Helps to improve eye health
- ☐ Glycaemic load of 3

So another humble but awesome vegetable that we can almost always get our hands on!

I will say though, I try to always buy organic carrots, because I learned that when farmers have soil that has become hard and not useful because of the buildup of fertilisers and chemicals etc, they grow carrots in it, because they soak up all of those things rendering the ground useable again.

While I don't get hung up on organic produce, carrots I tend too for this reason.

Casein

The protein component of dairy foods that can cause an immune reaction much like gluten.

The author of The China Study, Dr. T. Colin Campbell calls casein the most relevant cancer promoter ever discovered. In case you need an added incentive to help reduce your antibodies.

Cashews

These nuts are actually a seed from the inside of the cashew apple. Weird huh?

I have seen many documentaries now where it is said that cashews have the same therapeutic effect as prozac.

Let's look at the breakdown of 100g of cashews:

- □ 36% of DV in Protein (thyroid pathway)
- □ 13% of DV in Dietary Fibre (hormonal clearance, gut health)
- □ 4% of DV in Vitamin E (thyroid pathway, antioxidant)
- □ 43% of DV in Vitamin K (blood, bones)
- □ 28% of DV in Vitamin B1 (thyroid, hair)
- □ 3% of DV in Vitamin B2 (thyroid pathway)
- □ 5% of DV in Vitamin B3 (mental health)
- □ 9% of DV in Vitamin B5 (food conversion, energy production)
- □ 21% of DV in Vitamin B6 (mental health, progesterone)
- □ 6% of DV in folate (MTHFR, liver)
- □ 4% of DV in calcium (bones)
- □ 37% of DV in iron (thyroid, fatigue, gut acid)
- □ 73% of DV in magnesium (stress, sugar)
- □ 59% of DV in phosphorus (liver, bones)
- □ 19% of DV in Potassium (thyroid, fatigue, fluid)
- □ 39% of DV in zinc (mental health, thyroid, immunity, wound healing)
- □ 110% of DV in copper (skin, collagen, nerves)
- □ 83% of DV in Manganese (thyroid)
- □ 28% of DV in Selenium (thyroid pathway)
- □ 67% of DV in total fats
- □ Glycemic Load of 11

When you look at the mental health and thyroid connections, I can see how they might replace prozac. But please, talk to your health care giver, NEVER just go off medication for any kind of mental health issue without guidance.

Cat's Claw

An immune enhancing, anti-inflammatory, pain reducing bark that is used for chronic immune deficiencies and in diseases such as Rheumatoid Arthritis, osteoarthritis, chronic fatigue syndrome, fibromyalgia, lyme disease and autoimmune disease.

It is not to be used in pregnancy.

It is to be monitored closely if used with immunosuppressive drugs.

Caveman Diet

See Paleo Diet

Cayenne

A pungent circulatory and metabolic stimulant, cayenne is surprisingly a counterirritant, carminative and is used to help improve circulation, improve digestion (I know - weird right?) and assist in weight loss.

Cayenne is used topically for issues such as osteoarthritis, Rheumatoid Arthritis, Raynaud's Syndrome and diabetic neuropathy where the fingers and toes start to lose feeling.

It is not advised however to use if reflux or ulcers are involved and is to be avoided topically on broken skin.

Celeriac

I only started eating celeriac a few years ago as it is an ingredient in the Hippocrates Soup on the Gerson Therapy.

But I also now make a traditional French salad out of it which is julienned and combined with julienned apple and a light dressing. It is sooooo Yummy!

If you like celery, celeriac (being celery root) is just a milder version, but much more versatile. I read recently that celeriac is fantastic for balancing our electrolytes, which include potassium which we thyroid people struggle with, so it is a great vegetable to include in salads, soups and even in a stir fry.

Hidden behind 1 cup of that knobbly exterior is:

- ☐ 5% of DV in protein (thyroid pathway)
- ☐ 11% of DV in Dietary Fibre (hormonal clearance, gut health)
- ☐ 21% of DV in Vitamin C (thyroid pathway, antioxidant, adrenals)
- ☐ 3% of DV in Vitamin E (antioxidant, thyroid pathway)
- ☐ 80% of DV in Vitamin K (blood, bones)
- ☐ 5% of DV in Vitamin B1 (thyroid, hair, hyperthyroidism)
- ☐ 6% of DV in Vitamin B2 (thyroid pathway)
- ☐ 5% of DV in Vitamin B3 (mental health)
- ☐ 13% of DV in Vitamin B6 (mental health, progesterone)
- ☐ 18% of DV in Phosphorus (liver, bones)

- ☐ 13% of DV in Potassium (fluid, thyroid, fatigue)
- ☐ 12% of DV in manganese (thyroid pathway)
- ☐ 2% of DV in Selenium (thyroid pathway)
- ☐ 3% of DV in Zinc (immunity, thyroid, mental health, wound healing)
- ☐ 6% of DV in Iron (thyroid pathway, fatigue, gut acid)
- ☐ 8% of DV in Magnesium (stress, sugar)
- ☐ 7% of DVI in Calcium (bones)
- ☐ It has a glycemic load of 6

So this strange looking vegetable will help us with:

- ☐ supporting digestion
- ☐ Boosting cognitive function
- ☐ Improving bone density
- ☐ Reducing inflammation
- ☐ Improving skin health
- ☐ Improving heart health
- ☐ Improving wound healing
- ☐ Balancing electrolytes

There is no coincidence that this is a main ingredient in a soup that taken twice a day on a cancer healing diet such as The Gerson Therapy.

Celery

Poor celery is the not so loved member of the greens/salad/veg family. It's the last one picked on a crudité plate and often goes limp in the fridge before it is eaten. But it is so great for us.

1 cup of diced raw celery contains:

- ☐ 6% of DV in Fibre (hormone clearance, gut health)
- ☐ 1% of DV in Protein (thyroid pathway)
- ☐ 9% of DV in Vitamin A (Thyroid Pathway)
- ☐ 5% of DV in Vitamin C (thyroid pathway, adrenals, antioxidant)
- ☐ 1% of DV in Vitamin E (thyroid Pathway, antioxidant)
- ☐ 37% of DV in Vitamin K (Blood & Bones)
- ☐ 1% of DV in Vitamin B1 (thyroid, hair, hyperthyroidism)
- ☐ 3% of DV in Vitamin B2 (Thyroid Pathway)

- ☐ 2% of DV in Vitamin B3 (Mental Health)
- ☐ 4% of DV in Vitamin B6 (Mental Health)
- ☐ 9% of DV in Folate (MTHFR)
- ☐ 4% of DV in Calcium (Bones)
- ☐ 4% of DV in Copper (skin, collagen, nerves)
- ☐ 1% of DV in Iron (thyroid pathway, fatigue, gut acid)
- ☐ 3% of DV in Magnesium (stress, sugar)
- ☐ 5% of DV in Manganese (thyroid pathway)
- ☐ 11% of DV in Molybdenum (thyroid Pathway)
- ☐ 2% of DV in Phosphorus (bones, liver)
- ☐ 8% of DV in Potassium (Thyroid, fluid, fatigue)
- ☐ 1% of DV in Selenium (thyroid Pathway)
- ☐ 3% of DV in Sodium (adrenals)
- ☐ 1% of DV in Zinc (thyroid, immunity, mental health, wound healing)

This means that celery is helpful for:

- ☐ Digestive Health
- ☐ Cardiovascular Health
- ☐ Inflammation

Is it time to rock that Waldorf salad recipe now?

Celery Juice

Made famous by the Medical Medium Anthony William, celery juice now has a cult following and his latest book is all about just that.

Just searching #celeryjuice on instagram alone will find over 100k posts.

Anthony William states that 1 whole celery, washed, juiced and drunk on an empty stomach first thing in the morning will:

- ☐ Lower inflammation
- ☐ Support weight loss
- ☐ Heal Digestion
- ☐ Reduce bloating
- ☐ Helps Eczema & Psoriasis
- ☐ Fight infection
- ☐ Help prevent UTI's

- Help heal acne
- Prevent high blood pressure
- Help lower high cholesterol
- Help prevent ulcers
- Protect liver health

He believes this one practice will transform the gut like nothing else can.

Celery Seed

This amazing anti-rheumatic and anti-inflammatory is used extensively with osteoarthritis, rheumatoid arthritis, rheumatism and gout.

Like celery itself, celery seed is a diuretic so caution must be used in kidney disease.

Celiac Disease

An autoimmune response in the small intestine after ingesting gluten causing severe pain, cramping, bloating, nausea and vomiting.

There is a strong correlation between celiac disease and thyroid disease which finds many with celiac ending up with autoimmune thyroid disease.

This is because of the connection between leaky gut and autoimmune disease.

It is always good to remember that once you have one autoimmune disease you are predisposed to others if you don't get on top of the inflammation and reduce your antibodies.

Celloids

Also called Mineral Salts, celloids were developed by Maurice Blackmore (from Blackmores supplements) in the 1930's.

They are a safe, smaller doses of minerals but in more specific combinations for specific issues.

Some celloid examples include:

- M.P. (magnesium phosphate) calms the pituitary and the thyroid gland, balances calcium
- P.C. (potassium chloride) bile production, fluid retention, endometriosis, fibroids

- I.P. (iron phosphate) reduce inflammation, improve muscle tone, tonic to underactive endocrine glands, improves semen production
- C.P. (calcium phosphate) underactive thyroid, circulation, irritability, bones, kidneys, poor appetite

If you like this idea, look further into the work of Alfred Jacka, also Blackmores offers a short course on Celloid Minerals.

Cellulite

Most people understand that fat deposits under the skin, that forces its way through our connective tissue and forms the dimpled appearance of cellulite.

But what about the skinny girls that have cellulite?

In the health world cellulite is caused by hormones, particularly estrogen, insulin and thyroid hormones. Although what causes cellulite is actually based on theories or educated assumptions, the hormone connection explains why skinny girls get cellulite too.

There are ways to decrease it from the simple massaging to expensive treatments, but straightening out the hormones, losing weight and improving the integrity of the connective tissue is where the main game plan needs to be at.

Chamomile

The beautiful chamomile flower is widely available in tea and tincture form. It can be found in creams, balms, sprays and is a staple at most cafes with peppermint tea.

The reason this lovely gentle flower is so widely used is due to its anti-inflammatory, carminative, sedative, spasmolytic actions.

It is great for IBS, gastrointestinal distress, diarrhoea, peptic ulcers, restlessness, anxiety, insomnia and is the common ingredient in gripe water used for colic in babies.

Used extensively in topical creams for skin irritations, wounds and ulcers, this versatile and safe herb is fantastic to have on hand in any of its forms.

Change

Time for a little mindset understanding.

You know how we go on a diet and even though we never eat chocolate or maybe bread or whatever, suddenly it is all we want??

It's a mind thing - if we think we are going to lose something (ie weight, food, fun) then apparently we see it as a loss and our subconscious or ego does everything it can to resist that.

So it's not that we have no will power - we have to be kind to ourselves. There is so much more going on in our brains than we can ever hope to know.

Change simply represents a potential threat to our psyche, and our subconscious rebels. That's why we have become "creatures of habit", because change is uncomfortable. But we need to be uncomfortable if we are going to forge a life we love.

Try using one of the many techniques in this book to help you along that road such as EFT or the Ho'oponopono Prayer

Chaste Tree

Also known as Vitex agnus-castus, Chaste Tree is used extensively for hormonal balance in women.

Used for PMS, erratic ovulation, low progesterone, fibroids, endometriosis, ovarian cysts, postnatal depression and benign breast growths.

It is interesting to note though that it doesn't really work if you are also taking the Oral Contraceptive Pill and could interfere with progesteronic drugs so it is important to work with someone who specialises in reproductive hormones when using this amazing herb.

Chelation

The process of removing unwanted substances from the body.

The term is used when referring to heavy metals as the chelator will bind to a metal and then be excreted.

There are chemical chelators but the following examples are examples of natural chelators:

- Cilantro is a mercury chelator.
- Chlorella is an aluminium chelator
- Brazil Nuts are a mercury chelator
- Zinc is a cadmium chelator

Chemicals

One seminar I attended over the years announced at the beginning that the average woman is exposed to more than 500 chemicals before she even walks out the door of a morning.

This was rather shocking to me. But once the seminar got further in, it was actually easy to see how this can happen when every single body or hair product we absorb through our skin each has at least a dozen different chemicals in the ingredients list.

Our thyroid is a chemical magnet! So any way that we can reduce our chemical burden is going to help our thyroid function more efficiently.

Some ideas:

- ☐ Replace body and hair products for organic
- ☐ Replace makeup with organic or go without
- ☐ Replace nail varnish with a 10 free option or go without
- ☐ Organic food
- ☐ Remove pesticides and insecticides from the home
- ☐ Change cleaning products for natural alternatives or make your own
- ☐ Store food in glass or ceramic containers (no plastic) and don't buy takeaway in plastic containers
- ☐ Replace nonstick pans with cast iron
- ☐ Replace plastic shower curtains with fabric or PVC free
- ☐ Only buy tinned food with BPA free liners
- ☐ Don't handle cash receipts (phthalates) ask for them to be emailed

You can see from this list how easy it is for us to be consumed by chemicals at the start of our day.

It is not something we can generally afford financially to just swap out in a weekend, but it is something we can consistently work on for the sake of our thyroid.

Chia Seeds

These amazing little black seeds pack a huge punch in protein, fibre, fats and calcium.

You can turn them into jelly, pudding and add a teaspoon to a cup of water to fill you up with next to no calories. What's not to love about that?

100g Chia seeds contain:

- 31% of DV in Protein (thyroid pathway)
- 151% of DV in Dietary Fibre (hormonal clearance, gut health)
- 63% of DV in calcium (bones)
- 95% of DV in phosphorus (liver, bones)
- 5% of DV in potassium (thyroid, fatigue, fluid)
- 23% of DV in Zinc (thyroid, mental health, immunity, wound healing)
- 108% of DV in manganese (thyroid)
- 20% of DV in Omega 3s (joint health, mental health)

They help to:

- improve digestion
- reduce inflammation
- balance blood sugar
- balance cholesterol
- boost energy
- improve bone strength
- reduce weight
- inhibit cancer growth

One of the easiest jellies you can make is 2 cups of fruit pureed with 2 tablespoons of chia seeds, then let set in the refrigerator. My favourites here are raspberries and apricots.

Chlorella

A single-celled green algae that is considered a functional food as opposed to a supplement or vitamin. It grows in fresh water and is particularly helpful in removing toxins and heavy metals (including mercury and cadmium) from the body.

It is incredibly high in Vitamin A, B vitamins, iron, magnesium, and zinc which are all needed for the thyroid pathway, stress and mental health.

The first time I came across it was not as a naturopath but as a mom, when I was working with a doctor on reducing the aluminium load in my son's brain (they thought is was ADD, it was actually high aluminium). He gave my son Chlorella in liquid form to drink every day, which gently chelated the aluminium from his body. As a side note, within 6 months he was off medication and never touched it again and he is now 18.

Other benefits of regular Chlorella use:

- Immune system support
- Improved weight loss
- Regulates hormones
- Flushes out toxins
- Is Anti-ageing

Chloride

Chloride is a member of the Halide family (along with fluoride, bromide and iodide) on the periodic table and as such has the ability to block iodine in the body.

There is natural sources of chloride which are not harmful to the body and actually help us with fluid balance, and producing gut acid. This is found in foods such as tomatoes, olives, celery, lettuce and seaweed.

The concern for us with chloride is when it is used as a chemical or purifier. It is simply a matter of avoiding it wherever possible.

- Chlorinated swimming pools
- Tap & shower water (use a good filter)
- Cleaning products (bleach)

Cholagogue

An agent which stimulates or aids the release of bile from the gallbladder.

Examples Include: Barberry, Butternut, Cloves, Dandelion Root, Gentian, Globe Artichoke, Peppermint, Yellow Dock

Cholesterol

We can have cholesterol problems with both hyper and hypo situations.

In hypothyroidism low thyroid hormone means the body can't convert cholesterol into the hormones it is supposed to. (pregnenolone, progesterone, DHEA) which leaves excess of it in our body. It is also slow at clearing LDL cholesterol allowing it to build up in the blood.

In hyperthyroidism, quite the opposite occurs finding it being cleared out too quickly resulting in low cholesterol. Remember we do actually need cholesterol for the making of progesterone.

In either case it is the liver that helps process the cholesterol, and since liver is often a sluggish organ in thyroid disease, this is another contributing factor.

The first port of call is always straightening out the thyroid hormones first as they are likely the underlying cause, before heading for medication.

Chromium

Chromium is required for:

- Glucose metabolism
- Blood sugar regulation
- Reduces cholesterol

Deficiency Symptoms of chromium include:

- Anxiety & fatigue
- Poor balance, loss of feeling in hands/feet
- Atherosclerosis & Heart Disease
- High sugar levels
- High insulin levels
- High cholesterol

Factors that contribute to chromium deficiency:

- Excess refined foods
- Excess simple carbohydrates
- Diabetes
- Strenuous exercise
- Cardiovascular disease
- Estrogen therapy
- Physical trauma

Food sources of chromium include:

- Asparagus, mushrooms, potato
- Apples, prunes, raisins, grape juice
- Beer, Brewer's Yeast

- Lobster, oysters, shrimp
- Peanuts, nuts, egg yolk

Daily Requirements of chromium:

- Adult RDA - 50-200ug

Chronic Fatigue Syndrome

A disorder characterised by incredible fatigue, rendering patients unable to work or function for sometimes many months at a time.

With no known cause (although the Medical Medium states it is a symptom of the Epstein Barr Virus and therefore connected with thyroid disease) and no medical way of treating or managing it, sufferers are left in an awful limbo while their body fights it.

Herbs that may help include: Astragalus, Gingko, Hawthorn, Korean Ginseng, Licorice, Rehmannia, Rhodiola, and St John's Wort.

Chronic Thyroiditis

Another name for Hashimoto's Thyroiditis.

Cilantro

Also called coriander is one of those herbs that is an acquired taste! I promise! The more you have it, the more you want it! A bit like Olives and Avocado.

Cilantro has a chelating ability on heavy metals in our thyroid and body, particularly mercury that likes to hide in the thyroid.

It is said that 2 tablespoons a day over a few months will help to achieve this.

½ cup of cilantro provides:

- 32% of DV in Vitamin K (blood & bones)
- 4% of DV in Vitamin C (adrenal health)
- 10% of DV in Vitamin A (thyroid pathway)
- 2% of DV in Vitamin E (thyroid pathway)
- 2% of DV in Manganese (thyroid pathway)
- 1% of DV in Magnesium (sugar & stress)

- ☐ 2% of DV in Potassium (thyroid, fluid, fatigue)
- ☐ 1% of DV in Vitamin B1 (thyroid, hair, hyperthyroidism)
- ☐ 1% of DV in Vitamin B2 (thyroid pathway)
- ☐ 1% of DV in Vitamin B3 (mental health)
- ☐ 2% of DV in Folate (MTHFR & liver health)

Cinnamon

This tasty bark is incredible for balancing blood sugar so is a great spice to add to meals daily if you have diabetes, metabolic syndrome and insulin resistance due to its high chromium content.

In fact if you have any of these issues a great breakfast would be gluten free oats with cinnamon sprinkled on top every morning.

Cinnamon is also a carminative and can help to soothe nausea, diarrhoea, and improve digestive weakness.

It is to be used with caution though if you are already on diabetic medication because it works extremely well, so monitoring will be necessary as less medication would be required. It is important to understand though, that if you do use cinnamon daily, and you have reduced your medication because of it, you will need to keep consuming cinnamon.

Caution is needed in pregnancy and reflux.

Circadian Rhythm

This refers to the cycle of cortisol excretion from our adrenals that should be higher in the mornings and lower in the evenings.

This encourages alertness on waking and drowsiness at bedtime.

Being a night owl, and staying awake till 2 am, shows a sign of adrenal exhaustion and disrupted circadian rhythm which contributes to a decline in health.

People who work night shifts often suffer from chronic diseases due to the permanent disruption to their cycle.

Circulatory Stimulant

An agent which improves the circulation of the blood through the body.

Examples Include: Bayberry, Cayenne, Ginger, Ginkgo, Horseradish, Rosemary

CNS

Central Nervous System which is then broken down into the Sympathetic Nervous System (fight or flight) and the Parasympathetic Nervous System (rest & digest).

Coconut Oil

Full of medium chain fatty acids, this saturated oil has been declared the thyroid saviour for weight loss and thyroid function.

While coconut oil has many positive benefits, and I have read many glowing reports from people who eat it by the spoonful, I have a different story.

It actually makes me sick. Like nausea and vomiting kinda sick.

So this entry is not about telling you how amazing this is and you should take it, there are a thousand sites out there you can find to tell you that. I'm here to tell you, just because it works for someone else, and the science says it's so, doesn't mean it will do the same for you.

With so many amazing raw desserts floating around full of coconut oil, and recipes replacing butter with coconut oil it is not hard to suddenly get a lot of it in your diet.

Be open minded that this may, or may not, be helpful to you personally. That is all I ask. Keep a diary!

Cognitive Behavioural Therapy

Used by counsellors it is a treatment that helps interrupt and change negative thought patterns that lead to negative behaviour.

It is used in the treatment of depression, anxiety and addiction amongst other issues.

Cohen, Suzy

Known as "America's most trusted pharmacist", Suzy has written several books on various topics including the thyroid and diabetes.

I have her book "Thyroid Healthy" and it is one that I refer too often. Suzy has a great way of explaining things in a simple manor.

I highly recommend you get a hold of this book for your thyroid library.

Cold Intolerance

A very normal symptom of hypothyroidism as the thyroid is involved in temperature regulation, so people with low thyroid levels will experience cold weather a lot quicker than normal.

This usually presents initially with cold hands and feet, till eventually you are wearing 3 blankets in the height of summer. You get me.

Hypothyroid people often do better in warmer climates as hyperthyroid people do better in cooler climates. In most cases.

Keep in mind that Ginger is Nature's Blanket, and eating foods that have heat in them, plus making sure all your food and drink are warm not cold will help stoke the furnace which will help with cold intolerance.

Coleus

This is an herb root I take everyday. I take it in tablet form with a couple of other ingredients because the liquid version tastes absolutely ghastly (and I have taken some awful herbs)!!

The main reason I take it is for conversion. Coleus helps convert T4 into T3 but it also used for weight loss, metabolic syndrome, hypertension, heart health and digestive weakness.

Caution is required for those taking Blood Pressure medication due to its ability to lower blood pressure, it means you will likely need less medication so make sure you keep an eye on it if you use it.

It should not be used with low blood pressure and peptic ulcers.

Collagen

This anti ageing protein is a big component of our connective tissues, so it doesn't just keep our skin lovely, it keeps our joins smooth and strengthens the bones.

To make our own collagen we need:

- ☐ Vitamin C - citrus fruits, berries, tropical fruits, peppers
- ☐ Zinc - oysters, meats, pumpkin seeds, sunflower seeds
- ☐ Copper - avocado, shellfish, beans

Foods that are highly helpful in improving our collagen synthesis includes:

- ☐ Bone broth
- ☐ Chicken, fish, shellfish
- ☐ Egg whites

Colonic Irrigation

Also called Colonics, this is like an enema on steroids.

You have to book into a clinic somewhere for this procedure and there is always a trained practitioner there to administer it.

The process involves a tube up the rectum which is attached to a pump. Warm water is then pushed up into the colon to irrigate it.

There are pros and cons to this.

It is a great way to start enemas if you are a bit shy about doing an enema yourself, as a trained person does it for you.

However, enemas actually tone the bowel because it is gravity fed as opposed to water being forced up there if that makes sense?

Complementary Medicine

Complementary medicine is a modality, generally natural of ancient origin, used alongside allopathic (western) medicine to help with symptoms and healing.

Complementary medicines that may be of help in thyroid symptoms and disease are:

- ☐ Naturopathy
- ☐ Herbal medicine
- ☐ Traditional Chinese Medicine
- ☐ Ayurvedic Medicine
- ☐ Bowen therapy
- ☐ Kinesiology
- ☐ Iridology
- ☐ Chiropractor
- ☐ Colon Hydrotherapy

- ☐ Mindset / Life Coach
- ☐ Meditation
- ☐ Hydrotherapy
- ☐ Aromatherapy

Congenital Hypothyroidism

This is the term given to someone who has been born with thyroid disease. This is usually picked up via the Guthrie Test within the first 5 days of birth.

Connective Tissue Diseases

Rheumatoid arthritis, lupus, scleroderma, polymyositis and dermatomyositis are all examples of connective tissue diseases.

With no known cure for these diseases there is a higher prevalence of hypothyroidism in people that have them.

Herbs that help strengthen connective tissue include: Grape seed, Hawthorn, and Polygonum multiflorum

Constipation

A common issue in hypothyroid patients due to the overall slowing down of all bodily processes, it is also a common side effect of taking iron supplements.

It is important to increase water intake and fibre with lots of fruit and veg if this is an issue.

Enemas and colonic hydrotherapy can be of help in this area and get things moving again while you improve your diet and lifestyle habits.

Herbs to help move things along include: Aloe, Butternut, Damiana, Dandelion, Gentian, Globe Artichoke, Licorice, Marshmallow Root, Rehmannia, Rhubarb Root, Senna Pods, Slippery Elm, St Mary's Thistle, and Yellow Dock

Copper

Copper is needed in the body but it is unusual to have a deficiency. In most cases it is an excess that causes the problems, because the slower the metabolism the higher the rate of copper retention.

Add to that, copper and iron have an antagonistic relationship. When one is up the other is down. Since most thyroid people tend to have low iron, this also validates the excess copper.

Another interesting relationship is that of copper and estrogen as they tend to reflect one another. High estrogen levels are usually accompanied by high copper levels.

Copper is required for:

- Production of collagen
- Skin maintenance
- Bone & nerve function
- Regulates iron metabolism
- Wound healing

Sources of copper include:

- Green lip mussels, oysters, crab
- Avocado, broccoli, mushrooms
- Almonds, pecans, sunflower seeds
- Beans, dried legumes, whole-grain, buckwheat
- Lamb, pork, perch
- Copper water pipes

Daily Requirements of Copper:

- Adults RDA - 1-3 mg

Excess Copper

Symptoms of Excess Copper include:

- Fatigue, suppressing of thyroid function, hormone imbalance
- Hair loss, grey hair, early greying
- Fatty liver, sluggish bile, gallstones, gallbladder regulator
- Anaemia, iron deficiency
- Heavy and long menstrual cycle
- Allergies, Rashes, Easy bruising, flushed skin
- Syndrome X, Hypoglycaemia
- Viral infections, fungal infections, prolonged infections
- High risk of Epstein Barr virus

- ☐ High risk of Chronic fatigue syndrome
- ☐ Slow healing
- ☐ Excess copper levels block zinc, iron, folate, magnesium
- ☐ Postpartum depression
- ☐ Agitation, Depression, insomnia or;
- ☐ Emotional neediness or;
- ☐ Surly, aggressive, pushy, belligerent

Factors that contribute to Copper excess include:

- ☐ Low Vitamin C, zinc, molybdenum
- ☐ Low Cysteine, glutamine, histidine, threonine
- ☐ Copper water pipes for cooking, drinking, showering

Copper Deficiency

Deficiency Symptoms of copper include:

- ☐ Hair loss & grey hair
- ☐ Anemia, low white cell count
- ☐ Depression, poor coordination
- ☐ Slow healing
- ☐ High cholesterol
- ☐ High uric acid
- ☐ Ear infections, chest infections, sinusitis
- ☐ Thrush, boils, gastroenteritis

Factors that contribute to copper deficiency:

- ☐ Alcohol
- ☐ Excess sugar
- ☐ Pregnancy
- ☐ High fructose consumption
- ☐ Potassium deficiency

Corn Silk

You know the fine silky threads you pull off the inside of a corn husk before you cook it? That is corn silk and it is the most amazing ingredient for the urinary tract.

It is used for cystitis, urethritis, enuresis and urinary tract infections due to its diuretic and demulcent (soothing) properties.

It has no safety issues and is as easy as taking some silk and boiling it in some water to make a tea.

Or you could work with an herbalist and get the liquid tincture.

Cortisol

Secreted by the adrenal glands, cortisol is the hormone our adrenal glands produce in response to stress, regardless of cause. So physical, mental and emotional stress will all trigger our adrenals to produce cortisol.

We need cortisol..... in the right amounts.

The problem lies in the fact that we all seem to be under some form of stress 24 hours a day. Just having thyroid disease puts our body under physical stress and no doubt, for most of us, emotional stress too every minute of the day.

This leads to a chronic release of cortisol which does the following damage:

- Thyroid disorders
- narrowing of the arteries
- a flood of glucose into the body
- reduced insulin (the fat burning hormone)
- Increased risk of diabetes
- Weight Gain and obesity
- The suppression of the immune system, causing more autoimmune disease
- Indigestion
- Ulcers
- Cardiovascular disease
- Infertility
- Insomnia
- Chronic fatigue
- Dementia
- Depression

Unfortunately the only way to lower cortisol is the usual lower stress, improve the diet, take up a hobby... you know the drill!

Corydalis

This is a tuber with sedative and hypnotic actions that helps with headaches, insomnia, anxiety and emotional stress.

Corydalis is also used in pain management for issues like IBS, painful periods, due to its analgesic and spasmolytic abilities.

It is contraindicated in pregnancy.

Cosmetics

See chemicals

Couch Grass

Yes grass!!! Although the part used is the Rhizome or root not the grass.

This is another great one to have on hand if you are prone to Urinary Tract Infections. Team this with corn silk and Bearberry and it's great to relieve the symptoms of UTIs very quickly.

It is classed as a urinary demulcent, so soothing to the urinary tract and is also a mild diuretic.

Apart from UTI's it is also helpful for prostatitis and kidney stones and has no safety concerns.

Cracked Heels

A curse of many people but particularly thyroid sufferer's where dry skin is a common symptom.

With no oil ducts in the feet, moisturising daily is an absolute must to avoid this issue.

In Ayurveda it is a vata disruption (too dry) and can also be caused by wearing shoes with very thin soles or being barefoot a lot.

I am sorry to tell you that the hard work has to be done here to keep the cracks at bay. Forming a habit of massaging a non toxic cream or balm into the feet morning and night until you get on top of it and then every night is the only thing that keeps it from coming back. It doesn't matter what magical cream you use, if you stop using it, the dry cracked heels will appear again.

Cramp Bark

This bark is used for all things crampy.

Period cramps, endometriosis pain and also threatened miscarriage is a common use for this as it has spasmolytic and mild sedative properties to help calm the cramping.

Crampbark also has the ability to help lower blood pressure by dilating vessels.

Cramps

Most assume that cramps are caused from a lack of magnesium, but they can also be a lack of potassium which is more likely in thyroid disease.

When I am not paying attention to my nutrient intake, then I will experience the odd night leg cramp along with Restless Leg Syndrome. That is when I will add a potassium supplement to my diet for a while, and I up my magnesium and potassium foods too.

Herbs that help with leg cramps include: Ginkgo, Horsechestnut, Kava, and Prickly Ash

Craniosacral Therapy

A modality where different parts of the skull are palpated and massaged, releasing pressure and improving the circulation of the cerebrospinal fluid.

This helps to improve the functioning of the nervous system, relieve pain, improve skeletal traumas, improve learning disabilities and improve stress.

Cravings

The hardest part of any change in dietary regime.

Cravings can be caused by physical withdrawal to sugar or other substances and also deficiencies such as magnesium.

This is one of the reasons women often crave chocolate at "that time of the month" because somewhere in the depth of our knowing we knew that before chocolate was messed with it was high in magnesium (raw chocolate is packed with it)

Another deficiency that causes cravings is adrenal deficiency. It causes us to crave salty foods, so give it what it needs (Himalayan Salt).

Tips for combating cravings of any kind:

- ☐ Brush your teeth
- ☐ Do not use artificial sweeteners - they increase sweet cravings
- ☐ Eat more protein and fat
- ☐ Snack on sweet vegetables like carrot and sweet potato
- ☐ Do an activity
- ☐ Drink water
- ☐ Don't watch TV loaded with food adverts
- ☐ Don't keep sugary foods in the house
- ☐ Get some Gymnema from your naturopath - an herb that dulls the sweet taste

Supplements to help with cravings:

- ☐ Chromium (600-1000mg a day)
- ☐ Magnesium
- ☐ Zinc (deficiency causes lowered taste which encourages the craving for higher sugar and salt foods)

Cretinism

The old term for physical abnormalities and learning delays caused by severe congenital thyroid disease caused by iodine deficiency in the mother.

Severe forms of this is now a rare occurrence and the condition is now referred to simply as congenital hypothyroidism.

Crohn's Disease

See Inflammatory Bowel Disease

Crown Chakra

The Chakra located in the top of our head and is the place where we connect with pure consciousness.

- ☐ color - violet
- ☐ Key issues - inner wisdom
- ☐ Physiological system - CNS and brain

- Endocrine gland - pineal and pituitary
- Crystals - celestite, blue sapphire, sugilite, clear quartz and amethyst
- Aromatherapy - Ylang Ylang, rosewood, lime blossom

Cruciferous vegetables

See Brassica

Crying

Most people love a good cry and it is extremely cathartic releasing stagnant built up emotions.

Unfortunately with thyroid disease we tend to cry more than most.

Since there are so many T3 receptors in our brain, if our hormone levels are too high or too low it can cause an imbalance leaving us with mental health issues such as depression, anxiety, mood swings, irritability and so on.

And this then leads to us crying. A lot.

Please know that this is normal IF your thyroid is not in balance. Think of it as a big signal from our body that we haven't got our medication right yet.

Assuming you have gotten that part right, if you are still crying, it could also be down to blood sugar imbalance. So cut down the sugar, eat more fat and protein and see if the tears dry up a little.

Cucumber

Cucumber is a wonderful watery, cooling ingredient. High in silica and flavonoids, they are also anti-inflammatory, and who would have thought it contains iron??

A great vegetable to add to pretty much everything!

1 cup sliced cucumber contains:

- 1% of DV in Protein (thyroid pathway)
- 2% of DV in Fibre (hormone clearance, gut health)
- 3% of DV in Vitamin B1 (thyroid, hair, hyperthyroid)
- 2% of DV in Vitamin B2 (thyroid pathway)
- 1% of DV in Vitamin B3 (mental health)

- ☐ 2% of DV in Vitamin B6 (mental health, progesterone)
- ☐ 3% of DV in Biotin (Hair, skin, nails, sugar)
- ☐ 2% of DV in Folate (MTHFR, liver)
- ☐ 4% of DV in Vitamin C (thyroid pathway, adrenals)
- ☐ 1% of DV in Vitamin A (thyroid pathway, skin)
- ☐ 19% of DV in Vitamin K (bones, blood)
- ☐ 2% of DV in Calcium (bones)
- ☐ 4% of DV in Copper (skin, nerves, bone, collagen)
- ☐ 2% of DV in Iron (thyroid pathway, fatigue, gut acid)
- ☐ 3% of DV in Magnesium (sugar, stress)
- ☐ 4% of DV in Manganese (thyroid pathway)
- ☐ 12% of DV in Molybdenum (thyroid, excess copper)
- ☐ 4% of DV in Phosphorus (liver, bones)
- ☐ 4% of DV in Potassium (fatigue, thyroid, fluid)
- ☐ 1% of DV in Selenium (thyroid pathway)
- ☐ 2% of DV in Zinc (thyroid, immunity, wound healing, mental health)
- ☐ 98% Water

Cupping

This is another unusual therapy made famous by Gwyneth Paltrow a few years back and performed by a Traditional Chinese Practitioner. It involves using round glass cups that are applied to the skin in a way that forms suction.

The process leaves incredible large round spots on your back but helps with:

- ☐ reducing inflammation
- ☐ increasing blood flow
- ☐ relaxation and well being

It is essentially a form of very deep tissue massage that many love.

Curcumin

The active ingredient in turmeric that combats inflammation and targets cancer stem cells for destruction while making normal cells stronger.

See Turmeric for further information

Cysteine

A non-essential amino acid, however, is another one that becomes essential if we are sick or have a disease.

Cysteine is a sulphur containing acid that we use to make taurine (also an amino acid) but it is also involved in:

- Making insulin
- Skin and hair health
- Making CoQ10, biotin and glutathione
- Chemical detoxification
- Helps bile secretion
- Improves immune function
- Wound healing

Cytomel

A synthetic thyroid replacement hormone containing T3, the active thyroid hormone. It is often used in conjunction with thyroxine for people who struggle to convert their T4 into T3.

Cytotoxic T-Cells

Immune cells sent to destroy an antigen (toxin, virus or pathogen).

D

Determination

It is not for the faint hearted to decide they are going to reverse a disease, and possibly even do so in the more unusual natural ways.

Nothing is ever straightforward, least of all healing. So determination is required under all circumstances.

When I began administering regular coffee enemas, my husband was completely grossed out. And rightly so. I get it.

But I was determined to continue for the sake of my health, so I found ways to do it that would affect him the least, plus I always hid all of my "tools of the trade" away so he didn't see them.

On days that he wanted to sleep in, I would take all my equipment quietly and creep into the laundry, and do it beside the spare toilet.

Eventually my determination won him over and now he works around me.

Being determined to follow through no matter what the obstacles is an important requirement for feeling well when you have a chronic disease.

It doesn't mean you will never have hurdles, it means you are willing to accept them, take a breath and look for a way around them or over them.

It is determination that will keep you heading in the right direction.

D Vitamin

A story about Vitamin D before I get into the details. For most of my first 15 years with thyroid disease I consistently had low levels. Every now and then I would supplement but it really didn't change my test results.

When I started to naturally heal my thyroid pathway, as my other levels improved, my Vitamin D levels improved even though I was not taking any supplementation.

This I believe, is because Vitamin D, also called Calcitriol, is actually a hormone, so as my entire endocrine (hormone) system balanced out, so too did my Vitamin D levels.

Vitamin D is required for:

- ☐ Apoptosis (death) of colon, breast and melanoma cells
- ☐ Blood clotting
- ☐ Bone Strength
- ☐ Increases tyrosine activity (thyroid pathway)

Deficiency Symptoms of Vitamin D include:

- ☐ Bone pain, arthritis, osteoporosis
- ☐ Insomnia, nervousness
- ☐ Frequent or prolonged infections
- ☐ Autoimmune disorders
- ☐ Glucose intolerance

Factors that contribute to Vitamin D deficiency:

- ☐ Alcohol
- ☐ Ulcerative colitis, Crohn's Disease
- ☐ Pregnancy & lactation
- ☐ Autoimmune arthritis
- ☐ Hypoparathyroidism
- ☐ Insulin Dependant Diabetes
- ☐ Multiple Sclerosis, Schizophrenia
- ☐ High smog exposure

Sources of Vitamin D include:

- ☐ Sunlight on skin
- ☐ Fish liver oils
- ☐ Cod, halibut, herring, tuna
- ☐ Butter, egg yolks, milk
- ☐ Sprouted Seeds

Daily Requirements of Vitamin D:

- Adult RDA - 200-400IU
- Requires Boron to activate it in the body

Dairy

Dairy foods include milk, ice cream, yogurt, sour cream, and cheese.

Sadly, as nice as these foods are to eat, they can cause a reaction in many of us thyroid people, particularly auto-immune.

They have a similar molecular structure to gluten and so if gluten is an issue for you, removing dairy also can be helpful to lowering antibodies.

I have found that almond milk (particularly Almond Breeze) is the nicest alternative to milk and if you want a sour cream replacement, check out that entry.

Be careful with a lot of the plant based dairy alternatives on the market as a fair majority of them contain soy which can interfere with thyroid balance.

Damiana

This is the answer for you if you struggle with a low libido (low sex drive). Damiana is a tonic that helps with nerves, anxiety and depression it helps get you in the mood.

In college we made Bliss Balls with Damiana in them as an aphrodisiac. They were brilliant ... if you know what I mean!!

It has no safety issues, but it also has mild laxative properties so make sure you are following your herbalists script or your night in the bedroom could be transferred to the bathroom!

Dandelion Leaf

Those lovely weeds many of us pull out and throw in the compost has some amazing qualities.

The leaf (which you could throw into a salad) is a mild diuretic a mild laxative and helps if you are prone to gallstones.

This is a great way to help release excess fluid and lower blood pressure in a gentle way.

It has no major safety issues... except of course if you have put herbicide on your garden then you pick it for a salad! Don't do that ok? Same if you decide to go wild foraging for it, don't pick it from the sides of freeways where the toxins from traffic will have permeated it and made it more harmful than helpful.

Dates

Just to clarify, we are talking about those dried up pieces of fruit most commonly seen in either nana's Date Loaf, Sticky Date Pudding or in all those amazing raw desserts on Instagram NOT a hot night with our love (although that is good for the thyroid too).

Dates are packed with goodies that we need for our thyroid pathway but also are high in fructose. So if you are following a low fructose diet, leave these at the grocery store.

100g (about 4) of Medjool dates gives us:

- 27% of DV in Dietary Fibre (hormones, gut)
- 4% of DV in Protein (thyroid pathway)
- 3% of DV in Vitamin A (thyroid pathway)
- 3% of DV in Vitamin K (blood, bones)
- 3% of DV in Vitamin B1 (thyroid, hair, hyperthyroidism)
- 4% of DV in Vitamin B2 (thyroid pathway)
- 8% of DV in Vitamin B3 (mental health)
- 8% of DV in Vitamin B5 (food conversion, energy)
- 12% of DV in Vitamin B6 (mental health, progesterone)
- 4% of DV in Folate (MTHFR, liver)
- 6% of DV in calcium (bones)
- 5% of DV in Iron (thyroid pathway)
- 14% of DV in Magnesium (stress, sugar)
- 6% of DV in Phosphorus (bones, liver)
- 20% of DV in Potassium (thyroid, fluid, fatigue)
- 3% of DV in Zinc (thyroid, immunity, mental health, wound healing)
- 18% of DV in copper (skin, nerves, collagen)
- 15% of DV in Manganese (thyroid pathway)
- Glycemic Load of 39

DDT

An extremely toxic herbicide that can still be found in the ground of some countries even though it was banned in the 70s.

Anyone familiar with the Vietnam War will know it as Agent Orange, and is being blamed for many of the psychological and physical problems our soldiers returned with and often never recovered from.

Devils Claw

As scary sounding as the name is, this herb (root) is amazing for all things painful.

Rheumatoid Arthritis, Osteoarthritis, Rheumatism, Gout, back pain and myalgia all benefit from the anti-inflammatory, anti rheumatic, analgesic properties of this tuber.

The only caution is with peptic ulcers, so work with a qualified herbalist.

De Quervain's Thyroiditis

A viral infection that triggers the painful swelling of the thyroid. It is temporary and presents with fever, neck pain, jaw and ear pain.

DEXA Scan

A machine that measures the fat, bone and muscle ratio in the body.

It is easy to do, you just lie under a machine as the arm slowly waves over the top of you from head to foot scanning your body.

It is a great way of knowing just how much of your body is fat.

Dehydration

Everybody needs water, we all know that. I'm not going to bore you with a big long list of why our body which is almost 70% water needs.... well... water!

But what I am going to tell you is that our thyroid transport hormone actually can't get to thyroid receptors if we are dehydrated.

So drink up! If you don't like water, try flavouring it by adding some fruit and herbs to a large jug of filtered water.

My favourite combo is cucumber and orange. It makes the water taste so fancy, and you get an added boost of vitamins!

Dementia

A disease that causes loss of memory and judgement.

If hypothyroidism remains untreated or under-treated for a long period of time then dementia can develop.

Demulcent

An agent that is used internally to soothe, protect and lubricate irritated tissues and surfaces as well as relieve pain.

Examples Include: Chickweed, Comfrey, Fenugreek, Licorice, Marshmallow, Mullein, Ribwort, Slippery elm

Dental Health

Silver Fillings

Silver amalgam fillings used to be the standard, but as society learns better, we do better, and now they are banned in many countries and have been replaced by a composite filling (white ones).

The old silver fillings contain mercury, which continue to give off vapours for the rest of their days in your mouth.

Mercury has a particular love of attacking the thyroid which is what makes it so dangerous for thyroid people.

Now, it's not easy to rectify this situation. If you have been lucky like me and have only a few fillings you can have them removed and replaced. But please make sure you go to a dentist that knows how to do this safely! A rubber dam needs to be placed into your mouth so that you don't ingest the metal fragments as they are being removed. You may also want to load up on mercury destroying cilantro (coriander) both before and after the procedure.

This is not an easy undertaking for those of you with many of these fillings in your mouth, but still something you need to know.

Toothpaste & Mouthwash

Swap out your current toothpaste and mouthwash for a fluoride free option - *See Fluoride*

Root Canals

Root canals are the process of removing the root from a tooth, but leaving the dead tooth in place. This leaves a big whole under the tooth in the gum where infection can easily breed.

There are a few theories out there that root canals can contribute to breast cancer although the actual studies on that seem to be lacking.

I do believe the theory that a root canal can affect thyroid health, because anything that could cause an infection or bacteria to breed so close to the thyroid is bound to cause at the very least inflammation.

Deodorant

Deodorant impairs our thyroid in 2 ways.

Firstly, one of the active ingredients to stop the smell and sweat is Aluminium, which can cause mood swings, irritability in our brain and depletes calcium in our joints. Plus Aluminium blocks selenium, vitamin C and Vitamin B2 all of which we need in our thyroid pathway.

Secondly, it is actually designed to stop toxins getting out. That means the toxins will recycle in the body which puts a larger burden on our liver. We need a healthy liver to be able to convert our thyroid hormone into its active form.

So, while I understand there are times you can't go without it, I suggest a balance.

When you are home, don't wear anything - or use half a lime wiped over your armpit (works quite well). And when you have to be social or fancy, wear deodorant.

Balance in all things I believe, and when I find a natural deodorant that works for me, I will be happy, but so far none I love (yes even the crystal sticks don't really do it for me).

Depression

See mental health

Depurative

An agent which promotes the natural channels of elimination.

Examples Include: Black Walnut, Burdock, butternut, Echinacea Root, Globe Artichoke, Golden Seal, Nettle Leaf, Oregon Grape, Pau d'Arco, Poke Root, Red Clover, Sarsaparilla, Yellow Dock

Dermatitis

A broad term that covers all the types of skin inflammation including itchy rashes, blisters, reddened swollen patches or crusty and flakey patches. They all fall under the term of dermatitis.

A note here that almost all skin issues are a manifestation of gut health, so cleaning up the diet, removing chemicals and restoring the gut flora will help to get on top of dermatitis.

Causes:

- Nickel allergy
- Chemical sensitivity
- Stress
- B Vitamins deficiency
- Manganese deficiency
- Zinc deficiency

Topical herbs to help include: Agrimony, Calendula, Chamomile, Chickweed, Comfrey, Golden Seal, Gotu Kola, Licorice, Witch Hazel, Yarrow

Internal Herbs to help include: Albizia, Baical Skullcap, Blue flag, Burdock, Butternut, Clivers, Echinacea, Evening Primrose Oil, Nettle Leaf, Oregon Grape, Poke Root, Red Clover, Sarsaparilla, Yellow Dock

Desiccated Thyroid Hormone

See Armour

Detoxification

Officially the definition is to remove toxic substances from a living organism.

So to start with, let's not put any toxic garbage in. That will make the process so much easier.

Next, let's worry less about the big once a year detox and focus on how we can detox gently and slowly every single day.

- Sweat - move your body until you sweat, or sit in an infrared sauna. The skin is our largest organ, let's use it to our advantage. As a Hashimoto's person, I struggled to sweat for decades. Now, due to constant work and detoxing daily in some way, I can now break a sweat when I exercise. That is huge for me!

- □ Fiber- it clears our body of rubbish and helps with hormonal clearance.
- □ Enemas - plain water ones will help detoxify your colon and coffee enemas will detoxify your liver like nothing else.
- □ Organic - just the act of eating only organic foods will start a detoxification process in the body
- □ Juicing - vegetable and fruit juices will flush toxins from the cells.

Any small way we can detox day after day will have an additive effect on releasing toxins which will lessen the burden on our immune system and thyroid.

Detox Mask

To make a clay mask that helps to draw toxins out of the thyroid is a simple process once you have the ingredients.

You can use the same process on your armpits to help detoxify deodorant and antiperspirant ingredients that can contribute to breast cancer.

Ingredients:

- □ 1 tablespoon Bentonite Clay
- □ 1 teaspoon Apple Cider Vinegar
- □ 12 drops Essential Oils of choice *
- □ Water if necessary for a spreadable consistency

Method:

- □ Using a clay, ceramic or wooden bowl and spoon (no metals) stir the ingredients together and then spread onto either the neck or armpit.
- □ Leave to dry about 20 mins and then remove with paper towels and discard in the rubbish.
- □ Do not wash this down the drain as repeated use will cause clay to build up and block your pipes.

* The essential oils I use in my detox mask are frankincense, myrrh, lemongrass, peppermint, grapefruit & lemon myrtle

DHEA

A hormone secreted by the adrenal glands and is extremely abundant in the body. The main job of DHEA is to regulate cortisol when it gets out of control.

If there is more cortisol in our body than DHEA this can lead to autoimmune disease, inflammatory diseases, slow recovery, and rapid ageing.

DHEA serves to:

- ☐ Reduce the incidence of osteoporosis
- ☐ Reduce the incidence of heart disease
- ☐ Reduce the incidence of cancer
- ☐ Increase immune function
- ☐ Enhances weight loss
- ☐ Improves energy
- ☐ Improves Liver function
- ☐ Improves memory
- ☐ Maintains insulin levels

What contributes to Low DHEA levels:

- ☐ Ageing - by age 65 levels decrease by 80%
- ☐ High stress levels leading to high cortisol levels
- ☐ Excessive exercise
- ☐ Being overweight
- ☐ High consumption of refined carbohydrates
- ☐ High insulin levels (produces an enzyme that destroys DHEA)
- ☐ Oral contraceptive Pill
- ☐ Low Magnesium levels
- ☐ Poor Liver function
- ☐ Low Glutathione levels
- ☐ Excess Mercury

Like anything too much can be as bad as not enough. High levels of DHEA can lead to PCOS, acute stress, diabetes and heart disease.

What contributes to High DHEA levels:

- ☐ Adrenal tumor
- ☐ Excess bioidentical hormones

- ☐ Poor Liver function
- ☐ Low Glutathione levels
- ☐ Excess Mercury

Diabetes

A group of disorders where blood sugar levels and insulin become impaired.

Diabetes Type 1 is an autoimmune disease, so remember that when you have one, it is easy to get another.

- ☐ Type 1 Diabetes - autoimmune disease attacking the pancreas causing a block in the production of insulin - can't be reversed in the majority of cases
- ☐ Type II Diabetes - a chronic condition caused by a bad diet and lifestyle. Can be reversed, often found in hypothyroidism due to insulin clearance and sensitivity issues
- ☐ Gestational Diabetes - high blood sugar during pregnancy that usually corrects itself after the baby is born
- ☐ Type III Diabetes - I'll bet you haven't heard of this one (unless you follow Thyroid School) this is now what health practitioners are calling Alzheimer's due to the strong link between this disease and blood sugar

Diagnosis

Most thyroid people are diagnosed via a TSH blood test that shows their levels to be too high (indicating hypothyroidism) or too low (indicating hyperthyroidism).

Many people on Thyroid School have lamented to me that they can't get their doctors to diagnose them with thyroid disease, even though they have all the symptoms.

To be honest, in our current medical world, unless you literally cannot get out of bed or your heart feels like it is going to explode I would say don't force a diagnosis.

Once thyroid disease is on your medical record it stays there. It increases premiums and affects insurances. On top of that, taking thyroid replacement hormone makes your thyroid lazy and it is very hard to come off it again once your thyroid is used to having its work done for it.

But here's the thing. I have found that the people searching for somebody to diagnose them are simply using it as an avoidance measure. As long as they are not diagnosed, they do not need to follow the protocols that can help them feel better.

My advice would be to follow the thyroid wellness guidelines and see if you feel any better. It really is that simple.

Diaphoretic

An agent that increases perspiration and elimination through the skin, often used to reduce temperature in fevers.

Examples Include: Bayberry, Bupleurum, Cayenne, Chamomile, Elder Flower, Ginger, GoldenRod, Hyssop, Lemon Balm, Lime Flowers, Peppermint, Prickly Ash, yarrow

Diarrhoea

A common symptom in Grave's / hyperthyroidism. It contributes to the loss of nutrients and malabsorption in this disease.

Herbs to help: Bayberry, Chamomile, Cinnamon, Cranesbill, Fennel, Green Tea, Grape Seed, Meadowsweet, Raspberry Leaf, Rosehip, Thyme

Diary

I always recommend keeping a Thyroid Diary, in fact I even published one in 2017 but it wasn't popular enough to keep going.

I will bring it back one day though because I have always used one and it's the only way I can spot patterns and correlations in what I am doing and my current thyroid health.

I find them incredibly useful to go back over when I learn something new about thyroid disease to see if it checks out with my symptoms.

Even if you use an exercise book, I urge you to track symptoms, food, movement, social outings, the amount of medication and supplements you are on and glue an envelope to the back to keep copies of your blood test.

If you want to be the CEO of your health, you need to have immaculate bookkeeping skills ok?

Diet Soda

In the year prior to my thyroid "hitting the road" I had been living on Hamilton Island in QLD (I know, awesome right?) I had been trying to lose weight and ended up LIVING off diet cola. Like 10 cans a day.

Diet cola contains Aspartame as a sweetener and here are some of the nasty side effects of drinking beverages containing it:

- ☐ contributes to obesity (not kidding)
- ☐ contributes to sugar cravings
- ☐ increased risk of diabetes
- ☐ promotes inflammation
- ☐ Contributes to depression, mood disorders
- ☐ Increased risk of heart disease, stroke, cancer
- ☐ increased risk of dementia
- ☐ increased risk of kidney disease
- ☐ converts to formaldehyde in the body (would you drink that?)
- ☐ reduces serotonin levels
- ☐ reduces brain cells (it is an excitotoxin)
- ☐ Contributes to diarrhoea
- ☐ may contribute to fibromyalgia

So did I lose weight just drinking this? No. And although I cannot directly blame my liquid diet for my thyroid issues, I definitely don't dismiss it as a major contributor.

Over the years, since becoming a naturopath, I discovered many of my thyroid clients were also die-hard fans of diet drinks and sweeteners and it was and is always the first thing I try to convince them to change in their daily lifestyle.

It is always the little things that we do often that both help our thyroid or hurt our thyroid. Not the one off.

Dietary Fibre

We need fibre for so many things to keep our body running smoothly, reducing the excess oestrogen is just one of them. Other reasons include:

- ☐ lowering cholesterol levels
- ☐ keeping bowels regular
- ☐ preventing disease
- ☐ slows the absorption of sugar
- ☐ keeps you satiated (feeling full)

A study from the UK showed pre-menopausal women who ate at least 30g fibre daily, cut their risk of developing breast cancer in half. That's huge considering the rising incidence in this disease.

Let's have a look at a few foods high in fibre:

- 1 cup Navy Beans = 76% of DV
- 1 cup Lentils = 63% of DV
- 1 cup green peas = 30% of DV
- 1 medium pear = 22% of DV

If you are not used to eating fibre, go slowly, let your bowels adjust or you may end up regretting the whole fibre thing!

Differentiated Thyroid Cancer Cells

Both Papillary and Follicular thyroid cancer have these cells and it is the name for cells that look and act like normal thyroid cells but are cancerous.

Digestive Enzymes

Enzymes help us to break down and digest food. Can be purchased in supplement form if digestion is struggling.

Dill

This is not just a fabulous herb to make fish taste and look amazing!

The fruit of this herb is used in tincture form as a digestive and carminative.

A common ingredient in gripe water for infant colic it is useful for wind, bloating and a gripey belly.

Be careful using this if you have GERD.

Diuretic

An agent that increases the production and flow of urine.

Examples Include: Astragalus, Celery Seed, Corn Silk, Couch Grass, Dandelion, Globe Artichoke, Green Tea, Horsetail, Hydrangea, Shatavari

Diverticulitis

Small pouches that have developed in the large intestine. They cause no issues until they become inflamed.

Avoiding consuming small seeds that can become lodged in the pouches, causing inflammation is important.

Herbs to help: Echinacea, Garlic, GoldenSeal, marshmallow Root, Slippery Elm, Wild Yam

Dong Quai

This lovely root is anti-inflammatory and a uterine tonic so is used with issues such as endometriosis, irregular periods and for boosting after breastfeeding is finished.

Its antiarrhythmic action is also used for palpitations and cardiac arrhythmias.

Caution is required if using warfarin, or heavy periods and is not to be used in pregnancy.

Dopamine

An excitatory neurotransmitter that sends signals to parts of our body:

- tells nerve cells to move
- responsible for us feeling motivated
- it helps cognitive function like memory, learning, attention and concentration

To boost dopamine levels we need good levels of Tyrosine, which funnily enough is what we also need to make thyroid hormone. Enough said?

Down's Syndrome

Thyroid disease is not a cause of Down's Syndrome, however up to 50% of Down's Syndrome adults have hypothyroidism.

A small percentage of those are born with congenital hypothyroidism but the larger percentage have Hashimoto's Disease.

Dry Mouth Syndrome

A common symptom in both hyperthyroidism and hypothyroidism.

- □ hyperthyroidism - untreated or undertreated can cause dry mouth, but it will clear up once treatment is optimised
- □ hypothyroidism - a slow production of saliva can cause a dry mouth, again it is a sign that your levels need optimising

Durrant Peatfield, Dr Barry

Author of another one of my favourite thyroid books "Your Thyroid and How to Keep it Healthy" and another one to keep on your bookcase.

It is a little sciencey but if you like that kind of thing, this one's for you. He covers all forms of thyroid disease, where many books are only on Hashimoto's.

Dysbiosis

An imbalance in good and bad bacteria in the body.

Dysglycemia

The term for an abnormality in blood sugar.

Dysmenorrhoea

Painful periods usually involving heavy flow, clots and cramps. Often caused by fibroids, and endometriosis.

Dysthyroid Orbitopathy

See Graves Ophthalmopathy

E

Enemas

Before I began studying naturopathy, I knew what enemas were. In fact I had experienced a few colonic irrigations before then which is like the automated version of an enema. But it wasn't something I ever thought I would find myself doing on a regular basis... that was for hippies right? And, well, just plain weird!

In case you don't know, enemas are the act of inserting a thin tube into your rectum and allowing your colon to fill with liquid and then after holding it for a period of time you then release the liquid into the toilet.

Mostly enemas are used for constipation, but there is a particular kind using coffee that plays a part in helping to heal the liver.

I first discovered the coffee enema in college while sitting through a really interesting lecture about the Gerson Therapy. I listened in fascination as I learned that coffee, prepared in a particular way had the ability to travel up the colon and into the hepatic duct where it gave the liver a kind of dialysis.

You hold the solution in for around 15 mins which is enough time for all of our blood to travel through the liver 3-4 times. The coffee collects all of the toxins and pathogens and then pulls them out when released in the toilet.

While this was extremely interesting, I wasn't sure I would actually do it, but when you are studying Naturopathy you tend to be open to things you'll try. So like a good student I purchased an enema bucket and it sat in my bathroom cabinet for about 4 months.

It wasn't until I had my yearly blood tests that I discovered my ALT (liver studies) had crossed over into the red zone and my number was 31. This is the enzyme that tells us if our liver has become damaged and heading into cirrhosis.

That was all I needed to gain the courage to go home that day, learn how to prepare the coffee and then I lay down in my extremely small bathroom and got on with it! Afterwards I literally rolled my eyes and said "what was the fuss about" it really wasn't bad or hard or uncomfortable at all.

Fast forward a year and I had my yearly blood tests. My ALT? Now down to 20.... A year after that... 10... which is where it currently sits.

I believe it was through healing my liver that I was able to reduce my medication needs. I had been on 250mcg for close to 20 years. It is now down to 75 mcg and I am determined to remove it completely.

Do I still do coffee enemas? Yes! Until I have completely reversed the last of the medication my liver needs the help, after that I will be able to cut back to maybe once a week or month as a detox aid, because they increase glutathione in the body by 700%, which is our major antioxidant for all nasties inner body.

For those of you still thinking it's mad, here's a fun fact: Coffee Enemas were listed in the revered Merck's Manual up until the 70s as a treatment for physicians to use on patients.

E Vitamin

Also called Tocopherol, Vitamin E is required for:

- Major antioxidant (puts out fires in our body)
- Immune balancer
- Reduces decline from ageing
- Improves blood flow

Deficiency Symptoms of Vitamin E include:

- Poor taste & smell
- Fluid retention
- Anemia
- High Cholesterol
- Poor reflexes, poor balance
- Muscle wasting
- Ear infections, sinusitis, colds
- Delayed healing, prolonged infections

Factors that contribute to Vitamin E deficiency:

- ☐ Alcohol
- ☐ Celiac disease, Diabetes
- ☐ Gallbladder disease, Liver disease
- ☐ Pregnancy & lactation
- ☐ Heart Disease
- ☐ Crohn's disease
- ☐ Excess air pollution
- ☐ Ageing
- ☐ Excess Copper, Aluminium & Arsenic

Food sources of Vitamin E include:

- ☐ Almonds, nuts, hazelnuts
- ☐ Apricot oil
- ☐ Beef, egg yolk
- ☐ Safflower, sunflower, corn
- ☐ Wheat germ

Daily Requirements of Vitamin E:

- ☐ Adult RDA - 30 mg

Echinacea Root

Echinacea is probably one of the original herbs that started making its way into households to help lower the duration of the common cold.

It is immune enhancing, immune modulating, anti-inflammatory and a lymphatic.

It is used for infections, swollen lymph glands, respiratory conditions, skin conditions, gut issues, UTI's, tonsillitis, and long term infections such as chronic fatigue, fibromyalgia, glandular fever, ross river virus, mastitis, measles and mumps to improve immunity.

Ectopic Thyroid

The medical term for thyroid tissue that is not located within the thyroid, usually instead is at the base of the tongue. It is extremely rare and is mostly found in congenital hypothyroidism

Eczema

See Dermatitis

Edema

Edema is another word for fluid retention and is a condition where excess fluid is forced into the body's tissues and trapped there.

Fluid retention is commonly caused by low body temperature, which is experienced in hypothyroidism and Hashimoto's.

Ways to improve edema:

- normalise thyroid levels
- work towards normalising temperature levels
- Increase potassium and vitamin B6 levels
- Avoid refined carbohydrates
- Avoid white salt (only use Himalayan)

Herbs to encourage release of fluid include: Boswellia, Butcher's Broom, Dandelion Leaf, and Horsechestnut

EFT

Emotional Freedom Technique (EFT) is a way of using physical tapping movements on meridians in the body while talking about emotional issues.

The tapping is said to disrupt the belief pattern around what the topic is.

I actually use this technique a lot and can highly recommend it as a way of digging down into fears and blocks.

There are millions of Youtube videos on how to do it, but I particularly like the information by Carol Look as she explains it in a very simple manner.

You can find her at https://www.carollook.com

Egg Replacer

I love eggs!

They are so easy to use and quick if you need a meal in a hurry. I try not to eat too many of them though because they feed viruses and are one of the most common allergens and intolerances.

So what do we use instead when we are baking? Here are some handy substitutes for you:

1 egg =

- ☐ 1 tbsp ground flax + 3 tbsp water (let sit for 10 min)
- ☐ 1 tbsp chia seeds + ⅓ cup water (let sit for 15 min)
- ☐ 1 tbsp agar agar + 1 tbsp water
- ☐ ½ mashed banana
- ☐ ¼ cup unsweetened apple sauce
- ☐ 3 tbsp peanut butter

Plus don't forget you can actually buy egg replacements in the grocery store (although I'm not sure what the ingredients are so have a read first).

Electromagnetic Radiation

The radiation in the air from cell phones, wireless devices, microwaves, X-rays, and gamma rays.

There is growing evidence that suggests EMF can cause thyroid issues by damaging the hypothalamic-pituitary-thyroid axis.

ElderBerry

A lovely berry with anti-viral, antioxidant and immune enhancing qualities.

Great for colds and flus or other infections.

Elder Flower

Although store bought ElderFlower cordial tastes beautiful it probably no longer holds the diaphoretic and anticatarrhal properties the untouched flowers possess.

Used in colds, flu, sinus issues or anything with excess mucous, this lovely flower will help dry it up.

Elimination Channels

We have 6 elimination channels in our body with which to get rid of toxic matter. If one of them is blocked, then that puts a bigger load on the other 5. If 2 of them are blocked or not functioning optimally, then we are down to 3. Get the idea?

The elimination channels are:

- ☐ Skin - skin brushing, sweating, organic body products
- ☐ Lungs - deep breathing, meditation, exercise, yoga
- ☐ Bowel - colonics, enemas, psyllium, bentonite clay
- ☐ Kidneys - hippocrates soup, constant sipping of water
- ☐ Liver - silymarin, lemon water, coffee enemas
- ☐ Lymphatics - rebounding, exercise, skin brushing, massage

Emetic

An agent that induces nausea and vomiting for example Ipecac.

Endocrinologist

A doctor who specialises in the Endocrine System. Some countries refer thyroid patients directly to Endocrinologists, while others continue to see GP (in Australia we only see a specialist if we cannot get our disease under control, or request it).

Endocrine Disruptors

See Chemicals

Endocrine System

A system in the human body made up of endocrine glands that produce hormones. The endocrine glands and what they do include:

- ☐ Pineal Gland - biological clock
- ☐ Pituitary Gland - menstruation, growth, birth contractions, milk production
- ☐ Thyroid Gland - metabolism
- ☐ Parathyroid Glands - calcium & phosphorus regulation
- ☐ Thymus - white blood cells
- ☐ Adrenal Glands - fight or flight, body's pharmacy, anti stress
- ☐ Pancreas - blood sugar and insulin
- ☐ Ovaries - reproduction
- ☐ Testes - reproduction, male characteristics

Endometriosis

A condition where the endometrium (lining of the uterus) grows in places outside of the uterus, often causing pain, period problems and infertility.

Although the cause is unknown it is thought to be from excess estrogen.

In severe cases, laparoscopic surgery is performed to cut away the overgrown tissue, which I actually had done about 5 years before finally deciding on a hysterectomy, which solved the problem for good.

Herbs to help: Calendula, Chaste Tree, Cramp Bark, dong Quai, Ginger, Ladies mantle, Paeonia

Endoscopic Retrograde

An internal examination through the mouth using an endoscope that allows the surgeon to look at the pancreatic and bile ducts.

Endoscopic Thyroid Surgery

A new way of performing thyroid surgery that does not leave a scar across the front of the neck. Currently used for differentiated thyroid cancer.

Enemas

The act of inserting a tube into the rectum and allowing a sterile liquid (often water or coffee) to flow into the large intestine.

Different liquids achieve different health outcomes.

Water cleanses the bowel of faecal matter, coffee has the ability to enter the liver and pull out toxins. Chamomile tea is used for calming a painful spasming bowel.

Endemic Goiter

A goiter caused by iodine deficiency.

Energy Drinks

These dastardly drinks are full of caffeine and chemicals and really have no purpose in the thyroid world other than to make symptoms worse. Just don't do it.

English Spinach

This fabulous green leaf is a staple in our house. Strangely enough it is the one green leaf I can slip into my husbands food or rolls without him complaining. Go figure?

Plus it is so versatile. You can add it to salads, soups, pasta, eggs, sandwiches, rolls, smoothies, juices .... in fact I can't think of too many things you couldn't add it too!

Although many people avoid it due to the oxalate content, I find it ok for me and like all foods I try to eat a balance rather than an excess of anything in particular.

Here is the low down on why spinach is a great leaf to add to your salad every now and again.

1 cup English Spinach boasts:

- 2% of DV in Protein (Thyroid Pathway)
- 3% of DV in Dietary Fibre (Hormone Clearance, Gut Health)
- 56% of DV in Vitamin A (Thyroid Pathway, Skin Health)
- 14% of DV in Vitamin C (Thyroid Pathway, Adrenal Health, Antioxidant)
- 3% of DV in Vitamin E (Thyroid Pathway, Major Antioxidant)
- 181% of DV in Vitamin K (Blood, Bones)
- 2% of DV in Vitamin B1 (Thyroid health, hair health, hyperthyroidism)
- 3% of DV in Vitamin B2 (Thyroid Pathway)
- 1% of DV in Vitamin B3 (mental health)
- 15% of DV in Folate (MTHFR conversion, mental health)
- 3% of DV in Calcium (bones)
- 5% of DV in Iron (Thyroid Pathway, fatigue, gut acid)
- 6% of DV in Magnesium (stress, sugar)
- 5% of DV in Potassium (thyroid health, fluid retention, fatigue)
- 1% of DV in Zinc (Immune health, thyroid health, wound healing, mental health)
- 2% of DV in Copper (skin, nerves, bone, collagen)
- 13% of DV in Manganese (Thyroid Pathway)
- Glycemic Load of 0
- 41.4 mg Omega 3 Fatty Acids

How amazing is that lineup?

My favourite way of eating them is to lay out a bed of them on a plate, add 3 Zucchini & Carrot fritters on top and sprinkle with avocado salsa then drizzle with raw sour cream! Heaven!

Estradiol

Shortened to E2 this is the major form of estrogen our ovaries and adrenal glands produce, and is the most potent. It can induce uterine cancer.

Estriol

Shortened to E3, estriol is the waste product of estrange and estradiol metabolism. It is produced in the liver and the placenta. It has an anti-cancer action by binding to estrogen receptors before estradiol can.

Estrogen

The umbrella term for estrange, estradiol and estriol, this natural hormone promotes female characteristics in the body

Signs of excess estrogen:

- ☐ Fibroids
- ☐ Endometriosis
- ☐ Infertility
- ☐ xeno-estrogens
- ☐ Oral Contraceptive Pill
- ☐ High copper levels in the body
- ☐ adrenal fatigue
- ☐ low progesterone
- ☐ obesity

Ways to reduce excess estrogen:

- ☐ Chaste tree
- ☐ White peony
- ☐ Dietary fibre
- ☐ Infrared saunas
- ☐ Exercise metabolises excess estrogen
- ☐ Reduce coffee intake (4-5 cups a day can increase estrogen levels by 70%)
- ☐ Reduce inflammation

Signs of low estrogen:

- ☐ painful sex (dry vagina)
- ☐ irregular or missing periods
- ☐ breast tenderness
- ☐ mood swings, headaches, depression
- ☐ urinary tract infections
- ☐ hot flushes and night sweats
- ☐ fatigue and low concentration

Since low estrogen is usually only present once menopause hits, apart from HRT the only way to find relief is to improve adrenal health, as the adrenals are now responsible for producing the weaker form of estrogen.

Herbs to help: False Unicorn root, Korean ginseng, Shatavari, Tribulus, Wild Yam

Estrogen Modulating

An agent used to balance estrogen levels in the body.

Examples Include: Alfalfa, Aniseed, Black Cohosh, Fennel, False Unicorn Root, Hops, Paeonia, Wild Yam

Estrone

The estrogen present after menopause is estrone and it is weaker than estradiol, which is why many women feel the effects of lowered estrogen levels at this time.

Epinephrine

Also called adrenaline, this hormone is produced by the adrenal glands for the purpose of increasing cardiac output and raising glucose levels in times of need.

Epsom Salts

The common name for magnesium sulphate it is often used in baths to ease muscles and stress and is an easy way to get a quick hit of magnesium into our body.

See magnesium

Epstein Barr Virus

Also known as Glandular Fever, the Kissing Disease or Mononucleosis, Epstein Barr Virus (EBV) is a disease transferred by saliva and has been implicated as a precursor to Thyroid Disease.

As viruses like to hide in our organs until our immune system is weakened, in the case of EBV it likes to hide in the thyroid.

The immune system, in an attempt to kill the virus in the thyroid also damages the thyroid - collateral damage if you like.

When I was studying naturopathy, there was a theory presented to us that perhaps thyroid disease was caused by this virus, although this has not been proven.

Anthony William (see Medical Medium) does a lot of work around killing off the virus and actually refers to it as the thyroid virus. His information is channeled by spirit but pretty much all of it makes perfect sense and reading it, you tend to forget it is channelled (if you are not a believer of that kind of thing)

Herbs to help kill the Epstein Barr virus include: Andrographis, Echinacea Root, Elder Berry, Elder Flower, Myrrh, St John's Wort, St Mary's Thistle, Thyme

Erythrocyte Sedimentation Rate

ESR is a blood test that measures general inflammation in the body.

Essential Oils

Essential Oils are amazing. It takes 26 seconds for them to soak into your skin and get into your bloodstream and they offer support for physical, mental and emotional problems.

I use them all the time, particularly for the emotional aspect. If I am struggling with something I will reach for one of the emotional blends (these are doTerra blends) such as Forgive, Motivate (use this a lot while writing), Elevate and Balance.

I have diffusers all over the house which always has lavender and citrus type oils in them to make the house smell amazing and keep the peace. I often add Purify and Easy Air to help with keeping everybody at ease and to dispel stagnate energy.

Here are some particular favourites:

- Myrrh - cancer fighter, virus killer, worm and parasite killer, anti-inflammatory, antiviral and antibacterial, boost glutathione, clears xeno-estrogens by behaving like indole-3-carbinol

- ☐ Frankincense - balances hormones, promotes cell regeneration, immune boosting, wrinkle reducer, lessens scar formation, balances moods, reduces anxiety and stress, lowers inflammation
- ☐ Lavender - anti-inflammatory, antiseptic, reduces insomnia and anxiety, calms restlessness, soothes burns and bites, reduces diabetic symptoms (not kidding there was a study), promotes healthy hair, relieves headaches, reduces stress

I have a particular essential oil mix though that I use in my balancing balm and also roll it directly onto my neck (diluted with coconut oil). And because I love you... here is the recipe:

Thyroid Roller Oil

- ☐ 5 drops frankincense
- ☐ 5 drops myrrh
- ☐ 5 drops lemongrass
- ☐ 3 drops peppermint
- ☐ 3 drops lemon myrtle
- ☐ 3 drops grapefruit

Add these to a 10 ml roller bottle and top up with fractionated coconut oil or just leave them straight to add to a diffuser.

You can find more recipes on my website.

Essiac Tea

An herbal blend of burdock, slippery elm, sheep sorrel and Indian rhubarb used for clearing and draining lymph nodes, improve immunity, and decrease inflammation.

You can purchase it pre-made or the recipe is below:

- ☐ 1.5 pounds burdock root chopped
- ☐ 1 pound powdered sheep sorrel
- ☐ ¼ pound powdered slippery elm
- ☐ 1 ounce powdered Turkish rhubarb root
- ☐ Mix herbs together
- ☐ use 1 ounce of the blend for a quart of tea
- ☐ use 4 ounces of the blend for a gallon of tea
- ☐ bring water to the boil in a steel or cast iron pot only

- ☐ add herbs and boil for 15 mins
- ☐ cover with a tight lid and steep for 12 hours in a warm but not hot place
- ☐ the next day, reheat the water but do not let it come to a boil.
- ☐ let the herbs settle to the bottom and then strain the liquid and refrigerate
- ☐ for wellness, on an empty stomach combine ½ ounce of tea concentrate in 2 ounces of hot water daily
- ☐ for illness, on an empty stomach combine 1 ounce of tea concentrate in 2 ounces of hot water daily (you may need to build up to that from the ½ ounce)
- ☐ bedtime is a great time to drink this

European Thyroid Association

Thyroid Support Group and lots of information on all forms of thyroid disease.
https://www.eurothyroid.com

Euthyroid

A normal functioning thyroid

Euthyorid Graves Disease

A condition that presents with a normal thyroid function but the patient has thyroid associated ophthalmopathy (Graves eye disease)

Euthyroid Sick Syndrome

A condition where the thyroid appears to be functioning normally however the T3 and T4 levels are abnormal.

Usually found in critically ill patients (for example in intensive care) and starvation.

Evening Primrose OIl

An oil derived from the seed of the Evening Primrose plant which is used by many women who swear by it as a treatment for painful and irregular periods.

Other uses and benefits include:

- ☐ ease menopausal symptoms

- ☐ improve fertility by increasing cervical mucus
- ☐ skin conditions such as acne, dermatitis and eczema
- ☐ rheumatoid arthritis, dyspraxia, osteoporosis
- ☐ Alzheimers, schizophrenia
- ☐ high cholesterol and heart disease
- ☐ Multiple sclerosis, Sjogren's Syndrome, Raynaud's Syndrome, chronic fatigue syndrome
- ☐ obesity and weight loss
- ☐ improve hair growth (apply it as a mask for 30 mins then wash out)

Excess & Deficiency

This is a small piece of information that can change your symptoms forever.

An excess and a deficiency in anything,

often presents the same symptoms.

Read it again. I will wait.

So let's use iodine as an example. The symptoms you get from an iodine deficiency such as thyroid disease and goiter, you also get from having an excess in iodine.

It is the same with many other nutrients. So it is easy to quickly assume that you have low iodine when your thyroid is not functioning or you have low iron when you are tired, but an excess of these things can do the same, and if you are taking supplements it could be very easy to flip over into an excess.

Excitotoxins

Chemicals that excite the brain cells so much that they then are damaged or die.

Examples include: MSG, Aspartame, hydrolysed protein, aspartic acid, aspartate, casein

Exercise

My husband loves it, and says it is the answer to everything. I think healthy food is the answer to everything! So between us we have it right.

Here are a few different ways to look at exercise from a thyroid perspective:

- ☐ Intense exercise lowers adrenal function which affects thyroid function
- ☐ Exercising (not intensely) for 40 mins can reduce stress for up to 3 hours

- □ Our genome is wired for 18,000 - 22,000 steps a day. Our ancestors walked and walked and walked. Now we sit and sit and sit some more. Not on purpose, it is just the way our lives have changed since our hunter-gatherer days.
- □ Lifting weights builds muscle mass which burns fat

I don't do weird, strange out of my depth things, just basic stuff, like riding my bike, using a rebounder, walking to the shops, and using the bathroom step to go up and down, up and down, and with each passing day I get stronger and more motivated in general.

You just need to make the decision to do one small piece of movement everyday, then when that becomes a habit, add another. You will feel much better for it I promise, and who knows you may get to love it like I think I am beginning too (don't tell my husband).

Exogenous Hormones

Hormones not made by the body such as oral contraceptive pill or oestrogen creams

Eyebright

This herb is useful for allergies, hay fever, sinus, ear aches, asthma, dry eyes and conjunctivitis.

Its anticatarrhal, anti-inflammatory, astringent qualities paired with it being a tonic for mucous membranes is helpful to all things ear and nose.

This is a tincture for internal use though not topical.

Eyebrows

A common sign of thyroid disorder is the missing outer third of the eyebrows.

It is not known what causes this specifically however a general thinning of hair is a symptom.

F

Fritters

The most seriously underestimated of all dietary restricted foods! Yep, I believe this to be true.

Quite some time ago I needed a recipe that would cover a bunch of favourite people that were coming for brunch. Some were gluten free, some were dairy free, some were vegan.... you know how it goes.

I love all my friends and always (being the domestic goddess that I am) want them to eat what they like to eat, but also don't want to be making 10 different options.

Fritters to the rescue!! And I promise, even those that don't have dietary restrictions will LOVE these!

This recipe is so versatile you can add what you want! My recipe is Carrot & Zucchini (courgette) but be adventurous!

Carrot & Zucchini Fritters

- 1 cup Buckwheat flour
- 1 cup Chickpea (Besan) flour
- 2 eggs or egg replacer
- 1 cup plant based milk of choice
- 2 grated medium carrots
- 1 grated medium zucchini (courgette)

Method:

- Combine flours in a bowl (I find a whisk works well for this).
- In a seperate bowl combine egg or egg replacer and plant milk, whisking well.

- ☐ Add the milk mix to the flours whisking until smooth then set aside.
- ☐ Grate the carrot and zucchini and then squeeze out all extra liquid by putting in a clean cloth and ringing it out as tight as you can.
- ☐ Add the grated veg to the wet mixture, then add salt and pepper to taste.
- ☐ Using a little coconut oil in a pan, add tablespoons of the mix and cook until bubbles appear, then flip for a further min or two.

Serving:

- ☐ Get out as many plates as you need and spread out enough english spinach leaves evenly to cover it.
- ☐ Just before serving add 3-4 of the warm fritters overlapping each other in the middle of the plate
- ☐ Add a tablespoon or two of avocado salsa (chopped avocado, tomato, olives, spring onions) then drizzle with some raw sour cream and chopped cilantro.
- ☐ You can leave the final two ingredients in bowls on the table for people to help themselves if you wish.

Familial Dysalbuminemic Hyperthyroxinemia

FDH is a rare condition where an individual's albumin is abnormal and binds more T4 (sometimes T3) than usual.

It presents as higher T4 levels but normal FT4 levels

Fatigue

A common symptom of all thyroid disease states, although other causes can be implicated and should be checked out if thyroid levels are normal:

- ☐ Low iron levels - anemia
- ☐ Low Vitamin B12
- ☐ Low Potassium
- ☐ Low Biotin

Herbs to help with fatigue include: Astragalus, codonopsis, Kola Nut, Korean Ginseng, Licorice, Polygonum Multiform, Rehmannia, rhodiola, Sage, Sarsaparilla, Schisandra, Siberian Ginseng, Skullcap, St John's Wort, tribulus leaf, and withania.

Famine Pathways

Famine Pathways is a term I first heard used by Jon Gabriel where he explains how some external and internal influences can trick our body into thinking there is a famine and hold onto our fat reserves at all costs which clearly makes it difficult to lose weight.

Things that turn our famine pathways on:

- ☐ Inflammation
- ☐ Stress, trauma, turmoil
- ☐ Deprivation (restrictive diets)
- ☐ Starvation
- ☐ Lack of nutrients (different to restricted diets, you may be getting plenty of food and no nutrients)
- ☐ Bad digestion, causing malabsorption

Fat, Sick & Nearly Dead

A movie made by Joe Cross, that follows his journey of juicing a juice fast for 60 days to reverse his autoimmune disease and lose weight.

This was the first movie that inspired me to try a juice fast.

He refers to juice fasting as "Rebooting" our body so that we can both give it a rest and a tune up and enjoy eating more plant food at the other end.

Joe has made 2 follow up movies since then:
Fat Sick & Nearly Dead 2
The Kids Menu

He shares his daily lifestyle and juice habits on his social media platforms under "Reboot with Joe"

Fatty Liver

Sadly, the cases of Non-Alcoholic Fatty Liver Disease (NAFLD) is appearing even in our children.

It leads to liver damage and liver cirrhosis much like a liver that has been subjected to a lot of alcohol.

It is reversible, however a change in lifestyle, weight loss and liver support are all necessary for this to happen. Luckily all these things will also improve thyroid health.

Feedback Loop

There are many feedback loops in our very complex body. The thyroid pathway is a feedback loop that starts with the hypothalamus, works through the pathway and ends back at the hypothalamus.

Each step of the pathway gives feedback and is reliant on the next part working efficiently.

The thyroid pathway is a negative feedback loop which means it is self correcting to achieve a balanced thyroid hormone.

Positive feedback loops are self perpetuating, as in they encourage growth and amplification. Pregnancy is an example of this.

Feldenkrais

This is a method of exercise and movement developed by Mosh█ Feldenkrais, an Israeli Engineer

It uses movement, posture, breathing and sensations to bring about an improved lifestyle.

Practitioners are trained and use mindfulness techniques such as guided imagery with movement and touch to achieve lasting improvements.

Feldenkrais is useful for pain, coordination, injuries, emotional resilience, and neurological issues.

Fennel

The essential oils in fennel has many amazing qualities.

Fennel is a carminative, spasmolytic, expectorant, antimicrobial, galactagogue and is estrogen modulating.

These qualities directly help with issues such as upset belly, nausea and diarrhoea, colic, and wind.

It also helps with breastfeeding and helps to increase milk supply which is often lacking in thyroid mums.

This is another herb that is useful for drying up mucus in the nasal lining and in the chest so helps with bronchitis, bronchial asthma and coughs.

Caution must be used with GERD patients

Fenugreek

The Fenugreek seed is another one helpful for our thyroid mums to induce milk supply.

For the rest of us not having babies, it is anti-inflammatory, can help lower cholesterol levels and help lower sugar levels.

Having too much of this may leave you smelling a little like a fenugreek seed yourself and should be avoided with GERD but apart from that using it in a tea or tincture is helpful.

Fermented Food

Taking the natural grocery stores by storm, fermented foods are incredible at improving our gut microbiome or garden.

BUT, if you are not used to consuming these foods, they may render you in pain and discomfort if you start eating it by the tablespoonful.

Start extremely slowly, as in a little strand at a time and let the body adjust to the new bacteria, which will also let you gauge how it is affecting your thyroid health.

Fertility

See Infertility

Fibrocystic Breasts

The term given to lumpy breasts caused by small cysts or masses. It is not cancerous, do not increase the risk of getting breast cancer and is very common in many women.

There is a higher risk of developing fibrocystic breasts in Hashimoto's and Nodular Thyroid Disease.

It is thought to be caused by hormonal fluctuations, particularly estrogen plays a part in the development.

Fibromyalgia

I don't have fibromyalgia but my heart completely goes out to anyone reading that does. It sounds hideous and even more heartbreaking than thyroid disease.

This condition causes pain throughout the body and is considered incurable. It is thought to be caused by other autoimmune disorders such as Rheumatoid arthritis and thyroid disease.

It's important to understand that anything that causes us pain - physical, mental or emotional - increases our levels of RT3 which block our active thyroid hormone getting into our cells, so long term pain like fibromyalgia will have an ongoing affect on our thyroid function.

There are no tests to diagnose this disease however there are 18 points in the body that are painful when pressed, and doctors look for at least 11 of these to be painful for a diagnosis.

Since this is seen to be related to autoimmunity then feeling better or reversing it will depend on balancing the immune system and reducing inflammation, which will incidentally have a great effect on the thyroid also.

Herbs that may help: Astragalus, Bupleurum, celery Seed, ginkgo, Hawthorn, Korean Ginseng, Rehmannia, Rhodiola, St John's Wort, and Withania.

Fibroids

Benign growths consisting of fibrous tissue and must that grow inside the uterus.

They can cause severe abdominal and lower back pain, constipation and very heavy periods in the worst cases, although some are symptom free.

Thought to be caused by estrogen levels, reducing excess estrogen would be the starting point to reducing the fibroid. Meat, alcohol and caffeine may also play a role, but since these items are also either estrogen containing or estrogen mimics, it still comes down to the hormonal balance.

In worst case scenarios they are removed surgically.

Herbs to help reduce fibroids include: Chaste Tree, Echinacea Root, ladies mantle, Paeonia, Rosemary, Schisandra, and Thuja.

Fibrosis

An excess of connective tissue in an organ or tissue usually caused by scarring. *See Riedel Thyroiditis*

Fine Needle Aspiration

FNA is the procedure used to biopsy thyroid nodules.

Five Elements

In Traditional Chinese medicine everything is based around the 5 elements and their connections to the earth, emotions and our wellness.

- Wood Element - east, green, spring, wind, liver, gallbladder, eyes, anger, sour, tendons, nails, shouting, rancid, tears, soul, index finger, birth
- Fire Element - south, red, summer, hot, heart, small intestine, tongue, speech, joy, fright, bitter, blood vessels, complexion, laughter, burnt, sweat, spirit, middle finger, youth
- Earth Element - centre, yellow, late summer, damp, spleen, stomach, mouth, taste, worry, sweet, acrid, muscles, lips, singing, fragrant, saliva, intention, thumb, adulthood
- Metal Element - west, white, autumn, dry, lung, large intestine, nose, smell, sadness, grief, pungent, skin, body hair, crying, rotten, mucus, vitality, ring finger, old age
- Water Element - north, black, winter, cold, kidney, bladder, urinary system, ears, hearing, fear, salty, bone, head hair, groaning, putrid, urine, determination, little finger, death

I know when I look at this breakdown my imbalance def lies in the water element in that I have too much of it. So I would work on strengthening those aspects.

Flame Retardants

Flame retardants are a blessing and a curse. Yes they may stop the spread of a fire in a tragedy however they are full of nasty things that may be killing us slowly anyway.

One of the ingredients is Bromine which is an iodine blocker amongst other things.

Flame retardants are used on:

- Mattresses
- New carpets
- New soft furnishings

- ☐ Synthetic clothing (particularly pjs)
- ☐ Curtains and drapes
- ☐ Almost anything new and synthetic essentially

They can contribute to:

- ☐ thyroid disruption
- ☐ immune dysfunction
- ☐ hormonal dysfunction
- ☐ reproductive disorders
- ☐ cancer
- ☐ abnormal child brain development

How to avoid them? Go with natural products.

Flavonoids

See Bioflavonoids

Flaxseed

Also called Linseed, these little beauties are actually the only seed (used in oil form) that is used by the Gerson Therapy. They are that good.

Just 1 ounce (28g) of flaxseeds give us:

- ☐ 10% of DV in Protein (thyroid pathway)
- ☐ 31% of DV in Dietary Fiber (hormonal clearance, gut health)
- ☐ 31% of DV in Vitamin B1 (thyroid, hair, hyperthyroidism)
- ☐ 3% of DV in Vitamin B2 (thyroid pathway)
- ☐ 4% of DV in Vitamin B3 (mental health)
- ☐ 3% of DV in Vitamin B5 (food conversion, energy)
- ☐ 7% of DV in Vitamin B6 (mental health & progesterone)
- ☐ 6% of DV in Folate (MTHFR, liver)
- ☐ 7% of DV in calcium (bones)
- ☐ 9% of DV in Iron (thyroid, fatigue, gut acid)
- ☐ 27% of DV in Magnesium (stress, sugar)
- ☐ 18% of DV in Phosphorus (bones, liver)
- ☐ 7% of DV in Potassium (thyroid, fatigue, fluid)
- ☐ 8% of DV in Zinc (thyroid, mental health, immunity, wound healing)

- □ 17% of DV in Copper (skin, collagen, nerves)
- □ 35% of DV in Manganese (thyroid pathway)
- □ 10% of DV in Selenium (thyroid pathway)
- □ 266% of DV in Omega 3 fats (mental health, joint health)

So this translates into:

- □ Anti-inflammatory and Antioxidant
- □ Reduces the risk of hormonal cancers
- □ Improves microbiome and gut health
- □ Reduces menopausal symptoms
- □ Reduces blood pressure and cholesterol
- □ Improves hair, skin and nail health

Have you heard of a flax egg? This is a great egg alternative in baking. All you do is mix 1 tbsp of ground flaxseed meal with 3 tbsp of water. Let it sit for 20 mins or so until thick and goopy and egg like. This is the equivalent of 1 normal egg. You're welcome!

Float Tank

A float tank is an amazing cocoon of a bath that is so filled with magnesium that you can't possibly sink in it.

When you climb into one of these tubs, and pull down the roof, all senses are deprived so that you experience pure stillness, but you don't have to pull down the lid if you feel a little claustrophobic.

I remember watching a Simpsons episode years ago when Lisa and Homer were inside one, and of course Homer's float tank was picked up and moved and fell off the truck and all the things that can only happen to Homer, but he was blissfully unaware.

The pure hit of magnesium from a session in a float tank does so many amazing things for our body, nervous system, cortisol levels and thyroid. Give it a go as a gift to your thyroid. I highly recommend it!

Flower Essences

This is a modality that uses flower essences to bring about emotional change on an energetic level to help release patterns and habits that may be contributing to stress, chronic disease or a lack of harmony in life.

One of the ones I used extensively in both naturopathy and kinesiology are the Australian Bach Flower essences. They are the producers of Rescue Remedy, which is an essence that is made up of many different flower essences, that is said to calm the mind and soul from trauma, fright, shock, nerves, grief or any other emotion we need rescuing from.

I have to say, I keep a jar of the Rescue Remedy Lozenges on hand at all times.

Fluid Retention

See Edema

Fluorescent Lighting

I know this is an odd thing for a thyroid reference book, but bare with me.

Although we cannot force our workplaces to change their lighting for us, we can perhaps change our home lighting situation and who knows, maybe it's not such a bad thing if we change our actual workplace too.

Just the nature of how they work should ring alarm bells to our thyroids. An electric current excites mercury vapour in the tube. Scary!

Here are the dangers of this type of lighting:

- Causes eye strain and blurry vision
- Flickering fluorescent lights can cause headaches
- If broken, the powder inside contains mercury which could be inhaled
- Can potentially leak radiation causing UV exposure, this is more common in round fluorescent bulbs (ring bulbs)

Fluoride

This is a huge topic and there is so much you can find online about it if you want to dig deeper into the conspiracies and issues around this mineral.

But the basics are that fluoride blocks iodide in the thyroid and calcifies the pineal gland.

The first time I made a difference in my thyroid health and reduced medication was when I removed fluoride toothpaste. And yes, my teeth are still healthy with no extra fillings after 15 years of using organic, non-fluoride toothpaste.

We need to do our own research and reach our own conclusions. My husband still uses his usual brand and has the treatment at the dentist. I don't. And that's ok. We are all grown ups and can make our own decisions. I don't force anyone around me (no matter how much I love them) to do what I think is best for their health. It is their journey and we need to leave it up to them for the sake of our own stress levels. Got me?

So back to the fluoride, another big source of it in many countries, including mine is tap water. I use a distiller that removes it completely out of our water and I don't drink everyday black tea (often) because it is a naturally high source of fluoride.

So, before we reach for iodine supplementation, perhaps we need to remove anything that is blocking our natural sources of it first because our thyroid actually does not require much iodine to work.

Now, I know this becomes a grey area for the hyperthyroid people amongst us, and years ago fluoride was actually used to balance hyperthyroidism, but it does so many other nasty things inside too that I'm not sure I would be using this as a method to stabilise things.

Fluoride is also linked to:

- ☐ Disruption of the immune system
- ☐ Thyroid Disease
- ☐ Endocrine Disruption
- ☐ Calcification of the pineal gland
- ☐ Lowered synthesis of collagen
- ☐ Increased heavy metal absorption
- ☐ Increased tumour rate
- ☐ Kidney disease
- ☐ Cardiovascular Disease
- ☐ Increased infertility
- ☐ Muscle disorders
- ☐ Hyperactivity
- ☐ Bone Fractures & bone cancer
- ☐ Arthritis
- ☐ Dementia

It is as easy as starting with swapping out your toothpaste. But if you do, make sure you have a thyroid blood test 6 weeks after doing so as you may need to lower your medication needs.

And for those not willing to say no at the dentist when they want to give a fluoride treatment - I have been saying NO for about 10 years and my dentist only commented on my last visit how healthy my teeth are for "someone my age" (cough cough), after he practically forced me to have an X-ray (which I also put off as long as possible).

FMTV

Food Matters TV (FMTV is a subscription based television platform showcasing hundreds of health based documentaries, movies and how-to series by health professionals from all over the world.

Founded by James Colquhoun and Laurentine ten Bosch who led the charge with the game changing films Food Matters, Hungry for Change and now Transcendence, this platform is a place to find uplifting and motivating content no matter what your stage of health.

I watch something from this platform almost daily, and it always puts me in a great headspace and inspires me to keep going with my health, my dreams and my business.

It can be found at https://www.fmtv.com/

Folate

See B9 Vitamin

Follicle Stimulating Hormone

A hormone secreted by the pituitary gland to stimulate the making of an egg in women or sperm in men.

These levels can be low in hypothyroidism.

Follicular Cells

One of the two types of cells in the thyroid gland. Follicular cells secrete both T4 and T3.

The shape of the cells allow blood to flow in and around each cell which allows the hormones they secrete to go directly into the bloodstream.

Follicular Neoplasia

A medical term for a lump or tumor in the thyroid follicles. It may be benign or malignant.

Follicular thyroid Cancer

Also called Follicular Carcinoma, this is not as common as papillary carcinoma of the thyroid but is more aggressive.

It makes up about 15% of all thyroid cancers and is more common in older people (40-60) with women being 3 times more likely to get it.

The spreading of this type of cancer is more common than papillary carcinoma but it has a high cure rate of around 95% for people on the younger end of the range and decreasing with age.

It is usually treated with surgery (thyroid removal) and radioactive Iodine.

Food Colours and Their Benefits

The colours of the fruits and vegetables we eat give us clues as to how they can benefit us.

Knowing what each colour does for us means in times of need we can increase the ratio of the needed colour.

- Red foods - fight cancer, balance blood sugar, heart health, decreases risk of stroke, skin health, macular degeneration, free radical damage eg: raspberries, strawberries, watermelon, chili, tomato
- Orange & Yellow foods - Immune function, heart disease, eye health and vision, anti-inflammatory, healthy joints, skin protection eg: oranges, mangoes, sweet potatoes, carrots, lemons, pineapple, yellow peppers
- Green foods - immune system, reduces risk of cancer, detoxification, energy, vitality, tissue healing, digestive enzymes eg: kiwi fruit, spinach, courgette, lettuce, celery
- Blue & Purple foods - fight cancer, anti-inflammatory, anti-ageing, longevity, reduces risk of Alzheimers, memory boosting, slows progression of cancer eg: blueberries, plums, aubergine, blackberries
- White & Brown foods - cancer protection, bone health, heart health, lowers cholesterol, balances hormones eg: potatoes, onions, garlic, bananas

Food Colouring

Although many companies are starting to rethink the colours and additives they add to their processed foods, there are still plenty out there.

Here is a quick guide to some of them:

- □ Red 3 - Thyroid cancer, chromosomal damage
- □ Yellow 5 - Thyroid tumors, chromosomal damage, hyperactivity
- □ Yellow 6 - Adrenal Gland tumors, kidney tumors, hyperactivity
- □ Green 3 - Bladder tumors, testicular tumors
- □ Blue 1 - Chromosomal damage, asthma, kidney tumors
- □ Blue 2 - Chromosomal damage, brain tumors, bladder tumors

This list is a very good reason to make all our food from scratch and maybe give up those brightly coloured, oh so yummy, candy.

Food Combining

Food combining became popular in the 80s with the book "Fit for Life".

Although this was just prior to my thyroid going, I followed it and found I effortlessly dropped 2 dress sizes (although I wasn't what you would consider large at the time).

The premise is that certain foods don't mix well together as they create a surge of opposing enzymes in our gut which may cancel each other out. The other reason is that fruit, if eaten after a heavy meal, which only takes 15 mins to work through an empty stomach will sit on top of the starches or proteins and ferment, causing stomach discomfort.

The main rules are:

- □ Eat fruit on an empty stomach in the mornings only
- □ Do not eat starches with protein
- □ Do not eat fat with protein
- □ Do not combine different proteins in the same meal
- □ Do not eat dairy with other foods and eat only on an empty stomach

There are many scientific points that discredit the reasoning behind this diet, however I found personally that I felt really well and the weight dropping off was just a bonus.

Food Vibration

This may be a little woo woo for some, but if you are getting to know me even a little, then you will know I write about it for a reason. I believe in it.

Everything on the planet has a vibration or energy that can be measured in MHz including us and the food we eat.

I feel that the frequency of the majority (we need balance too) of the food we eat directly affects our mood, mental health and wellness.

Here is a list of vibrations for you:

- □ 52-320 Essential Oils
- □ 90 Raw vegetables
- □ 72-90 Human Bain
- □ 75 Fresh Fruits
- □ 67-70 Human Heart
- □ 62-68 Humans
- □ 62-68 Thyroid Gland
- □ 58 Disease begins
- □ 58 Coffee
- □ 52 Epstein Barr Virus
- □ 42 Cancer
- □ 25 Onset of death
- □ 2 Meat
- □ 0 Processed or canned food

You can see from the list if you have a life filled with takeaway processed foods, lots of meat and coffee, then our bodies are going to match the vibration, manifesting in possible depression, anxiety and other chronic diseases

How to Raise your vibration quickly:

- □ Positive thoughts raise 12 MHz within 12 seconds; negative thoughts lowers the same amount in 3 seconds
- □ Prayer raises by 15 MHz

Frozen Food

I have always been an organised person and I grew up in a family where Grandma would stock up our freezer with school lunches and pre-prepared home cooked meals to make life a little easier for my mom.

As a wife and mother myself, having home-cooked meals ready to go was just normal for us and stopped us from eating take-away too often.

After learning more about Ayurveda and attending the hospital in India, I learned that once food is frozen it retains the "cold energy" even after it is reheated.

Because I have a Kapha dominant body according to Ayurvedic medicine it means I am already cold, damp and wet, so the food I need to eat must be warm, hot and drying to counteract it.

Frozen foods do not do that. They keep putting cold energy into my already cold body. According to their philosophy I will never lose weight if I continue to do this.

When I thought about it, I pretty much ate most meals from my freezer. It may or may not be an issue, but I have since stopped this practice and cook fresh. I have lost 10kg since India.... you be the judge.

Fructose

A naturally occurring sugar found in fruits, vegetables, sugars and honey.

When consumed in excess it is converted directly into fat and stored in the liver.

High Fructose Corn Syrup is a common ingredient in many processed foods and may be a contributor to Non Alcoholic Fatty Liver Disease (NAFLD).

Sarah Wilson's I Quit Sugar program (which she is no longer running) was based on removing fructose from the diet.

Foods to **absolutely avoid** if you think fructose is an issue for you include:

- ☐ Fruits - All dried fruit, apples, apricots, Blackberry, Blood Orange, boysenberry, cowberry, gooseberries, grapes, guava, honeydew, kiwi, lychee, mango, mirabelle plum, nacho pear, nectarine, peach, pear, pineapple, plums, pomegranate, raspberry, redcurrant, reship, sour cherry, sweet cherry, camarillo, watermelon
- ☐ Vegetables - artichoke, autumn turnip, beetroot, beans, broccoli, Brussels sprouts, cabbage, carrots, cauliflower, chickpeas, eggplant, field beans, green beans, kidney beans, kale, lentils, leeks, mung beans, onions, oyster mushrooms, paprika, peas, pickles, radicchio, radishes, red cabbage, red pepper, savoy cabbage, sauerkraut, shallots, shiitake mushrooms, bring onions, sunroof,

sweet potatoes, turnips, tomatoes, water chestnut, white cabbage, yellow capsicum, zucchini

- ☐ Grains, breads & flours - wheat, bulgur, couscous, wheat germ, semolina, whole grain flours, soy flour, baguettes, crisp bread, pumpernickel, wholemeal rye bread, pita bread, breakfast cereals
- ☐ Legumes, nuts & seeds - peanuts, soybeans, all nuts, peanut butter, coconut & coconut products
- ☐ Dairy Products - sweetened Ice cream, sweetened and fruit yogurts, sweetened and flavoured milk
- ☐ Spices, seasonings & condiments - Cayenne, chervil, chili, dill, garlic, paprika, tomato paste, vinegar (balsamic & distilled), agave nectar, high fructose corn syrup (HFCS55), honey, maple syrup, molasses, sucrose, soy sauce, pesto, chutney, commercial sauces such as teriyaki, ketchup, bbq sauce
- ☐ Alcohol - champagne, cider, dessert wine, cider, egg liquor, glogg, honey wine, rosé wine, port wine, sparkling wine, white wine
- ☐ Drinks - all fruit juices, ice tea, multivitamin juice, smoothies, milk / soy sweetened drinks, tomato juice, almond milk, sodas (included diet and zero), energy drinks, ovaltine, protein shakes, oat milk,

Now because some of us would look at that list and go "But what CAN I eat???" I am going to follow this list with the list of *completely safe* and almost safe foods:

- ☐ Fruits - *avocado, jackfruit, kumquats, lemon, lime, loganberry, plantain*, ripe bananas, blueberry, cranberry, grapefruit, mandarin, oranges, passionfruit, starfruit, strawberries
- ☐ Vegetables - *asparagus (cooked), bamboo sprouts, celery, chanterelle mushrooms, chinese spinach, cress, daikon, endive, fennel, frisee lettuce, ginger, horseradish, lettuce, lotus root, nori, olives, pak choi, potatoes, pumpkin, radish, rhubarb, spinach, swiss chard, white turnips,* asparagus (raw), button mushrooms, carrots (cooked), chicory, chinese cabbage, corn, cucumber, dandelion greens, mixed lettuce, morel mushrooms, okra, parsnip, watercress
- ☐ Grains, breads & flours, legumes, nuts & seeds - *amaranth, barley, brown rice, buckwheat, corn, oatmeal, popcorn (plain), quinoa, white rice, rye, rice flour, cornmeal, almost all seeds*, wheat/rye bread, cornflakes, spelt, wheat bran, pumpkin seeds
- ☐ Dairy Products - *butter, buttermilk, cheese, coffee cream, condensed milk, cream, crème fraîche, curd, kefir, mascarpone, milk (non sweetened), milk powder, sour cream, whey, whey powder, natural yogurt*

- ☐ Spices, Sweeteners & condiments - *baking powder, fish sauce, mayonnaise, oyster sauce, Worcestershire sauce, rice syrup, dextrose, cider vinegar, red wine vinegar, white wine vinegar, most seasonings (cinnamon, cumin etc),* brown sugar, coriander
- ☐ Alcohol - *Cachaca, gin, ouzo, sambuca, tequila, vodka, whiskey,* beer, cognac, guinness, malt beer, red wine, rum, sherry, vermouth, wheat beer, dry white wine
- ☐ Other drinks - *coffee, espresso, mate, mineral water, rice milk, tea (black, herb, oolong, rooibos, green),* carrot juice, lemon juice, mandarin juice
- ☐ All fats & Oils are fructose free, and all meats, fish and seafood are fructose free as long as they are not marinated in something that may contain fructose.

Phew! It is easy to see though, how overloading our liver with fructose could happen so easily, even if we are eating a healthy diet.

For example my lunch today was red and white onion (no list), red and yellow peppers (no list) with 2 baked potatoes (thankfully on the yes list). I grated fresh garlic into the lightly stir fried onion and peppers (again on the no list). So although it looked healthy, if I was avoiding fructose, I would have failed miserably!

G

Gimmicks

There are so many gimmicks and fads and trends out there. Most of them are completely harmless simply because they don't do anything, but some of them may make your health worse, and of course you may just find the one "thing" that reverses your disease.

I am not immune to the gimmicks, in fact I've probably tried more than most. When you have a chronic disease, often you will do absolutely anything to get rid of it which will mean trying things that may seem insane (think coffee enemas). Some will help, some will not.

If you want to try the latest gimmick or trend, you absolutely can, but you just need to be open minded and a bit smart about it.

Start with always keeping a diary. You always need to know where you are BEFORE you start something new, and don't do anything else during that trial time so you can honestly and fairly judge if it has helped you or not.

A good trial time for any new protocol is 4-8 weeks. Anything less than 4 weeks will not tell you anything, because if you are removing something from your diet you will likely feel the withdrawal and detox effects for the first week or two and then your body needs time to adjust.

If after a couple of months though, you don't feel any better, and there are no changes to symptoms or you feel worse, then maybe it's not for you. Move on and don't feel bad about it. Just congratulate yourself for trying something and staying the course.

Gabriel, Jon

Author of "The Gabriel Method", Jon lost 226lb (103 kg) by going back to basics.

When he started on his weight loss journey he began by simply adding a salad to everything he ate. So pizza was cut up and thrown into a salad as an example. He gradually crowded out the bad foods with good food.

Jon was left with no loose skin, he believes, due to his visualisations of how he wanted his body to look. Jon says our mind understands pictures, so by showing his mind a picture of how he wanted to look, he achieved his goal.

Galactagogue

An agent which increases or promotes the flow of breast milk.

Examples Include: Fennel, Milk Thistle, Goats rue, Fenugreek, Chaste Tree, Aniseed, Shatavari

Gallbladder

A small organ attached to the liver that stores and secretes the bile that our liver makes.

In the Traditional Chinese Medicine Clock, it is believed that if we wake regularly between 11pm - 1am then it may indicate that our gallbladder needs support.

Since people with thyroid disease (more so hypothyroid patients) have an altered cholesterol metabolism, this can cause a build up of bile possibly leading to stones.

But it is avoidable, as a study published in the American Journal of Gastroenterology showed a 17% decreased risk of gallstones in women who ate good amounts of insoluble fibre, which we need for estrogen clearance and gut health anyway, so win win right?

Nutritional support for healthy bile secretion and flow includes:

- ☐ Dandelion root
- ☐ Globe artichoke
- ☐ Milk Thistle
- ☐ Ginger
- ☐ Peppermint
- ☐ Taurine
- ☐ Betaine

- □ Vitamin C
- □ Lecithin

Herbs that help with gallstones include: Barberry, Corydalis, Dandelion Leaf, Dandelion root, Fringe Tree, Globe Artichoke, Greater Celandine, Peppermint and St Mary's thistle.

I have never experienced gallstones as such, however, a few years ago I was on an apple juice (green apples) fast for 3 days. Whenever I do any juice fasts, I always do coffee enemas with them to help with the toxic load the juice releases from my cells.

After the second day I looked into the toilet to see hundreds of little green round balls.

After staring unbelievably I took to google and my text books and what I think happened was this.

The malic acid in apples softened the stones and the coffee enema (which has the ability to go up into the liver) cleared the stones.

It only happened one more time during that fast and has never happened since. If you think you want to have a go, please talk to someone about it first ok?

Garlic

There are many people out there (I used to be one of them) that becomes quite nauseous after eating garlic. This actually indicates a sluggish liver which is common in thyroid disease.

Garlic is well known to be an all round human wellness boosting bulb. It is known to reduce cholesterol, reduce blood pressure, is an antioxidant, anti parasitic, anti fungal, antibacterial and antiplatelet.

I remember sitting in a nutrition class years ago and a lovely old man was sitting there eating garlic sandwiches. He had cancer and was eating truckloads of garlic and the bread helped him to get it down.

Being high in sulphur compounds it helps the liver pathway that is also responsible for converting our thyroid hormone along with other members of that family such as onion and leek.

Garlic can help reduce heavy metals, kill intestinal worms and parasites.

It must be used cautiously with blood thinning medication such as warfarin as it directly changes the dosage requirements.

Gelatin

Gelatine is full of collagen which is a powerhouse of healing for our gut in particular.

Since most thyroid disease is caused by auto-immune disease and most auto-immune disease is caused by leaky gut, and add to that 20% of our inactive thyroid hormone (T4) is converted into active form (T3) in the gut, then the importance of healing it is really obvious right?

Gelatine is derived from the bones of animals, so bone broths that have been simmered over 24 hours are one of the quickest ways to get gelatine into your body (recipe under bone broth).

Gelatine is helpful for:

- ☐ gut health
- ☐ joint inflammation (arthritis)
- ☐ bone health (osteoporosis)
- ☐ strengthening fingernails
- ☐ improving hair quality
- ☐ improving leaky gut
- ☐ improving autoimmune diseases

If you are vegetarian and thinking you will use agar agar instead, sorry it does not contain collagen. Although it is really good for you and has fiber and other great nutrients, it does not actually contain the gut healing attributes of gelatine.

Generic Medication

Many medications have the original brand and then a generic version which is cheaper but "just the same" we are told.

I have a story that says otherwise.

My hubby takes a particular kind of medication which he has taken for well over a decade now. When generic options came in, we eventually decided to try one (yes, we are brand snobs).

It took a couple of months before hubby realised the medication was the cause of his sudden bouts of insomnia, which had never happened before (he can sleep any time any where that man).

Through trial and error we discovered that only the original medication and one of the generic versions is ok for him to take.

The point of this is for you to know that although the active ingredient may be the same, the excipients (fillers) may not be and can cause problems where there weren't any previously.

Just something to look out for.

GMO's

The word "GMO's" is infiltrating our social media, the news and current affairs.

It stands for Genetically Modified Organism. It is referring mostly to our food and means that many of our regular foods have had their DNA altered via genetic engineering in some way.

Generally this is done to make the plant more resistant to disease and pests, but many believe that the process of doing this is contributing to our growing health problems and diseases.

Wheat is an example of this. Many centuries ago our wheat contained far more chromosomes than it does today. It leads you to wonder if that is our major issue with wheat as opposed to gluten?

In France, they still use very old wheat that has not been tampered with, and I have heard of many people that cannot digest bread easily here, able to happily eat croissants and baguettes when they are visiting this beautiful part of the world. So you be the judge for yourself and decide if you wish to eat these kinds of altered foods.

It will be obvious to you in the fruit and vegetable section, they are the ones like "tomatoes for sandwiches" (because they have been engineered to have less pulp).

Genetic Susceptibility

An inherited risk of developing a disease.

Thyroid disease is said to be a genetic susceptibility.

GERD

Gastro-Esaphageal Reflux Disease (GERD) is a disorder of the digestive system where the lower oesophageal sphincter (valve) is faulty allowing food and gastric acid to return back up the oesophagus causing pain and burning.

There is a link here for patients with Hashimoto's as it can cause issues with oesophageal motility that results in reflux symptoms.

It can also be caused by a hernia pressing on the valve causing it to be weak.

It is an extremely common affliction and is treated with lifestyle and dietary changes, and if that fails, medication is used to lower acid secretion completely.

Gerson Therapy

Dr Max Gerson developed a protocol over 100 years ago to treat his own debilitating migraines.

After discovering an eating regime that kept them away, he started trialling it on some of his patients. Over time, as his patients returned to him saying that the diet had also cured them of other disease, Dr Gerson began to realise the diet was one that just helped the body to heal from whatever was going on.

The Gerson Institute is situated in Mexico and receives many cancer patients and chronic disease patients.

The protocol consists of:

- Fresh raw juices every hour
- Vegetarian diet
- Hippocrates soup for lunch and dinner
- Coffee enemas for detoxification
- Many supplements for liver healing and thyroid support
- Is very pro-thyroid in general

Patients follow the diet and protocol for 2 years during which time the Liver is said to completely regenerate.

I followed a reduced version of the therapy for quite a while and it helped me to reduce my medication, which is still low even though I no longer follow the protocol.

Gestational Thyroid Disease

Thyroid disease brought on by pregnancy. It can be hyperthyroid, or hypothyroid and often corrects itself after the baby has been born.

Treatment is the same as it would be if you were not pregnant, although levels will be monitored more closely for the health of the baby.

Ghee

Ghee is a clarified butter that is used in India and southeast Asia for both its medicinal qualities and in religious ceremonies.

The process of making it involves slowly boiling butter on the hotplate until the milk solids are separated from the fat. The resulting ghee is pure fat that contains no dairy useful for cooking all kinds of recipes.

In Ayurveda medicine ghee is used as a carrier medicine for people with a Pitta Dosha, as it helps whatever herbs they are using to get into the tissues more effectively.

There are many Youtube videos showing how to make this yourself at home, because store bought versions are rather expensive.

Ghrelin

Ghrelin is the opposing hormone to Leptin, and is our hunger hormone. It stimulates appetite and promotes fat storage.

It is secreted when the stomach is empty and tells the hypothalamus it's time to eat.

If you find you are someone who is constantly hungry, even though you just ate, your plan of attack would be to increase foods to increase your Leptin (the satisfied hormone). *See Leptin*

Ginger

When I was a child I tried glacé ginger and thought it was horrid and therefor associated any other kind of ginger (except for gingerbread) with that taste.

Fast forward a gazillion years and when I started juicing, one of the first green juices I ever made was the Mean Green from the movie Fat Sick & Nearly Dead by Joe Cross which contained fresh ginger.

It turned out I love fresh ginger and as time has progressed, our ginger ratio is getting larger! I also now grate it on top of fruit salad, oatmeal and stir-fry veggies.

Ginger is like Nature's Blanket and warms us from the inside out. In my research, many experts recommend eating ginger for so many reasons and ailments. Here are just a few:

- Anti-inflammatory, carminative, digestive
- Increases circulation (particularly to the hands & feet)

- ☐ Raynaud's syndrome
- ☐ Osteoarthritis & Rheumatoid Arthritis
- ☐ Bronchitis & Asthma
- ☐ Irritable bowel syndrome
- ☐ Endometriosis
- ☐ Acute infections
- ☐ Nausea, vomiting, motion sickness, morning sickness (it opens our pyloric valve to let the contents out)
- ☐ Protects stomach lining against NSAIDS & alcohol
- ☐ Kills salmonella & Staph bacteria
- ☐ Blood Thinner (beware if taking warfarin, see your doctor as your medication will be affected)
- ☐ Will help prevent and lessen headaches and migraines
- ☐ Pain Relief

In thyroid terms it can:

- ☐ Improve heat levels in the body
- ☐ Lower fasting glucose
- ☐ Reduce Inflammation
- ☐ Reduce food sensitivities
- ☐ Improve Digestion

Since ginger is something we only eat a little at a time it is hard to show you just what goodies are kept inside these strange looking tubers. So I am using a larger amount, because this amount I would easily consume over a week.

100g Ginger gives us:

- ☐ 8% of DVI in Vitamin C (thyroid pathway, adrenals, antioxidant)
- ☐ 1% of DVI in Vitamin E (thyroid pathway, antioxidant)
- ☐ 2% of DV in Vitamin B1 (thyroid, hair, hyperthyroid)
- ☐ 2% of DV in Vitamin B2 (thyroid pathway)
- ☐ 4% of DVI in Vitamin B3 (mental health)
- ☐ 8% of DV in Vitamin B6 (mental health, progesterone)
- ☐ 3% of DV in folate (MTHFR, liver)
- ☐ 2% of DV in Calcium (bones)
- ☐ 11% of DV in Magnesium (stress & sugar)
- ☐ 8% of DV in Iron (thyroid pathway, fatigue)

- ☐ 3% of DV in Phosphorus (liver, bones)
- ☐ 2% of DV in Zinc (thyroid pathway, healing)
- ☐ 12% of DVI in Potassium (thyroid, fatigue, fluid)
- ☐ 11% of DVI in Manganese (thyroid pathway)
- ☐ 11% of DVI in Copper (skin, collagen nerves)
- ☐ 8% of DV in Dietary fibre (hormone clearance, gut health)
- ☐ 4% of DV in Protein (thyroid pathway)

When I spent time in an Ayurvedic Hospital in India, twice a day, everyday we were brought a thermos of hot ginger tea, so its healing properties are used across the world.

Ginger is an amazing little miracle!

Gingko Biloba

This is the most beautiful tree. If you have never seen one, google it. Not only is it pretty, the leaf is powerful in all things brainy.

Gingko is cognition enhancing, neuroprotective and a circulatory stimulant, so it is used in the prevention and treatment of Alzheimer's disease, dementia, dizziness, vertigo, concentration, memory and cognitive performance.

I have started taking it for vertigo that I have had a few bouts of over the years. I will be tracking it to see if I get any bouts while taking it.

It is starting to gain traction as a use for tinnitus and hearing loss.

The only caution is with people taking anticoagulant drugs, but the risk is minimal.

Glandular Fever

See Epstein Barr Virus

Gliadin

The portion of gluten that causes an immune reaction in those with gluten intolerance or celiac disease.

Globe Artichoke

This is known to herbalists as the "go-to" herb for the liver. The Medical Medium has it as the "go-to" food for thyroid health. So either way, I think it's good for us!

It lowers cholesterol, protects and restores the liver, is a mild bitter tonic, diuretic, and depurative.

The key uses for the tincture are helping the liver to restore, Gallstones, gall bladder dysfunction, elevated triglycerides, constipation, flatulence, bloating and food sensitivities.

Although the tincture would clearly be stronger, there is a lot to be said for eating the whole food on a regular basis.

Glucosamine

This nutrient is becoming very well known as the "joint nutrient". There are a million different glucosamine supplements on the market now because of its amazing relief in our connective tissues, but it is also required for:

- liver detoxification
- protection of the stomach lining
- cartilage metabolism
- increases leptin production in the body (the hormone that tells us we are full)
- improves chemotherapy outcomes
- leaky gut syndrome
- osteoporosis
- bone healing
- ulcerative colitis
- gastric ulcers
- arthritis and back pain

The strange thing here is, that all the medications we take for these kinds of ailments (NSAIDS, aspirin etc) actually inhibit our body making glucosamine for ourselves, which leaves us with no option but to purchase the supplemental variety (made from shark cartilage and the shells of shellfish or synthetic).

Daily Requirements of Glucosamine:

- Adults 600-3000mg

Glucose

Main energy source of our body which converts to glycogen.

A naturally occurring sugar in plants and fruits, the human body can also make it when needed.

Glutamine

Another non-essential amino acid that becomes essential when we are sick or diseased.

Glutamine is important for us in times of stress (so all of us!) and helps our gut function and immune system.

This amino acid also helps with:

- Making glutathione (master antioxidant)
- Making DNA
- Immune enhancer
- Increases our IgA levels in the gut (gut immunity)
- Involved in energy production
- Helps balance our pH

Having any kind of gut issues such as leaky gut syndrome, celiac disease and poor immunity then adding glutamine rich foods is a good start.

Glutamine rich foods include:

- Beans and legumes
- Dairy products, cottage & ricotta cheeses
- Ham, sausage meat, most proteins
- Rolled oats

Glutathione

Our body's master antioxidant. The fireman chief if you like. Glutathione is required for:

- immunity boosting
- killer of free radicals
- immune regulation
- modulates DNA synthesis
- protects cells against oxidation
- protects mitochondria (energy)
- protects red blood cells
- reduces replication of HIV virus

- ☐ required for vanadium metabolism (required in thyroid pathway)
- ☐ detoxifies DDT
- ☐ recycles vitamins E and C (his fire crew who also put out spot fires)

Deficiency Symptoms of Glutathione include:

- ☐ cancer
- ☐ heart disease
- ☐ chemical sensitivity
- ☐ immune dysfunction
- ☐ cognitive decline
- ☐ poor balance
- ☐ premature ageing

Factors that contribute to Glutathione deficiency:

- ☐ alcohol consumption
- ☐ aspirin, oral contraceptives
- ☐ excess unsaturated fat consumption (avocado, nuts, olive oils, vegetable oils, some meats)
- ☐ low protein intake
- ☐ copper deficiency
- ☐ autoimmune disease
- ☐ heavy metal exposure
- ☐ high blood sugar
- ☐ high pollution, smoking
- ☐ rheumatoid arthritis
- ☐ Down's Syndrome

Food sources of Glutathione include:

- ☐ Asparagus
- ☐ avocado
- ☐ eggs
- ☐ garlic
- ☐ walnuts
- ☐ whey protein

Another unusual source of Glutathione is from coffee enemas which increase the production of glutathione by 700%

Daily Requirements of Glutathione:

- Adults 100-500mg

Gluten

Gluten is a protein found in wheat and wheat-like grains that give it strength and elasticity.

The studies are showing that we ALL (meaning all humans) have an immune response when we eat gluten, so the theory goes if we ingest gluten and the immune system goes after it to destroy it then it will also go after the thyroid in a case of mistaken identity.

This is the major reason behind the advice from the experts to remove gluten when we have thyroid disease.

It doesn't matter which kind of thyroid disease we have - hyper, hypo or regardless of us knowing if we have autoimmune disease or not, removing gluten from our diet then gives our thyroid a free pass from possible further attacks.

Gluten is in wheat, rye, barley and oats, however the gluten molecule in oats is slightly different to the others and some people find they have no problems with it, like me.

As a side note, I have read many times during my research that little bumps on the upper arms could indicate a gluten intolerance.

Going Gluten Free

It is really important to understand that if we want to go gluten free to reduce our antibodies, then doing it means going without it completely for 6 months before all traces of gluten and its response are out of our body.

If you get 3 months in and even a crumb from the butter your kids have used gets onto your gluten free toast, that is enough to start the reaction all over again.

The other thing I want to mention here is the sheer number of "Gluten Free" items we can purchase from the grocery store now. And most of them chock full of chemicals and sugars (because they are gluten free).

Suddenly, the person who never ate a cookie for morning tea before, is eating gluten free cookies that some lovely soul has bought for them thinking they were doing something nice for them.

We have to get smart and understand if we are removing gluten, we are taking something away, not suddenly adding in whole food groups we never ate before simply because it has the magic words "Gluten Free" branded across its shiny packet. Are we good?

Cross Reactive Grains

Have you gone gluten free but still don't feel any better? There are many grains that actually behave like gluten in the body so can cause a similar reaction. And many of them are the ones we use to replace our beloved glutenous foods in the first place.

How many of these do you eat:

- ☐ Dairy - milk, butter, cream, ice-cream, yogurt, sour cream
- ☐ Corn - all varieties, cooked and raw
- ☐ Millet
- ☐ Oats - see above
- ☐ Rice - yep... the thing we turn too! All varieties, even brown rice
- ☐ Yeast - the yeast in our gluten free baked goodies may cause a reaction

Glycemic Index

A number given to a food based on how much it raises blood sugars two hours after consuming it. The number is out 100 and the lower the number the better.

Glycemic Load

This is worked out on the quantity of the food.

Glycemic Load =
GI x Carbohydrate (g) content per portion ÷100

For example let's take a potato:

- ☐ Glycemic Index (GI) of 85
- ☐ Carb content of 14g
- ☐ GL = 85 x 14/100 = 12

The Glycemic Load is classified into

- ☐ Low - less than 10
- ☐ Medium - 11-19
- ☐ High - 20 or more

Glycine

A non-essential amino acid that becomes essential when we are sick and diseased, glycine is the most versatile and in demand of all the amino acids due to the number of functions it performs.

We need glycine for:

- Making collagen
- Making glutathione
- Improve Human Growth Hormone release
- Improve clearance of uric acid from the kidneys
- Involved in making bile salts
- Involved in liver detoxification
- Involved in salicylate clearance
- Improves triglyceride levels
- Anti-inflammatory properties
- Immune modulating properties
- Improves memory recall

This amazing little amino acid helps therapeutically with arthritis, autoimmune disorders, atherosclerosis, cancer, chemical sensitivity, fatigue, gout, kidney failure, myasthenia, nail growth, digestion, seizures, and wound healing.

Food sources of Glycine include:

- Most protein / animal sources
- Beans and nuts
- Brewers yeast
- Eggs and whey protein
- Fish and seafood

Goiter

A painless swelling of the thyroid gland that results in difficulty breathing, swallowing, talking and coughing.

While lack of iodine is a cause of goitres, so too is an excess of iodine and surprisingly, it does not always mean that the thyroid gland is no longer working.

Causes include:

- ☐ Graves Disease causing overstimulation of the thyroid which induces the swelling
- ☐ Hashimoto's causing an elevated TSH which can induce swelling
- ☐ Nodules on the thyroid begin to swell
- ☐ Thyroid Cancer, although not common
- ☐ HCG the pregnancy hormone can cause swelling of the thyroid
- ☐ Inflammation can cause swelling

Treatment includes:

- ☐ Medications to stabilise thyroid hormone production and inflammation
- ☐ Radioactive Iodine if the gland is overactive
- ☐ Surgery to remove all of part of the thyroid

Goitrogens

See Brassica

Goji Berries

This incredible little Berries from Tibet are incredibly high in protein and fibre, taste amazing and are great for the thyroid!

100g of Goji Berries contain:

- ☐ 22% of DV in protein (thyroid pathway)
- ☐ 32% of DV in Dietary Fibre (hormonal clearance, gut health)
- ☐ 180% of DV in Vitamin A (thyroid pathway, skin)
- ☐ 32% of DV in Vitamin C (thyroid pathway, adrenals, antioxidant)
- ☐ 10% of DV in Vitamin B1 (thyroid, hair, hyperthyroidism)
- ☐ 75% of DV in Vitamin B2 (thyroid pathway)
- ☐ 10% of DV in calcium (bones)
- ☐ 50% of DV in iron (thyroid pathway, fatigue, gut acid)
- ☐ 24% of DV in Potassium (thyroid, fatigue, fluid)
- ☐ 18% of DV in Zinc (thyroid, immunity, mental health, wound healing)
- ☐ 100% of DV in Copper (skin, nerves, collagen)
- ☐ 91% of DV in Selenium (thyroid pathway)
- ☐ Glycemic Load of 7

Since thyroid people struggle to convert beta-carotene into Vitamin A, this little berry is fantastic as it is already converted into Vitamin A form, plus the huge amount of selenium, potassium and zinc make this a must have snack item for thyroid nutrients.

Warning: these belong to the nightshade family, so in the same family as potatoes and tomatoes.

Gotu Kola

This lovely herb is a healing promoter. It is particularly valuable for venous insufficiency, varicose veins, haemorrhoids, wounds, ulcers and burns.

It is anti-inflammatory and a nervine tonic so has also been used for anxiety, concentration and cognitive performance.

Grains

There are lots of opinions out there on grains and there is really no "one right answer".

I have come across many thyroid people that have cured their disease from a plant based, grain heavy diet.

I have come across many thyroid people that have cured their disease by removing all grains, even pseudo grains such as buckwheat and quinoa from their diet.

There are some great books such as "Grain Brain" by David Perlmutter and "Against all Grain" by Danielle Walker.

This one is going to be down to you to decide if it plays a part in your diet and lifestyle.

I personally tend to not eat a lot of grains as they sit heavily on me and bloat me. If I sit down to a plate of baked potatoes (no fat) I feel great. So for me it is not the starch but the grain that doesn't sit right.

Like everything else, it is up to you to trial this for yourself. Although most thyroid practitioners will likely have you off grains, it is not a given outcome that it will reverse your antibodies and make you feel better. So keep that in mind when you trial it. Be open to all eventualities.

Often, when you repair your gut health, you can tolerate any kind of grains with no problem, so that may be an area I still need to work on.

Grapefruit (pink)

I love pink grapefruit juice! I love the tartness and yet weird sweetness and the color! How could you not love the color right?

Grapefruit has been linked over the years to reducing cellulite and weight loss. Who remembers the Grapefruit Diet?

So let's have a look at what is in an average sized grapefruit:

- ☐ 4% of DV in Protein
- ☐ 16% of DV in Fibre (Hormone metabolism)
- ☐ 2% of DVI of Vitamin E (Thyroid Pathway)
- ☐ 128% of DV in Vitamin C (Adrenal health)
- ☐ 56% of DV in Vitamin A (Thyroid Pathway)
- ☐ 8% of DV in Vitamin B1
- ☐ 4% of DV in Vitamin B2 (Thyroid Pathway)
- ☐ 2% of DV in Vitamin B3 (mental health)
- ☐ 6% of DV in Vitamin B6
- ☐ 8% of DV in Folate (Liver & MTHFR)
- ☐ 6% of DV in Calcium
- ☐ 6% of DV in Magnesium (Stress & Sugar)
- ☐ 10% of DV in Potassium
- ☐ 2% of DV in Manganese
- ☐ 2% of DVI of Zinc (thyroid pathway)
- ☐ 2% of DVI of Iron (thyroid pathway)

So that all adds up to a fruit that is:

- ☐ extremely high in antioxidants
- ☐ inhibits tumour formation
- ☐ inhibits breast cancer
- ☐ lowers cholesterol
- ☐ prevents kidney stone formation
- ☐ protects against colon cancer
- ☐ repairs DNA damage
- ☐ strengthens blood vessels
- ☐ improves Digestion
- ☐ aids weight loss

- reduces plaque in the arteries
- reduces appetite
- alleviates Insomnia

Finally, let's talk about the dangers. Grapefruit has an additive effect on some medications and on others it can make it difficult for the body to process and excrete, keeping the medication in the body for a lot longer than designed.

So if you are on medication, talk to your doctor first. If it has been suggested that you should take a statin for your cholesterol and you haven't started yet - perhaps try having a RUBY grapefruit juice (freshly squeezed) every morning for a month and then retest your cholesterol before deciding on medication.

As for the mix with thyroid medication, it may have a decreasing effect in the bloodstream, meaning you may need more medication. However, I have been eating grapefruit daily for years (about an hour or two AFTER my medication) and I have reduced my medication substantially not increased it. So I guess it is up to you to talk to your doctor or try it out for yourself.

Grass Fed Animals

Since the rise of the paleo movement, so to the rise of Grass Fed Animals have come with it.

The reason they are promoted over commercially grain fed animals is in the meat. Studies have shown that meat from a commercially raised animal is inflammatory to our arteries and heart.

Meat from grass fed animals do not have that effect on us, and as an added benefit contain higher levels of fatty acids including Omega 3s and one called conjugated linoleic acid (CLA) which does not contribute to disease and helps prevent other diseases such as diabetes and obesity.

Gratitude Journal

Made famous by Oprah, the gratitude journal has been around for many years.

The idea is that you write daily the things you are grateful for to help keep you focused on the positive aspects of your life.

Everybody that follows this has a different process, but the easiest way to start would be to simply write down 5 things every day that you are grateful for.

I use the Abraham Hicks method "Rampage of Appreciation" which means I write for pages everything that I appreciate in that moment. I find it uplifts me like nothing else, it just takes a little time.

Graves Disease

The autoimmune disease causing hyperthyroidism.

While Hashimoto's slows everything down, Graves makes everything go faster.

Symptoms include:

- ☐ feeling hot when others are not
- ☐ increased perspiration, sweaty palms
- ☐ weight loss (sometimes weight gain)
- ☐ diarrhoea or frequent stools
- ☐ low cholesterol levels
- ☐ brittle nails, hair loss, dry skin, hives, itchy skin
- ☐ bulging eyes, staring eyes
- ☐ shakiness, tremors, nervous fighting
- ☐ hyperactive, fast speech, racing thoughts
- ☐ talkative, ambitious, impulsive
- ☐ anxiety, nervousness, depression, mood swings, panic attacks, insomnia, irritability, emotional and behavioural issues, poor focus, aggression
- ☐ fatigue, exhaustion, wired and tired
- ☐ high sex drive, light or no periods, PMS, infertility
- ☐ muscle weakness, cramps
- ☐ racing pulse, heart palpitations, chest pain
- ☐ increased appetite, increased thirst

Treatment can include a variety of approaches, but due to the dangers of everything in the body being permanently on high speed, doctors don't like to leave Graves' Disease to go unbalanced for longer than 2 years, and many end up having the thyroid removed or killed.

Treatments include:

- ☐ Anti-thyroid medication
- ☐ Radioactive iodine therapy

- ☐ Beta Blockers
- ☐ Surgery

Graves, Robert

An Irish Doctor who first discovered the collection of symptoms in several patients in the mid 1800s.

Graves Ophthalmopathy

An added symptom with approx 50% of people suffering from Graves' disease is vision problems and Grave's eye disease.

This presents in many degrees and is graded according to vision, inflammation, alignment and appearance.

It can go away after a few years but most sufferers don't wait that long and seek treatment which is generally corticosteroids or in more severe cases, surgery and radiotherapy of the eyes.

Green Beans

Green beans are often seen as a boring side veg, but once you see how many amazing thyroid nutrients they contain, I'm sure you will start adding them to your cart with more regularity.

100g of green beans contains:

- ☐ 4% of DV in Protein (thyroid pathway)
- ☐ 14% of DV in Dietary Fibre (hormonal clearance, gut health)
- ☐ 14% of DV in Vitamin A (thyroid pathway, skin)
- ☐ 27% of DV in Vitamin C (thyroid pathway, adrenals, antioxidant)
- ☐ 2% of DV in Vitamin E (thyroid pathway, antioxidant)
- ☐ 18% of DV in Vitamin K (blood, bones)
- ☐ 6% of DV in Vitamin B1 (thyroid, hair, hyperthyroidism)
- ☐ 6% of DV in Vitamin B2 (thyroid pathway)
- ☐ 4% of DV in Vitamin B3 (mental health)
- ☐ 4% of DV in Vitamin B6 (mental health, progesterone)
- ☐ 9% of DV in Folate (MTHFR, liver)
- ☐ 4% of DV in calcium (bones)

- ☐ 6% of DV in iron (thyroid pathway, fatigue, gut acid)
- ☐ 6% of DV in Magnesium (stress, sugar)
- ☐ 4% of DV in Phosphorus (bones, liver)
- ☐ 6% of DV in Potassium (thyroid, fluid, fatigue)
- ☐ 2% of DV in Zinc (thyroid, mental health, immunity, wound healing)
- ☐ 11% of DV in Manganese (thyroid pathway)
- ☐ 1% of DV in Selenium (thyroid pathway)
- ☐ Glycemic Load of 3

That all adds up to

- ☐ Improved immunity
- ☐ More balanced blood sugar
- ☐ Reduced risk of heart disease
- ☐ Reduced risk of diabetes
- ☐ Reduced risk of colon cancer
- ☐ Better bone health
- ☐ Helps lower cholesterol
- ☐ Improved fertility
- ☐ Improved digestion

All that from humble, ordinary green beans! And they are inexpensive, and if you want to go the extra mile, they are easy to grow!

Green Tea

Green tea is the same type of plant as black tea and oolong tea, but they have not been fermented which gives them a high level of antioxidants.

Health benefits include:

- ☐ Lowered risk of heart disease
- ☐ Lowered risk of atherosclerosis
- ☐ Lowered risk of cancer
- ☐ Lowered risk of stroke
- ☐ Lower blood pressure
- ☐ Lowered risk of diabetes
- ☐ Lower cholesterol levels

- ☐ Improved management of Thyroid Ophthalmopathy
- ☐ Improved bone density
- ☐ Improved memory
- ☐ Improved cognition
- ☐ Improved weight loss outcomes
- ☐ Reduced signs of ageing
- ☐ Reduced tooth decay
- ☐ Reduced depression and anxiety
- ☐ Anti-viral and antibacterial

This particular beverage also comes with some downsides, so make sure you are aware of them before you help yourself to that 23rd cup today.

- ☐ Can decrease T4 & T3
- ☐ Can elevate TSH
- ☐ Can be antithyroid
- ☐ Contains Fluoride (like black tea)
- ☐ Can increase the risk of thyroid cancer
- ☐ High in caffeine
- ☐ Thins the blood
- ☐ More than 2 cups a day may increase the risk of miscarriage
- ☐ May reduce iron absorption

I know many of you are crying right now. I'm sorry.

Grounding

Also called earthing, grounding is the process of walking barefoot on the earth or beach and receiving the negative ions into our body.

Since we are an electric body full of energy, we actually need recharging so to speak.

The place with the highest amount of negative ions is along the ocean edge where it hits the beach and is all foamy, but anywhere we can be in nature, preferably without the pollution and shoes so we can be in contact with the earth is fantastic for us.

Grounding helps us to:

- ☐ reduce inflammation
- ☐ reduce chronic pain

- ☐ reduce muscle tension
- ☐ improve sleep
- ☐ improve energy levels
- ☐ lower stress
- ☐ calm the nervous system
- ☐ regulate blood flow
- ☐ regulate hormones
- ☐ speed healing and recovery
- ☐ reduce jet lag
- ☐ protect against EMF's

Unfortunately most of us are wearing shoes around the clock and walking on tiles, carpet, cement, anything but the earth, that is why we need to make a particular effort to take those shoes off and get our toes dirty or sandy!

Growth Hormone

See Human Growth Hormone

Gua Sha

This is the Chinese practice of scraping or spooning a smooth object over the skin. It may cause slight bruising or purple and red spots.

It is used to unblock stagnant chi which can cause illness or chronic disease.

Benefits include:

- ☐ stimulating the immune system
- ☐ reducing pain
- ☐ reducing inflammation
- ☐ anti ageing

I experienced this once when I was seeing a Traditional Chinese Doctor and getting acupuncture. It was actually quite a pleasant experience.

Guggulu

A resin harvested from a variety of Myrrh tree, guggulu (meaning "protects from disease") has been used in India for centuries as a treatment in Ayurvedic medicine.

It's benefits include:

- ☐ increases thyroid hormone production
- ☐ lowering cholesterol
- ☐ weight loss
- ☐ reducing acne
- ☐ reducing pain in arthritis
- ☐ clear sinuses
- ☐ soothe joints
- ☐ relieve chronic skin diseases including vitiligo
- ☐ blood detoxifier
- ☐ reduces fluid retention and edema

It is really a perfect hypothyroid supplement, however if you want to work with it, find a really good Ayurvedic Practitioner who can make sure it works with your unique history.

Guthrie Test

A heel prick blood test routinely carried out on newborn babies within a few days of birth.

It picks up on disorders such as congenital hypothyroidism, cystic fibrosis, and phenylketonuria (a condition where too much phenylalanine has accumulated in the brain).

Gut Thyroid Connection

Did you know there are more bacteria in our gut than human cells in our body?

For our body to get the activated thyroid hormone it needs it first has to be converted into its usable form and 20% of that happens in our gut by the good guys (bacteria).

In Hashimoto's disease it is believed one of the root causes is a leaky gut, causing the immune reaction.

So while gut health seems to be everywhere in health circles right now, it is particularly important for us thyroid people to pay attention to it.

We need good gut health for:

- ☐ strengthening the immune system
- ☐ lowering inflammation

- ☐ heart and brain health
- ☐ digesting fiber
- ☐ weight control
- ☐ blood sugar
- ☐ mineral absorption

Improving our gut microbiome includes doing things like:

- ☐ Taking a probiotic everyday
- ☐ Eating the rainbow - a diverse diet
- ☐ Eating fermented foods
- ☐ Drinking Kombucha
- ☐ Having bone broth regularly
- ☐ Eating prebiotic foods daily
- ☐ Avoiding all junk food and processed foods.
- ☐ Removing artificial sweeteners
- ☐ Avoid antibiotics where possible
- ☐ Include herbs such as chamomile, fenugreek, marshmallow, and slippery elm

If you currently have a less than lovely gut-garden, please don't go planting lots of new things (fibre, ferments etc) until you have weeded and cleared things out. The gut will react poorly if you start throwing a huge amount of fibre and probiotics at it that it is not used to. A little at a time, and more importantly, remove the bad stuff first.

Gymnema

Gymnema was the first herb that we tasted in class when I was studying Western Herbal medicine.

This herb is used for sugar imbalance and has the ability to numb the sweet taste buds on the tongue. If you squirt some of this amazing herb onto your tongue prior to eating candy, it will remove the sweetness leaving you feeling like you just ate some lard.

It also helps regulate blood sugar and reduces the risk of diabetes, so it is a valuable ally when it comes to cravings and giving up sugar.

Its actions are anti diabetic, hypoglycaemic, hypocholesterolemic (lowers cholesterol), hypolipidemic (lowers triglycerides) and anti-obesity.

Gymnema is used in Diabetes, insulin resistance, metabolic syndrome and weight loss.

H

Habits

Did you know it takes 21 days to break a habit and 66 days to form a new one? So patience is required, determination a must and you will need courage to see it through.

My previous book is called Thyroid Habits and is 50 little habits you can do either everyday or week to help improve thyroid health.

Our daily habits are what make the biggest difference in our thyroid health. It is not the grand trips to an Ayurvedic Hospital in India (although completely amazing) or the raw juice fast you do once a year that moves the needle in the right direction the quickest.

The big things will certainly get you started but it is the little things we do day in and day out that make the most profound difference.

How do we start? The best way is to attach a new habit to an existing activity that you already do everyday. For example, every time you are about to have a shower sit with your legs up the wall for 5 mins before you do so.

I have a client who formed the habit of using mint to signal to herself it is the end of the meal. In an effort to stop eating dessert with her family, she started eating a couple of mint leaves after her meal and kept telling herself, the meal was finished now. Well it worked for her! Never again did she crave dessert after having her mint leaves! Genius!!

So make sure your daily habits are tilted towards thyroid health, attach them to an existing habit and you will see a difference.

Hair

Commercial shampoo is another sneaky little assault on our thyroid every day or every few days depending on our washing frequency.

Commercial shampoos contain a huge array of chemicals and hormones that disrupt our endocrine system. In some cases it has been referred to as "a placenta in a bottle"!!!

Add to that we are putting it on our bodies when they are heated, so our pores are open and even more receptive to sucking up the toxins and then as we rinse it all out, it is running directly over our neck and thyroid.

It may take a while to find an organic shampoo you like, but keep searching, because this is one of those things that is easily changed and can reduce your chemical load incredibly.

Hair Loss

Both hypothyroid and hyperthyroid diseases cause hair loss. Hypothyroid tends to experience thinning all over, and hyperthyroid often has patchy bald spots.

Apart from calming the immune system, balancing hormones (big jobs) and nutritional supplementation with biotin, vitamin B1 and silica, there is not much else that can be done except for removing the chemicals and dyes.

Grey Hair

Many people with thyroid disease will find that we have early grey hair. By that I mean as early as our 20's. (I think I was in my early 30's)

If we look at Traditional Chinese Medicine it could be due to the kidney deficiency that is associated with thyroid disease and the kidneys appear to be the governor of grey hair.

So from this point of view then, supporting the kidneys is probably as important as supporting the thyroid pathway. Let's face it, symptoms such as grey hair is really just a message from our body after all.

Hair Dye

For those of us that wish to cover those early greys (although, I think now for me it's not considered early any more; cough) hair dye is actually really toxic and full of chemicals that can reduce thyroid function and conversion. I love that it exists but I hate that I feel the need to use it!

And no that doesn't mean hyperthyroid people can justify using it. It is toxic to all of us.

Traditional Hair Dye contains tin (to make our hair shiny) which stops the conversion of our inactive T4 thyroid hormone into T3 our active hormone. So constantly putting it into our body is clearly going to have an ongoing affect to our thyroid health.

I have done the chemical dyes, the not-so chemical dyes, henna and now I have found organic.

The Henna that I did myself, ended up causing a build up in my hair and giving it a really unhealthy appearance, so after using that for a while I went back to the store-bought not so chemical dye that still contained tin.

Then one day I was at my organic beauty salon and in between waxing the left eyebrow and the right eyebrow, my waxer told me about a hair salon AROUND THE CORNER that was fully organic.

Jumping for joy I made an appointment that day. And that is what I will continue to use until I get brave enough to reveal the greys.

Hair Mineral Analysis

This is a fabulous test that I have used many times with clients, family, friends and myself.

It is the process of cutting off a very small section of hair across the back of the head which gets sent to a lab to analyse.

Our hair contains the history of what has gone into our body, so an analysis will tell us both what's in the store cupboard (nutrients such as B12 and potassium) and also what's in the junk room (toxic metals such as mercury and aluminium).

It is a great scientific way of seeing exactly what you need to work on and most naturopaths will either offer it or be able to point you in the direction of where you can have one done.

Hand Washing

This is a sneaky way we end up with far more chemicals in our body than we need to.

How many times a day do you wash your hands? Particularly if you are cooking. I know for me, if I am in the kitchen I can wash my hands dozens of times if I am handling meat products etc.

That is why the soap I keep in the kitchen is pure liquid Castile soap, with no fragrances or numbers or chemicals. I just purchase a huge container of organic soap and decant it into smaller pump bottles that I have at every sink.

It really is a simple way to reduce the toxic load.

Hashimoto's Thyroiditis

An autoimmune disorder in which the immune system attacks and destroys the thyroid gland.

Signs and Symptoms include:

- ☐ Weight gain, fatigue, laziness
- ☐ Dry skin, coarse dry hair, brittle soft nails
- ☐ slow weak pulse, low body temperature
- ☐ decreased perspiration, slow reflexes
- ☐ loss of eyebrows, hair thinning
- ☐ irregular heartbeat, high cholesterol
- ☐ feeling cold, heat intolerance
- ☐ low muscle tone, muscle weakness, cramps
- ☐ low immunity, joint pain, aches and pains
- ☐ digestive issues, leaky gut
- ☐ insomnia, sleep apnea, tinnitus
- ☐ social isolation, depression, anxiety, irritability, manic behaviour, phobias, nightmares, panic attacks, personality changes, excessive crying, lack of confidence, no motivation, indecision, angry about little things,
- ☐ poor memory, concentration, slow speech, slow thinking, headaches
- ☐ carpal tunnel syndrome, bursitis, numbness and tingling in fingers and toes
- ☐ infertility, low libido, heavy long periods, breast discharge

Treatment from doctors involves bringing the thyroid levels up and rarely includes anything that helps the immune system to calm down.

For people with Hashimoto's it is about:

- ☐ Reducing inflammation
- ☐ Reducing stress
- ☐ Healing the gut
- ☐ Detoxifying the liver
- ☐ Improving lymphatic flow

Hashitoxicosis

When a Hashimoto's patient swings into hyperthyroidism caused by inflammation which irritates the thyroid follicles causing them to release more hormone.

Hawthorn Berries

This is another bottle of herbs I am never without personally.

It is a heart protector. I don't have heart issues, but as someone with thyroid disease I am at higher risk, so I use it regularly as a preventative.

Hawthorn Berries main uses include mild congestive heart failure, arrhythmias, angina, cardiomyopathy, heart attack prevention, hypertension and palpitations.

It also has the ability to calm mild anxiety, which I have used it for often and it works well.

Although I take it in a general mix of herbs on a regular basis, I also take a one off acute dose if I am feeling any palpitations or anxiety. It doesn't happen often, but this stops it really quickly and gently.

Hayfever

Hayfever and allergies are a common issue I have found in thyroid people. And there is a really obvious connection.

Most allergies are derived from a lack of zinc and an overload of copper. Also a common thyroid issue.

So up the zinc and if you have copper water pipes (usually the cause of excess copper) then get a water filter or distiller, and see if that reduces your symptoms.

Herbs to help: Albizia, Baical Skullcap, elder Flower, Eyebright, Garlic, Golden rod, Golden Seal, Ground Ivy, Horseradish, Nettle Leaf, Ribwort

HbA1c Blood Test

A blood test that gives an average of the last 3 months blood sugar levels. It is used for diabetes patients to check the general management of the disease.

HCL

Hydrochloric acid or stomach acid.

We need it to turn on methyl groups which turn on good genes, like tumour suppressing genes, and turn off bad genes that cause cancer.

Low gut acid is common in thyroid disorders but can be improved by eating fermented vegetables, chewing your food really well and drink a tablespoon of apple cider vinegar in water before meals.

There are also many digestive enzymes on the market to help.

Headaches

There is no clear correlation that thyroid disease cause headaches other than, many thyroid people get headaches. So I have never found solid research over the years to tell people why we get them.

Although, from my experience, I only get them when I have run myself too thin and am not taking care of my thyroid pathway.

Herbs that help sinus Headaches:elder Flower, eyebright, Golden Seal, Horseradish, Peppermint, Ribwort

Herbs to help tension headaches: California Poppy (I can vouch for this one completely), Corydalis, Feverfew, Hawthorn, Hops, Jamaica Dogwood, Lime Flowers, Passionflower, Rosemary, Valerian, Willow Bark, Wood Betony

Heat Therapy

The act of using heat to decrease pain and inflammation, relieve spasms and increase blood flow to the area it is applied.

It is useful for chronic pain such as arthritis and sore joints.

There are fancy blankets and gadgets that do this, but I just use a hot water bottle. It works a treat if I have been sitting and writing too long, and I often sit with a hot water bottle in the small of my back like a cushion.

Heart Chakra

The Heart Chakra is located at the centre of the chest and represents love and passion for others and also for ourselves. Working with the heart chakra triggers creativity which we need in our daily lives.

- Color - green, pink, red, white
- Key Issues - passion, rejection
- Body System - Circulatory, lymphatic, Immune
- Endocrine Gland - thymus
- Crystals - peridot, pink topaz, pink kunzite, rhodonite, rose quartz, rhodochrosite
- Aromatherapy - Rose, Melissa, Neroli

Heart Disease

See Cardiovascular disease

Heart Palpitations

The sensation that occurs when it feels like your heart has skipped a beat then has to beat quickly for a couple of seconds to catch up.

It is a common symptom in thyroid disease as the thyroid helps regulate heart function.

Here is a list of herbs that help, and I can specifically say that Hawthorn Berries work extremely well here: Corydalis, Dan shen, Dong Quai, Hawthorn, Lime flowers, Motherwort, passionflower, Polygala, and Zizyphus

Heat Intolerance

Like cold intolerance, heat intolerance can be a big issue with thyroid people.

Any extremes in temperature should be avoided. If it cannot be avoided and the new environment will be around you for more than a week or two, then a tracking of your thyroid levels are a must.

For example, by the time this book hits bookstores, I will have moved to a much hotter town in Australia. A town that "enjoys" over 100 f daily through summer. One would call that extreme right? Well, I know this is going to mean I will need to further reduce my medication, so I will have tests every 6 weeks for at least 6 months after moving to keep an eye on things.

Hemp Seeds

Also called Hemp Hearts, Hemp Seeds used to be illegal, but luckily that nonsense has been sorted out and we can all benefit from the amazing nutrients they have to offer.

And no, they do not make you high but they are particularly great for thyroid people which is kind of a natural high right?

1 ounce (28g) contains:

- 77% of DV in Vitamin E (thyroid pathway, major antioxidant)
- 22% of DV in Iron (thyroid, fatigue, gut acid)
- 75% of DV in Magnesium (stress, sugar)

- 41% of DV in Phosphorus (bones, liver)
- 34% of DV in Zinc (thyroid, immunity, mental health, wound healing)
- 140% DV in Manganese (Thyroid pathway)

This adds up too:

- better hormone balance
- less joint and muscle pain
- natural appetite suppressant
- prebiotic food for our gut
- improved hair, skin and nails

And look at the zinc and iron content!! Is it any wonder it's great for thyroid disease!

I often have Hemp seeds on my oats in winter along with 2 chopped brazil nuts and a kiwi fruit. Drizzled with some Jarrah raw medicinal honey and I'm good to go!

Hepatoprotective

An agent that helps protect the liver.

Examples Include: Bupleurum, Globe Artichoke, St Mary's Thistle, Rosemary, Schisandra

Herb Tea

Many of you have purchased my herb teas over the last few years and I am now happy to share the recipes with you.

These teas are a really great way of getting healing herbs into our body without taking more supplements. They are gentle and easily absorbed, plus personally I think they taste amazing.

I purposely did not go for a recipe that was full on and tasted ghastly. It's more valuable to have a tea that tastes good that you will drink everyday.

Thyroid Everyday Tea*

- 2 tablespoon Nettle
- 3 tablespoon Lemongrass
- 3 tablespoon Ginger
- 5 tablespoons Rosehips
- 6 tablespoons Hibiscus

All of these are loose and dried. So the ginger is actually dried pieces NOT powder.

Combine them all and store in a tin. Use a tablespoon or two in a teapot depending on the size you make.

*Use this tea on a daily basis for all round thyroid goodness.

Thyroid Calming Tea*

- 10 tablespoons Peppermint
- 10 tablespoons Hawthorn Berries

Combine them and store in a tin. Use a tablespoon or two in a teapot depending on the size.

*Use this tea when you are overwhelmed and need to think more clearly.

Herbicides

Like pesticides and insecticides, herbicides are designed to attack endocrine systems of bugs often through contact or consumption.

What it damages in the bugs, it can damage in us over a long period of time.

As talked about in Chemicals, our thyroid is a magnet to them, so reducing them in any way is in our thyroid's best interest.

HGH

HGH is Human Growth Hormone. It's the stuff Sylvester Stallone got into trouble with bringing it into Australia many moons ago (funny the things you remember).

HGH is secreted by our Pituitary Glands and it stimulates our liver to make IGF-1 (Insulin Growth Factor 1).

We need IGF-1 for our Sulfation Pathway in our liver. What does this pathway do? Processes and activates our Thyroid Hormone!!

It also helps with the regulation and balance of:

- regulates body fluid
- sugar metabolism
- fat metabolism
- bone and muscle growth
- stimulates protein synthesis in muscles
- speed up healing after injury

- ☐ boost metabolism and energy
- ☐ weight loss from burning fat
- ☐ regulates body composition
- ☐ anti ageing to the skin
- ☐ Improves hair growth
- ☐ regenerates cells and tissues

Since we want pretty much all of these actions going on in our body and it is illegal unless prescribed by your doctor in very special circumstances we need to look at how we can stimulate it naturally.

Here's the tips:

- ☐ High Intensity exercise such as weight lifting with short rest periods
- ☐ Intermittent fasting
- ☐ Reduce sugar
- ☐ Eat a very low sugar light dinner well ahead of bedtime
- ☐ Be in bed before 10.00pm - the release of GH occurs in waves prior to midnight
- ☐ Take melatonin to help regulate sleep patterns
- ☐ Laughter - watch some comedy
- ☐ Supplements to increase GH - glycine, creatine, glutamine

Are you ready to turn back the ageing clock?? I am not too shy to say I wanna do that!!!

High Fructose Corn Syrup

A nasty cheap ingredient in a lot of processed and packaged foods comprising of 55% fructose and 45% glucose. *See fructose*

Histidine

This essential amino acid needs to come from food sources as our body is unable to make it, and if you want to know the main reason we want this little beauty..? It improves sexual pleasure when combined with Vitamin B3 and B6. Now who wouldn't want that right? Oh and I guess the thyroid benefits are good too!

Apart from that little piece of gold we need histidine for:

- Involved in making Thyrotropin releasing hormone (made by the hypothalamus)
- Increases zinc absorption
- Involved in making collagen
- Involved in making histamine
- Decreases heavy metal toxicity
- Increases protein digestion
- Anti-inflammatory properties
- Improves memory

Food sources include:

- Bananas
- Chicken, eggs, fish and meat
- Legumes and wheat germ
- Cottage Cheese and whey protein

Homocysteine

An amino acid that raises in our blood when we are deficient in Vitamins B6, B9 (folate) and B12.

High levels in the blood can indicate heart disease, low thyroid levels, and damaged arteries.

Checking it requires a simple blood test and should be added to the yearly health check for thyroid patients.

Homeostasis

A state of balance and good health in the body.

Ho'oponopono Prayer

An ancient Hawaiian Prayer that believes all situations stem from ourselves. The prayer: "I'm sorry, Forgive me, Thank you, I love you" is intended to be said to oneself.

- I'm Sorry (for bringing this situation into life)
- Forgive Me (for thinking I needed to learn this)
- Thank You (for letting go of this situation)
- I Love You (transcends all)

Dr Hew Len, who brought this prayer to the mainstream, likens it to cleaning out our email inbox. All of our beliefs, traumas and blocks are emails sitting waiting to be opened, but often we have so many that we fail to recognise the ones that will make a difference in our lives.

He believes that saying this prayer over and over when focusing deletes or "cleans" out our inbox.

You can find more information around the history and teachings of the Ho'oponopono Prayer at

https://www.zero-wise.com/mess...

Homeopathics

A system of medicine where the theory that "like cures like" is utilised as treatments for physical and emotional problems.

Homeopathic medicine is extremely safe as it contains "the energy of the item".

So for example if you were to have a fever, a good homeopathic treatment would be Belladonna because ingesting this item would actually cause a fever. So the "energy" of this plant but no longer contains any actual belladonna.

There is a homeopathic called Thyroidinum which has been said to have cured many with primary hypothyroidism. If your thyroid disease is autoimmune derived though, this would not be an appropriate treatment.

Honey

Did you know that processed honey contains essentially no nutrients or health fighting benefits?

Get yourself some raw honey though and we are talking a whole other story. Finding a local beekeeper (often at markets) near you is a great option because if you eat honey made from the pollen of the trees around you, it will lessen any environment allergies you may have to those trees and plants. Cool huh?

Benefits of raw honey:

- major source of nutrients
- boosts the immune system
- speeds wound healing (topically)
- boosts energy

- protects the respiratory system
- weight loss if used instead of sugar
- improves pollen allergies
- promotes sleep
- natural cough syrup

If I am at an Expo for Thyroid School, I always take honey with me to help soothe my throat from talking too much. If I didn't do that I would lose my voice with in a couple of hours.

Hops

Most of us know that beer comes from Hops, but did you know it is referred to as one of the sexiest plants on the planet visually?? Go ahead... check it out!!

Considered a hypnotic, mild sedative, spasmolytic, bitter tonic, estrogen modulator and a libido reducer in men its key uses are for sleep, anxiety, restlessness, panic attacks, excitability and tension headaches, although it is contraindicated in depression.

Also useful for menopause symptoms and androgen excess due to its oestrogen modulating ability. Because of this action it is to be avoided in estrogen sensitive breast cancers.

Hormone Replacement Therapy

A therapy used in menopause to replace hormones (usually estrogen and or progesterone) and reduce symptoms.

This type of treatment has many pros and cons and a lot of conspiracy theory attached so research carefully before you decide to go down that road.

One major downside to it is that it reduces thyroid function. So that may work in hyper people, but will need to be monitored in hypo people.

Keep in mind also that if you are suffering major menopausal symptoms it is a sign your adrenal health is not up to scratch, so perhaps you could work on that while you research HRT?

Horse Chestnut

The seed of this herb is used in edema (fluid retention), as a venous tonic and anti-inflammatory.

Helping with issues such as varicose veins, venous insufficiency, lymphedema, spider veins, capillary fragility, and easy bruising.

It can be helpful where excess fluid retention in the tissues push down on nerves causing sciatica, carpal tunnel and Bell's Palsy.

Hot Flushes

A sudden increase in temperature that is extremely uncomfortable and different to just being hot. I have never experienced one, but have been told that you would never mistake it for just a case of overheating.

It is a symptom of menopause and is often a sign of struggling adrenals. Our adrenal glands take over the production of hormones after menopause, so if they are struggling, then symptoms like Hot Flushes show up regularly. The key here is to improve Adrenal health.

Hot Nodules

Nodules that grow on the thyroid are made up of two kinds - hot and cold. Hot nodules are almost always benign (non-cancerous).

HPA Axis

Hypothalamic-pituitary-adrenal axis.

HVP

Hydrolyzed Vegetable Protein. A flavour enhancer that is high in MSG.

Hydrotherapy

The act of alternating hot and cold water, either in baths or showers or as a thyroid treatment, using hot and cold towels on rotation around the neck, starting with hot and finishing with cold.

Three cycles of three minutes of each temperature can have the benefits of :

- ☐ Lowering thyroid antibodies
- ☐ Improve thyroid function
- ☐ Lowering the size of nodules

Hypertension

The medical term for high Blood Pressure

See Blood Pressure

Hyperthyroidism

When the thyroid is overactive or being stimulated to make too much thyroid hormone.

Can be caused by a deficiency in calcium and magnesium but the most common cause is Graves Disease

Herbs to help calm the thyroid include: bugleweed, motherwort

See Graves Disease

Hypotension

The medical term for Low Blood Pressure

See Blood Pressure

Hypnotherapy

A modality that involves the recipient being lulled into a trance like state where they are extremely suggestible.

Many people have claimed it has helped them to

- Quit smoking
- Lose weight
- Let go of phobias
- Cure anxiety
- Release bad habits

Hypochlorhydria

A condition where the stomach produces too little stomach acid or hydrochloric acid (HCl)

Hypoglycemia

The term for chronically low blood sugar, common in hypothyroidism or Hashimoto's

Treatment includes balancing thyroid levels, cleaning up the diet of excess processed foods, trans fats and sugars (particularly fructose).

Nutritional support should include:

- ☐ Chromium
- ☐ Choline
- ☐ Inositol
- ☐ L-carnitine
- ☐ CoQ10
- ☐ Rubidium
- ☐ Vanadium

Hypoparathyroidism

Lowered parathyroid hormone production which results in low calcium and increased phosphorus.

People with this disorder will need to take supplemental calcium and phosphorous possibly for life.

Causes include:

- ☐ Damage to the parathyroid gland during surgery on the thyroid gland
- ☐ Autoimmune disease
- ☐ Hereditary or congenital (born with no parathyroid gland)
- ☐ Radiation treatment on the face or neck
- ☐ Radioactive iodine treatment on the thyroid
- ☐ Low levels of magnesium

Symptoms include:

- ☐ Fatigue and weakness
- ☐ Depression and anxiety
- ☐ Dry skin, brittle nails, patchy hair loss
- ☐ Muscle aches, cramps, twitches and spasms
- ☐ Tingling or burning sensation in the fingertips, toes and lips

- Difficulty breathing
- Seizures
- Heart arrhythmia, fainting
- Kidney malfunction
- Teeth deformities

Hypotensive

An agent that lowers blood pressure by dilating vessels.

Examples Include: Astragalus, Black Haw, Coleus, Cramp Bark, Evening Primrose Oil, Garlic, Hawthorn, Motherwort, Olive Leaf, Zizyphus

Hypothalamic Pituitary Dysgenesis

A problem between the hypothalamus and the pituitary gland axis.

Hypothalamus

A tiny cone shaped part of the brain that communicates between the autonomic nervous system and the endocrine system and controls metabolic processes

The hypothalamus starts the Thyroid Pathway by measuring how much thyroid hormone is in the blood and then sending out Thyroid Releasing hormone to the Pituitary Gland.

Hypothyroidism

When the thyroid is underactive or not producing enough thyroid hormone.

Causes include

- Congenital thyroid disease (born with it)
- Primary hypothyroidism (the thyroid is being stimulated but is failing to produce hormones, so the thyroid is the source of the issue)
- Secondary hypothyroidism (the thyroid is not being stimulated by the pituitary, meaning that is the source of the issue)
- Hashimoto's Thyroiditis (the thyroid is being attacked by the immune system) This is the most common form of hypothyroidism

Herbs that help increase thyroid function include: Bacopa, Bladderwrack, Coleus, Withania

See also Hashimoto's Thyroiditis

Hysterectomy

The removal of the uterus and or the ovaries and fallopian tubes generally due to damage, endometriosis, fibroids or other issues that cause permanent pain and bleeding issues.

I had one in 2015 (aged 43) after years of endometriosis issues. It was honestly the best thing I have ever done. I did not suffer from any side effects, hormonal drops, low libido. Nothing, and still nothing 5 years later.

I was actually surprised that the whole procedure these days only involved 3 days in hospital (although hubby required 4 weeks holiday, oh I mean carer's leave, to look after me) and no lifting anything "heavier than a teacup" for a month.

To those suffering I can only tell you my experience. The rest is up to you.

I

Imagine

What would your life be like without thyroid disease?

I was 21 when I was diagnosed and only just starting my adult life. Now at almost 50 it has become my business.

There have been so many times in the early years, that like so many of you I believed that yes, I would be taking that little white pill and feeling horrid for the rest of my life.

But I would like for you to imagine something different. Imagine something better for your life and health.

If you no longer have a thyroid, and truly are on medication for life, imagine a life free from symptoms.

If you take medication, imagine a life free from that, where you don't have to remember if you took it that morning, or pack them when travelling.

Imagine a life where the word thyroid does not enter your daily vocabulary in a negative way.

Imagine a life where you do not have to pretend to your family and loved ones that you are feeling great when underneath you feel like you are drowning.

Imagining is the first step. Something must be first imagined before it can become real, before a plan can be made and carried out.

And maybe some where along the way you may like to imagine helping others with thyroid disease.

Anything is possible when you first imagine.

Iatrogenic Hypothyroidism

This is the term used for hypothyroidism that is caused either by a treatment, such as radioactive iodine, surgery to have the thyroid removed or some medications such as amiodarone (a potassium channel blocker).

Immune Depressant

An agent used to calm an overactive Immune System.

Examples Include: Hemidesmus, Tylophora

Immune Enhancing

An agent used to increase Immune response.

Examples Include: Andrographis, Astragalus, Cat's Claw, Echinacea Root, Elder-Berry, Pau d'Arco, Poke Root

Immune Modulating

An agent used to keep an erratic immune system balanced.

Examples Include: Korean Ginseng, Reishi, Shiitake, Siberian Ginseng, Withania

Iodine

Iodine is tricky when it comes to thyroid disease.

Yes it is something our thyroid needs, however too much of it is just as dangerous as too little. For my final paper before I graduated as a naturopath I chose "thyroid & iodine" as the topic. It turns out, half the goitres out there were caused by too little and half were caused my too much iodine.

Our body though is really smart, so if it can't find what it needs to function it will find the closest thing that looks like it and give that a go.

In the case of our thyroid and iodine, if there is not enough of that (please remember there is a fine line between too much and too little) then it will turn to one of the other Halides in that chemical group.

Unfortunately for our thyroid these replacements can gradually destroy it.

So that means:

- Chlorine / chloride
- Fluorine / fluoride
- Bromine / Bromide

We need to avoid excess of these 3 Halides wherever we can.

- Sources of Chloride: tap water, pool water, cleaning products, the sweetener Splenda
- Sources of Fluoride: toothpaste, mouth wash, dental treatments, foods such as rice and black tea
- Sources of Bromide: bakery products, some white flowers, chemicals in spa baths

Now that we have looked at what can block our iodine, let's talk about supplementation with it.

I have many people approach me that want me to endorse or sell their iodine products. But the issue I have with taking iodine on its own is that when we isolate an ingredient or vitamin and take it on its own it doesn't pay off because everything works together in synergy. So taking iodine drops for example may (or may not depending on the individual) send you the other way to where you are now, which can clearly be dangerous.

Food is the best medicine. Always. Bar none. Full stop.

Food sources of iodine will also contain other minerals that it needs to be absorbed well. Here are some common and less known sources of iodine:

- Kelp (obvious one)
- Jerusalem Artichokes and potato
- Pineapple (who doesn't love this?)
- Celery (bring on the celery juice)
- Pears
- Romaine Lettuce (put it in everything!)
- Irish Moss (awesome for belly problems too)

Ionic Silver

For years colloidal silver has been readily available at health food shops and said to be full of antibiotic, antimicrobial, antibacterial properties.

And that's true. The problem with Colloidal Silver is that it can drop out of suspension, meaning the silver particles can start to accumulate in the body.

A new comer to the table is Ionic Silver which does not drop out of suspension and still has all the amazing abilities that colloidal silver does.

I always have a product called Hydrocell in my house, which is a combination of ionic silver and oxygen, and while I take 10ml of it daily (because I have no time to be ill frankly), the second someone walks into my home with a cough or illness I'm dosing them up!

It kills everything! I take it to Bali with me too, and also took it on the cruise hubby and I went on at the beginning of the year. On holidays we both take it every day because the last thing you want is to be sick on holidays right? And when I say it kills everything, I'm talking about anything from tummy bugs to colds and flu.

In case you go looking for it though, Hydrocell is for adults because of the oxygen component, but the plain ionic silver is perfectly fine for children.

Indole 3 Carbinol

This is the result of a reaction when veggies from the brassica family have been processed (chewed, cooked etc) that can also be mimicked in a laboratory.

It is used by our body to facilitate the following:

- ☐ blocks estrogen receptors (inhibiting cancer)
- ☐ decreases carcinogenic activity
- ☐ improves phase II detoxification in the liver
- ☐ induces apoptosis (death of cancer cells)
- ☐ induces glutathione production (major cancer fighting antioxidant)
- ☐ converts estrange to 2-hydroxyestrone (dangerous estrogen to one that can be processed and cleared)

We find this incredible cancer-fighting, hormone clearing substance in broccoli, cabbage, cauliflower, kale and Brussels Sprouts. And yes I know, they are the things that cause us problems with thyroid disease!

If deciding to take this as a supplement, then I would look at risk versus benefit. If you believe you are at a high risk of say breast cancer and you know your thyroid levels and iodine intake is good then the benefit would outweigh the risk. Talk to your natural health practitioner to figure out if it is something you should be trying.

Infertility

Unfortunately infertility is a common story amongst thyroid women, and as I learned recently, also men who have thyroid disease can often be the infertile one.

I'm glad I didn't know this when I started trying for our first baby, because mindset may have played a part in me getting pregnant. I just assumed I would, and I did.

But I never fell again, so we are eternally grateful for a perfectly happy and healthy 18 year old (at the time of writing).

Let's look at how thyroid issues can interfere with our fertility:

- Impaired ovulation - in both hypo and hyper there can be an issue with ovulation, or the release of the egg. In both cases it revolves around luteinizing hormone (LH), which is the signaller to the ovaries to release the egg. In hyper it remains elevated when it should come down, and in hypo not enough is produced.
- Excess estrogen levels - if excess weight is an issue, then there will be excess estrogen in the system. Estrogen is what the Oral contraceptive pill is made from. Therefore excess estrogen will act as birth control when we don't want it.
- Hormonal issues - often endometriosis, PCOS and fibroids are an affliction in thyroid disease, namely due to the excess oestrogen or impaired insulin action. Working on correcting these imbalances may improve your fertility.

Don't forget if you do fall pregnant (my heart is bursting for you if you do) then be sure to have extremely regular thyroid tests throughout your pregnancy.

Inflammation

I have said many times over the years - Thyroid Disease is an inflammatory disease. It both causes inflammation and is made worse by inflammation.

For thyroid hormone to get into our cells it needs to have a receptor on the cell (or lock on the door), so think of the hormone as the key and the receptor is the lock.

When we are inflamed, the locks disappear so even if we have lots of keys (thyroid hormone) there are not enough locks for them, leaving us feeling unwell.

Inflammation is one of the key issues we must always be working on. It's about the Little Things remember, so here are some that you can try to do everyday:

- Remove Sugar
- Remove Gluten, Soy, Dairy

- Don't eat junk food
- Don't eat food from packets with lots of numbers in the ingredients
- Get some movement in every day
- If we sit for work, get up and move as often as possible. At least every hour.
- Take Turmeric or Boswellia daily
- Eat lots of orange veg (anti-inflammatory)
- Eat lots of green leafy veg
- Increase Omega 3 intake
- Include Ginger in our diet
- Be well hydrated! (non fluoride water)
- Reduce as much stress as possible

I am constantly working on inflammation because I am always trying to whittle away at my medication. So the less inflammation the less medication I need.

The best anti-inflammatory foods include: turmeric (curry), berries, fatty fish, avocados, peppers, green tea, tart cherries, mushrooms, green leafy veg, and olive oil.

Inflammatory Bowel Disease

This is an umbrella term for two bowel disorders.

- Ulcerative colitis - ulcers and inflammation of the colon and rectum lining
- Crohn's Disease - an inflammation of the lining of the entire digestive tract

Both conditions are painful, life altering and cause severe pain, fatigue, fever, weight loss, and diarrhoea that sends the sufferer to the bathroom many times a day.

With both diseases nutrition and hydration requirements are more than others due to the loss of nutrients through diarrhoea. Since absorption is problematic, liquid herbals instead of supplements would be a much better way to increase nutrient status, so finding an herbalist that is experienced in this field is important.

There are a few studies that have shown a link between inflammatory bowel disease and congenital thyroid disease.

Infrared Sauna

Infrared saunas are different to regular saunas, as they are able to penetrate deeper into our skin and help detoxify us.

Here is how they help us:

- help induce sweating in hypothyroid people
- help remove bad oestrogen
- help reduce inflammation
- help sweat out arsenic, cadmium, lead, DDT and mercury
- decreases muscle and joint soreness
- may help reduce blood pressure
- help improve skin conditions
- help with weight loss
- Antiageing as it stimulates autophagy (cell cleanup)
- may improve mental health & cognitive function (stimulates the growth of brain cells)

Buying one of these baby's is on my wish list, as you can get them small enough to put on a balcony if you don't have space inside. Until then I will continue to treat myself to hiring a 30 minute session whenever I can at my local spa.

Keep in mind that saunas will also sweat out our beneficial electrolytes, vitamins and minerals so it is vital to up your intake of these or consume a lovely vegetable juice while sitting in the sauna to counteract that affect.

Insecticides

Insecticides, like pesticides are considered an endocrine or hormone disruptor.

Many of them are designed to attack the reproductive system of an animal so that it also kills any eggs or larvae along with the insect.

One could argue that contact with these chemicals over a lengthy period of time could render a similar effect on our own endocrine system.

Natural alternatives:

- Fly swatter - give it to the kids and pay them per fly!
- Fly catcher - my husband has this thing he purchased from the hardware store that hangs outside of the shed. It is then filled with a really nasty smelling substance which attracts flies. Once they fly into this trap they can't get out. I am always amazed by the number of flies it catches daily.

- ☐ Insect repelling plants - marigolds, lemon grass, citronella, garlic, chilli, basil, and catnip are just some of the amazing plants we can keep around the home to use instead of the chemicals

Insomnia

Insomnia is more of an issue for hyperthyroidism due to the overstimulated nervous system.

If you have hypothyroidism and experience insomnia from time to time, and assuming it is not caused by something external, then I would suggest that maybe you have swung into hyperthyroidism as we tend to do, particularly with Hashimoto's.

The first step is to optimise the thyroid and your medication as that may solve the issue.

After that, it would be worth trying the many different natural ways of addressing it before hitting the hardcore medication or alcohol to knock you out.

Although some ideas may seem obvious and you roll your eyes, but have you tried them in conjunction with balancing your thyroid hormone?

These may just work given some time and patience:

- ☐ Remove the screens at sunset. This is a tough one, but as a species we were not meant to look at bright lights well into the night. it completely upsets our circadian rhythms.
- ☐ Some herbs are amazing if you find the mix that works for you. Great ones for insomnia include liquorice, bacopa, rehmannia, passionflower, valerian and zizyphus
- ☐ Make sure your nutritional intake is amazing and cut back on stimulating foods such as chocolate, sodas and sugars after lunch.
- ☐ Have a nightly ritual. It's called sleep hygiene and is used to teach babies how to sleep, but we should be doing the same for ourselves. Having a routine such as a bath, herb tea and maybe listening to some soft music, meditation or even an audio book if you are not woo woo will eventually trigger your brain that it is bedtime.
- ☐ Don't have naps during the day. I knoowwww you're tired, but this will continue the pattern.
- ☐ Get up and go to bed at the same time every day. Again, this is getting your body used to it.

- ☐ Re-decorate your bedroom - this is your permission! I did this a little while ago now, and removed the television from our room and turned it into more of a sanctuary. I breathe out just entering that room now, and my brain knows that its purpose is for sleep (and you know, that other fun thing wink wink)

Sweet Dreams x

Insulin

The first thing we need to commit to our foggy memories about insulin is this:

INSULIN IS A FAT STORING HORMONE

Any time we have excess insulin in our blood we are going to store anything we consume as opposed to using it for fuel.

Let's look at some of the reasons we may have excess insulin in our blood:

- ☐ Hyperthyroidism - due to a fast metabolism, insulin can be cleared too quickly causing a build up of sugar and a larger requirement for insulin. It is this lack of insulin in the hyperthyroid body that contributes to the usually slimmer body shape.
- ☐ Hypothyroidism - due to a slow metabolism, the clearing of sugar out of the blood is slow causing the insulin to stay in the blood longer, causing a sensitivity to insulin.
- ☐ Excess sugar or carbohydrates - it is up to insulin to deal with these foods, the more we have in our blood, the more insulin we will have in our blood. If there is too much sugar for the insulin to deal with, it will simply store it as fat for later (wink wink)
- ☐ Stress - high levels of stress triggers insulin release in our body. Another reason why stress needs to always be on our list of "how to lower it today"

Insulin Resistance

When our cells refuse entry to insulin and therefore glucose, which results in high blood sugar. This then triggers a higher TSH.

Nutritional support we need for healthy insulin / blood sugar balance:

- ☐ chromium - to balance blood sugar (cinnamon is a great source)
- ☐ magnesium - the valve that lets insulin into the blood to deal with the sugar (nuts, seeds and green leafy veg)

- ☐ vanadium - balances blood sugar (black pepper, seafood, parsley)
- ☐ biotin - glucose metabolism (egg yolk, oats)
- ☐ zinc - supports insulin synthesis (meat, oysters, sunflower and pumpkin seeds)
- ☐ inositol - helps insulin to be more productive (made in the gut, citrus, lentils, pork, nuts and seeds)
- ☐ gymnema sylvestre - a herbal plant that dulls the taste of sugar on the tongue (great for quitting sugar) and balances blood sugar

Intestinal Permeability

see Leaky gut

Intrinsic Factor

This mysterious sounding name is responsible for us being able to make our own Vitamin B12.

If you know your nutrition, you will know that our biggest source of B12 is through animal products. This is because they make it in their gut. We just tend to forget that if we are healthy, then we make it in ours too!

Intrinsic factor is made by parietal cells in the stomach however autoimmune issues can cause a lack of it as is the case in pernicious anaemia.

You can have an antibody blood test for this just as you can for thyroid disease (IF antibody) and the treatment is Vitamin B12 injections.

Inulin

Inulin is a type of fermented fibre known as Fructo-oligosaccharides (FOS) this fibre is found in onions, garlic, hickory, burdock, Jerusalem artichokes, legumes, wheat, oats and rye and is required for:

- ☐ food for our gut (prebiotic)
- ☐ alkalises the gut
- ☐ improves liver function
- ☐ increases lactobacillus
- ☐ increases bifidobacterium

This particular fibre is one of the no-no's on the FODMAP diet however if you have no intestinal issues with it, then all the foods containing inulin is a fantastic way to increase your gut health and combat things like candida, leaky gut and any other diet derived gut issues.

Iridology

I love iridology! It is literally a science, did you know that? It is the science of the eyes in reflection to the health of our body and is scarily accurate.

Our iris is like our fingerprint, completely unique to us and it is the most complex structure in the human body, with a connection via the nervous system to every organ and tissue. This is why it can reflect the health of what is going on in there.

When I first began studying I had my iris photos taken and it revealed many stress rings. After much effort and extra magnesium, the next photos showed the rings had magically vanished!

Blue Eyes overview (this is me, and it is so true!):

- ☐ Lymphatic Issues
- ☐ Ear Nose & Throat sensitivities
- ☐ Inflammation
- ☐ Skin Weaknesses
- ☐ Respiratory illness
- ☐ Immune system imbalance
- ☐ Musculoskeletal issues with age
- ☐ Thyroid & Parathyroid imbalance
- ☐ Fluid Retention
- ☐ Energy Depletion
- ☐ Circulation Deficiency
- ☐ Not great with Dairy Products
- ☐ Mucous production increased with Acidic foods
- ☐ Often deficient in Iron, Calcium, Magnesium & Zinc
- ☐ Life Lesson: Love the skin you're in.

Brown Eyes overview:

- ☐ Digestive Disorders
- ☐ Flatulence

- ☐ Impaired bile production
- ☐ Liver congestion
- ☐ Glandular disorders
- ☐ Impaired circulation
- ☐ Haemorrhoids
- ☐ Unstable blood sugar
- ☐ Benefit from a B-Vitamin daily and a Vitamin E
- ☐ Life Lesson: Exchange negative obsessive thoughts for more constructive positive ones. Think before acting.

Green/mixed eyes overview: (in iridology there are only three colours, so if you are not blue or brown you fall into this category)

- ☐ Gastrointestinal weakness
- ☐ Constipation
- ☐ Flatulence
- ☐ Liver & Gallbladder issues
- ☐ Enzyme deficiencies
- ☐ Diabetic tendency
- ☐ Physical tension when under stress
- ☐ Alcohol & coffee tend to be too stimulating
- ☐ High fat foods including meat, dairy & rich sweet foods can be too taxing on the liver
- ☐ Slow uptake of fat soluble vitamins: A, D, E, B12, K
- ☐ Life Lesson: Listen to the people that love you when in two minds about making decisions, as you are often in two minds.

If you want to look into this modality further, this information is from the work of Toni Miller who teaches iridology and has written books and programs about it.

Irritability

Are you always irritable? This is a particular concern for hyperthyroid people. It goes along with the anxiety, restlessness and nervousness.

This can be due to a nutritional issue, because hyperthyroid people burn through nutrients that much quicker.

Possible nutritional causes include:

- ☐ Vitamin B5 deficiency
- ☐ Vitamin B6 deficiency
- ☐ Vitamin B12 deficiency
- ☐ Magnesium deficiency
- ☐ Molybdenum deficiency

Go to these entries to find the foods you need to double down on.

Herbs that can help with irritability include: Lemon Balm, Mexican Valerian, passionflower, Polygala, Skullcap, St John's Wort, Valerian, Vervain, and Zizyphus.

Irritable Bowel Syndrome

An uncomfortable issue where the bowel spasms and unevenly contracts causing pain and bloating.

Although there is no link to thyroid disease, often symptoms crossover leaving a patient with a diagnosis of IBS when in fact the symptoms were actually thyroid derived.

Possible causes include stress, bacterial infection, or food intolerance, but is not dangerous (just uncomfortable) and not a risk factor for other bowel diseases.

Symptoms include:

- ☐ pain
- ☐ bloating
- ☐ constipation / diarrhoea
- ☐ wind

Herbs that support and calm IBS include: Chamomile, Corydalis, Cramp Bark, Globe Artichoke, Greater Celandine, Marshmallow Root, Meadowsweet, Peppermint, Skullcap, slippery Elm, St John's Wort, and Valerian.

If this is you, it may be worth checking out the FODMAPs protocol which was developed for this very purpose. Your welcome!

Iron

Iron is required for:

- ☐ Plays a part in converting phenylalanine to tyrosine which is required in the thyroid pathway
- ☐ Immune resistance

- ☐ Respiration
- ☐ Skin & nail formation
- ☐ Oxygen transport
- ☐ Making of red blood cells

Deficiency Symptoms of Iron include:

- ☐ Low T3 levels (iron is needed to get into cells)
- ☐ Anaemia, breathing difficulties
- ☐ Heavy periods
- ☐ Muscle fatigue, restless legs
- ☐ Disrupted sleep, fatigue, Depression
- ☐ Dizziness, headaches
- ☐ Brittle nails, Hair loss, acne
- ☐ Cracks in corners of mouth, sore tongue, mouth ulcers
- ☐ General itching all over the body
- ☐ Sinusitis, colds, ear infections
- ☐ Thrush, Chronic herpes

Factors that contribute to Iron deficiency:

- ☐ Dairy products reduce absorption
- ☐ Tea consumption can reduce absorption
- ☐ Antacids reduce absorption
- ☐ Heavy periods
- ☐ Pregnancy
- ☐ Haemorrhoids, stomach ulcers
- ☐ Bruising, Blood noses
- ☐ Molybdenum deficiency
- ☐ Excess copper - iron and copper are antagonistic, where one goes up the other goes down
- ☐ Excess mercury & lead

Food sources of Iron include:

- ☐ Almonds, pine nuts, sunflower & pumpkin seeds
- ☐ Apricots, avocado, parsley
- ☐ Clams, Oysters, Beef, Poultry, Liver, Kidneys
- ☐ Wheat Germ, yeast

Daily Requirements of Iron:

- Adult RDA 10-20mg

Islets of Langerhans

This magical sounding place is actually areas in our pancreas (yes, not as magical I know) which produce hormones such as insulin, ghrelin, glucagon and somatostatin.

For the most part, this is of importance in diabetes. If the Islets of Langerhans don't produce enough insulin then there will be too much glucose in the body which is what happens in Diabetes Type 1.

Studies show that thyroid hormone has a role to play in the development of this tissue and so may be a contributing factor in the connection between diabetes and thyroid disease.

Isoleucine

An essential amino acid, meaning we need to get it from food, isoleucine's main function is to help the body recover from strenuous exercise.

Since thyroid issues often come with weak muscles, this is helpful not just for the athletes.

The other jobs for this amino acid include:

- Lowering glucose levels in the blood
- Improve endurance
- Reduces muscle breakdown in high altitudes
- Reduces fatigue and depression
- Reduces sugar induced irritability
- Helps athletes recovery
- Improves stress response

Food sources include:

- Almonds, pumpkin seeds, nuts
- Beef, chicken, eggs, fish
- Legumes, soy beans
- Milk and whey protein

J

Jigsaw

I read recently a quote about imagining our life as a jigsaw.

When we purchase a jigsaw, we have faith that all the pieces of the puzzle are inside the box and only when we complete the puzzle do we get to see where each piece fits.

I love doing jigsaw's and usually get one every Christmas. The dining table is then covered in puzzle pieces until I have found the right place for each and every one of them.

The satisfaction I get when one little piece finds its perfect space after endless attempts of "not quite right" lights me up.

But in life how often do we stop to feel lit up when we make something fit instead of longingly trying to see the finished picture?

The fun is in the individual pieces not in the finished product. We are so eager to know the outcome, know how it is all going to turn out that we miss out on feeling the joy of discovery and the joy of the little wins.

I completely put my hand up and admit to not celebrating the little wins. In fact many of my friends had no idea I had 4 other thyroid books until this one came out. I tend to finish it and move on to the next piece instead of allowing myself that little buzz of excitement and satisfaction.

So let's all remember the picture of our life would never come together unless we felt the joy of each individual piece, which makes us want to find another individual piece and another.

Jar Food

Thyroid Jar Food was my second book.

It came about, as most of my books do, as an easy way for me to store my recipes.

At the time of writing that book, I was a wife, mother, full time student and business owner. I had a LOT on my plate.

Jar Food is very popular now, but my Thyroid Jar Food book was simple recipes and a way of eating that kept me healthy and organised at the time. I still utilise my jars (I have about 100 of them) and keep everything from home-made chia jam in them to raw sour cream, to full single meals that I eat when I am the only one home.

Now that our son is an adult and rarely home, hubby works away that is a common situation for me.

As a thyroid person, one of my symptoms is lack of appetite. When I am banging away on the keyboard, I can actually forget to eat all day which is really bad for us. It switches on the famine pathways which makes our body hold onto excess fat.

Jaundice

So much of our thyroid health is tied up in our liver health and jaundice is an issue with our liver and gallbladder.

It is caused by reduced bilirubin excretion from our body, and hypothyroidism can see a decrease of up to 50% excretion in both bilirubin and bile from the gallbladder.

It presents as a yellowing of the skin, whites of our eyes and body fluids.

Doctors will order liver tests to check the levels of bilirubin before deciding on a cause of action, which will be based around the cause. If it is thyroid disease causing it, looking at the thyroid pathway, conversion, liver and gut health will help to improve the issue.

JERF

An acronym for Just Eat Real Food, JERF is a great website and online platform created by Sean Croxton and simply encourages us all to eat real food.

He believes that if we just go back to basics and make everything ourselves from scratch and eat as much as we can in its natural form that many diseases will abate and weight will normalise.

So in JERF terms, you don't say NO to the Apple Pie, instead you make one from scratch with quality ingredients.

Jerusalem Artichoke

Jerusalem Artichokes are root vegetables that look a little like ginger.

The first time I experienced them was in a fancy hotel and I ordered scallops on potato & jerusalem artichoke smash. I was feeling adventurous at the time and wow it was delicious.

They have a slightly sweet flavour that lend themselves to all sorts of dishes, plus they are high in a fibre called inulin which is both a prebiotic (feeds our good gut flora) and also is amazing at regulating blood sugar, so good for diabetes.

1 cup of sliced Jerusalem Artichokes contain:

- ☐ 10% of DRI in Vitamin C (Adrenals)
- ☐ 1% of DRI in Vitamin E (Thyroid Pathway)
- ☐ 20% of DRI in Vitamin B1 (Thyroid Health)
- ☐ 5% of DRI in Vitamin B2 (Thyroid Pathway)
- ☐ 10% of DRI in Vitamin B3 (Mental Health)
- ☐ 6% of DRI in Vitamin B6 (mental health)
- ☐ 5% of DRI in Folate (MTHFR, liver health)
- ☐ 2% of DRI in Calcium (bones)
- ☐ 28% of DRI in Iron (Fatigue)
- ☐ 6% of DRI in Magnesium (stress, sugar)
- ☐ 12% of DRI in Phosphorus (bones, liver)
- ☐ 18% of DRI in Potassium (thyroid health)
- ☐ 1% of DRI in Zinc (thyroid, immunity, wound healing, mental health)
- ☐ 10% of DRI in Copper (skin, nerves, bone, collagen)
- ☐ 4% of DRI in Manganese (thyroid pathway)
- ☐ 2% of DRI in Selenium (thyroid pathway)
- ☐ 10% of DRI in Fiber (hormone clearance, gut health)
- ☐ Glycemic load of 11
- ☐ A rich source of prebiotics
- ☐ High in Inulin (dietary fibre, prebiotic, sugar balance)

So if you haven't tried these, I urge you to give them a go. I love them just baked in the oven (like a potato) but they are amazing in soups too.

Joint Pain

Caused by inflammation, joint pain can be arthritis, damage or what some people simply call "their dodgy knee".

Regardless of the category the course of action is working on reducing inflammation. Thyroid disease is an inflammatory disease, so that inflammation can spread quickly when not kept under control.

See *Inflammation* for ideas on reducing it.

Juice Fasting

I love juicing!

In fact - juice fasting has been the only way to date that I have been able to lose significant amounts of weight.

BUT.... that's not why I consider it my thyroid's best friend!

Fresh, cold pressed fruit and vegetable juice is like medicine to our cells.

Now, we are talking about juice here - NOT a smoothie which is made in the likes of a nutribullet or blender. Still great - but it is not juice.

Here is the difference so it is easy to remember:

Juice is medicine

Smoothie is food

With thyroid disease, we are often also plagued with digestion issues, fatigue and our body struggling to get nutrients from our food regardless of what kind of thyroid disease we have.

When we drink juice - particularly on an empty stomach, all those vitamins and minerals and enzymes go directly into our cells. Our body doesn't have to work hard to get them, nor does it have to process a synthetic version of these nutrients in supplement form.

It's just in there instantly - BAM - Nutrients!!

So if we want to give our thyroid a rest, and get the nutrients we need without adding a burden to our digestion or liver function, then juicing is amazing!!

It is important to note though, that if you are going to embark on a juice fast you do it under supervision. The first extended fast I did, I continued taking my thyroid medication at my usual dose. On day 17 I started experiencing extreme hyperthyroid symptoms because everything was working better, so I needed less medication. At the time I didn't know better.

I encourage you to work with somebody if you are going to do this and as an added insurance, take your temperature daily to keep an eye on your levels.

Even if I am not juice fasting, I will ALWAYS have green juice in my fridge. My thyroid depends on it I believe!

K

Kind

This is a tough gig this thyroid disease. If we are not kind to ourselves during this journey we are going to never feel good.

Practicing to speak to ourselves in a kind manner is tough to do. We are so used to criticizing ourselves and being so quick to put ourselves down.

I found it hard to stop this, and still struggle with it every day.

But I found that if I purposefully found reasons to be kind to OTHER people then it had a knock on effect to me.

It started with me simply finding reasons to compliment strangers when I was out and about....

"I love your dress"
"Your skin is gorgeous"
"Gosh I love your hair"

It doesn't have to be grand, just a quick word as you walk past the lady that is struggling with her 2 year old, will bring a smile to her face that will last longer than you know.

After awhile I found myself saying those things to myself when I looked in the mirror. It was quite the revelation the day it first happened, and I laughed because I felt so happy that I had complimented myself.

Try it and see if it happens to you too. At the very least you will make someone's day when you compliment them.

K Vitamin

Vitamin K is required for:

- ☐ Blood clotting
- ☐ Bone health & calcium metabolism
- ☐ Brain tissue repair
- ☐ Reduces wrinkles

Deficiency Symptoms of Vitamin K include:

- ☐ Birth defects
- ☐ Cognitive impairment
- ☐ Lowered vitality
- ☐ Easy to bruise
- ☐ Low bone density
- ☐ Osteoporosis, osteopenia
- ☐ Early ageing

Factors that contribute to Vitamin K deficiency:

- ☐ Calcium supplements
- ☐ Celiac disease, Crohn's disease, ulcerative colitis
- ☐ Irradiated food (canned foods, animal products, seafood, fresh fruits & vegetables)
- ☐ Extensive surgery
- ☐ High salicylate diet
- ☐ Rheumatoid arthritis
- ☐ Gallbladder and liver disease

Sources of Vitamin K include:

- ☐ Bacterial production in the gut
- ☐ Asparagus, broccoli, cabbage, kale, lettuce, spinach
- ☐ Camembert, eggs, pork
- ☐ Oats
- ☐ Kelp

Daily Requirements of Vitamin K:

- Adult RDA - 70 - 15ug per kg / weight

Kefir

This is a fermented milk drink which is used for gut health.

Originally from Eastern Europe, this thin, yogurt type drink is made using "grains" as the fermenting agent and can be purchased in health food shops.

Although it is made using milk traditionally, thyroid peeps would be better using coconut milk, almond milk or other plant based milk if consuming regularly due to the possible interaction between dairy and autoimmune disease.

Kale

Kale is a cruciferous vegetable, meaning it can cause goitres if consumed in large quantities as it blocks iodine in the thyroid.

While Kale is an extremely nutritious green, because of the goitrogens, it is not the best option on a regular basis in our diets.

Many people begin juicing and due to the popularity of the "Mean Green" in Joe Cross's movie start loading up on Kale. Then they wonder why they feel awful and stop juicing.

I use the Mean Green recipe, but I swap out Kale for Romaine Lettuce which is extremely thyroid healthy, so that may be an option if you want to try juicing again.

If you like eating Kale in general, try cooking it first. It is said that cooking cruciferous vegetables reduce the goitrogens considerably.

Kava

If you have ever been to Fiji, this is the sacred drink offered in ceremonies that is hypnotic, a mild sedative, muscle relaxant, analgesic, anaesthetic and anxiolytic.

It tastes ghastly so lucky it comes in supplement form now.

Useful with anxiety, panic attacks, emotional stress and insomnia, it also is a great pain reliever for toothaches, leg cramps, tired muscles and headaches.

Not easily obtained, caution must be used in pregnancy, lactation and in Parkinson's Disease.

Kelp

I remember when I was younger my mom would sprinkle dried kelp into her juice. I didn't know at the time that she also had thyroid disease (since she was 11) and going back 40 years this was about the only natural treatment option if you were into the natural type of treatments.

Kelp has an amazing array of nutrients and 100g gives us:

- ☐ 2% of DV in Vitamin A (thyroid pathway)
- ☐ 5% of DV in Vitamin C (thyroid pathway, adrenals, antioxidant)
- ☐ 4% of DV in Vitamin E (thyroid pathway, antioxidant)
- ☐ 82% of DV in Vitamin K (blood, bones)
- ☐ 3% of DV in Vitamin B1 (thyroid, hair, hyperthyroid)
- ☐ 9% of DV in Vitamin B2 (thyroid pathway)
- ☐ 2% of DV in Vitamin B3 (mental health)
- ☐ 45% of DV in Folate (MTHFR, liver)
- ☐ 17% of DV in calcium
- ☐ 500% of DV in Iodine (thyroid pathway)
- ☐ 16% of DV in Iron (thyroid, fatigue, gut acid)
- ☐ 30% of DV in Magnesium (stress, sugar, fatigue)
- ☐ 4% of DV in Phosphorus (bones, liver)
- ☐ 8% of DV in Zinc (thyroid, mental health, immune, wound healing)
- ☐ 10% of DV in Manganese (thyroid pathway)
- ☐ 5% of DV in Dietary Fibre (hormonal clearance, gut health)
- ☐ 3% of DV in Protein (thyroid pathway)

While you can get it dried still, these days there are so many other ways to get this sea vegetable and I have seen many recipes on line where it is added to soups and stews.

Because it is so high in iodine, don't have it too often as too much iodine can cause just as many issues as not enough.

Ketogenic Diet

The Keto Diet, as it is referred to, is a high fat, moderate protein, low carb diet which puts the body into a fat burning mode instead of glucose burning.

There are many studies around its effectiveness, particularly with Type 2 Diabetes (although patients may need to stay on it to stop it returning). But studies also show it benefits people with heart disease, cancer, PCOS, brain injuries, Alzheimers and Parkinson's Disease.

A standard keto menu would look like:

- 75% Fat
- 20% Protein
- 5% Carbohydrates

The type of foods eaten on this diet include:

- Fats - Avocados, nuts, seeds, butter, cream
- Protein - Meat, eggs, fish
- Carbs - Green veggies, tomatoes, onions

If you like your high fat foods and do well with them, this may be a great option for you.

Ketosis

The state of fuel burning the body goes into when most of its energy or food is fat based instead of glucose based (carbohydrates).

Kharrazian, Dr Datis

The author of the book "Why Do I Still Have Thyroid Symptoms? When My Lab Tests are Normal" Dr Kharrazian is a leading expert in treating chronic disease without medications.

This book is a must read for all thyroid patients, even though it is aimed at Hashimoto's and hypothyroidism.

It has been my favourite book so far in learning how to connect the dots for myself.

Kidneys

Although I have not included many other organs in this book, according to Traditional Chinese Medicine (TCM) the kidneys are directly linked to thyroid health, so I decided it was important to add what I do know about kidneys here.

This is what I know or have found in my research so far:

- ☐ Kidney issues are the hardest to fix
- ☐ Electrolytes are the hardest elements to stabilise in the body
- ☐ Once the sodium:potassium ratio is low it will be a struggle to ever get it up again. It will take a lot of hard work
- ☐ Taking Algotene for life would be helpful (due to its high potassium levels and it is a functional food not a supplement)
- ☐ Low Kidney Yin (TCM) is responsible for early grey hair, dry mouth, night sweats, low urination, dizziness, tinnitus, diabetes, UTI's, constipation, hair loss, weak muscles, sleepiness and lower back pain. Sounds very thyroidy right?

If we follow TCM guidelines for improving kidney deficiency we could incorporate the herbs Rehmannia and Schisandra and eat more of the following:

- ☐ Protein, eggs, duck, beef
- ☐ Black sesame seeds, walnuts
- ☐ Asparagus, string beans, celery, parsley
- ☐ Sweet potato, potato, squash
- ☐ Adzuki Beans, black beans, kidney beans
- ☐ Grapes, plums, berries
- ☐ Sea salt, kelp

Kinesiology

I love Kinesiology and studied it for a few semesters until I realised I wanted to be able to travel with my work. I decided after that the thousands of dollars I would have spent on schooling, was better spent on actually going to a great kinesiologist!

So what is it? Kinesiology is a modality that uses muscle movement and monitoring to get to the route of a person's well being. It is non invasive and often brings out the emotional cause behind diseases and disorders of the body.

In short it is a weird way of having the best counselling session you have ever had.

A session would include laying on a bed (fully clothed) while the practitioner moves your arm and monitors the response to questions asked. When the arm "locks" it usually indicates a stress around whatever is being asked or stated.

I have seen incredible and meaningful breakthroughs using this modality, so if you know you have a lot of baggage to work through, this is an awesome way of doing it.

Kombucha

Kombucha is a fermented drink that is taking the world by storm in a promise to improve our gut health.

It is made using green or black tea and a "Scoby" which is the culture or bacteria that turns the tea into a fermented drink. Other flavours are generally added to achieve different flavours.

The thing with Kombucha is that it is based on tea, which is a natural source of fluoride. Like anything, having one every now and then wouldn't be a problem but because this is touted as the best thing going for gut health, often people are making it at home and drinking it many times a day.

Konmari

If you have not gotten on board the Konmari train yet, let me introduce you to something that will change your world and help you enormously on those brain fog days!!

No it's not a supplement! It's a woman named Marie Kondo and she is storming through the world in her very gentle way showing people how to organise their homes and cupboards.

Her ethos is that if an item "does not spark joy" then it does not belong in your home.

At first I found this tricky in my wardrobe, because many of us in the thyroid world, purchase clothes that fit us and hopefully makes us look slim. That's it! No joy sparked there really!

But as time went by and as I culled all the excess "stuff" in our home I found shopping easier. Because if it didn't light me up or fill me with joy, I didn't buy it. Not only did this mean less stuff, but I felt more calm every time I looked inside my closet.

I urge you to check out her netflix series and all the videos on Youtube where people are showing their transformed drawers. They are quite something, and I have to say, yes, mine look like that too now!

Korean Ginseng

There are many varieties of Ginseng, all with their own actions and purposes.

The Korean Ginseng is about building up. It is an adaptogenic, tonic, immune modulator, cardio tonic, male tonic, cancer preventative and cognition enhancer.

Anywhere that someone needs nourishing and building up this ginseng is your friend.

Useful for emaciation, chronic immune deficiency, fatigue, physical stress, recovery from illness, during chemo or radiotherapy, and after viruses such as chronic fatigue.

Avoid with warfarin and antidepressants.

Krebs Cycle

This is the fancy medical name for the way our body makes energy for us.

It is a series of chemical reactions that need to happen which results in the making of ATP (energy).

Kruse, Jack Dr

If you are a bit of a science nerd then Dr Kruse's book "The Epi-Paleo Prescription" is simply incredible.

Although his prescription to life is paleo based, the other things he does for good health and the reason behind them are just a great read, and much of the information is very pro-thyroid.

L

Loved Ones

Our loved ones always want what is best for us through their eyes. When they don't understand what we are doing because it is not the "norm" then they can sometimes be challenging to cope with.

The thing to remember is this.

They are really and truly only concerned with how this new thing we are doing is going to affect them.

That's it.

Are we going to make them eat like us?

Are we going to start looking and feeling better than them, and therefore make them feel bad about themselves?

Are we going to want to stop doing fun things with them like going to restaurants?

I find a way around these issues is to NOT announce we are trying a new diet or following the latest health regime. Instead, when I catch up with girlfriends for example, I order a peppermint tea and rave about how much I have been craving them lately and comment on how weird that is.

Because they think it is something I really want instead of something I am "settling for" they are happy, roll their eyes and order their own coffee.

At home, go ahead and make your salad or veggies that nobody else will eat, and announce happily you ate this at a cafe the other day and can't stop thinking about it, does anybody else want to try it? It's sooooo good and I really don't want to share it, but if you wanna bite I'll let you!!

Take the focus off it being a negative, but also be careful not to push it onto them.

Lactobacillus

A type of friendly bacteria in our gut that can help with:

- ☐ Allergies
- ☐ Skin conditions such as eczema
- ☐ Cold and flu
- ☐ Weight loss
- ☐ Vaginal candida caused by antibiotics
- ☐ Irritable Bowel Syndrome
- ☐ Reduce diarrhoea caused by bacteria
- ☐ Reduces cholesterol levels
- ☐ Reduces lactose intolerance

There are a lot of different strains of probiotics on the market now, so make sure you speak with somebody who knows what each strain is for.

Lactose

The natural sugar in dairy products, lactose is comprised of one glucose monosaccharide bound to one galactose monosaccharide.

Latent acidity

This is the term used to describe a body that is well on its way to becoming acidic.

If you keep your blood tests (and you should) then you can work out your levels with this nifty equation:

(sodium + K) - (Bicarbonate + chloride) = anion GAP

- ☐ Optimum level is 9-11
- ☐ Higher = latent acidity
- ☐ Lower = abnormal proteins

Lavender

Who doesn't love the beautiful, calming fragrance of lavender? I love it and we grow it in front of our bedroom window at every house we live in.

I do however draw the line at putting it in food. Apart from a little rosewater in Turkish Delight, I struggle to eat food that smells like perfume. But that's just me!

Lavender is a carminative, spasmolytic, antidepressant and anxiolytic. So all things calming.

Used in anxiety, insomnia, nervousness, depression, colic, IBS and tension headaches it is one of the most gentle ways to help these issues.

The oil is actually amazing for skin burns, as long as it is the first thing applied to the burn.

Laxative

An agent used to induce bowel movement.

Examples Include: Blue Flag, Dandelion, Rhubarb Root, Senna Pods, Slippery Elm

Lead

Since the removal of lead paint from the hardware store and lead from our gasoline, lead exposure has reduced and is not a big an issue as it used to be.

There are still homes out there though with lead paint on the walls that young children may be licking or scratching or one of those other random things that young children do, so here is how it can damage our body:

- ☐ Syndrome X
- ☐ Hardening of the arteries
- ☐ High Blood Pressure
- ☐ Kidney Damage
- ☐ High cholesterol
- ☐ Makes you feel dull
- ☐ Gives a fear of being poisoned
- ☐ Red blood cell (RBC) production disrupted
- ☐ Affects the central nervous system resulting in neuropsychiatric symptoms
- ☐ Blocks or inhibits iron, molybdenum, calcium, manganese, selenium, sulphur, vitamin B12, chromium, melatonin,

To help combat lead toxicity we need:

- ☐ Vitamin C
- ☐ Glutathione
- ☐ Iron
- ☐ All of the nutrients mentioned above.

a lot of algotene

Leaky Gut syndrome

When the lining of the intestinal wall is damaged allowing undigested food and other substances to leak into the bloodstream where they shouldn't be causing an immune reaction.

Considered by many health professionals to be one of the causes behind Hashimoto's.

The damage is often caused by substances like:

- ☐ neurotoxins
- ☐ GMO
- ☐ Antibiotics
- ☐ Poisons
- ☐ Prescription Drugs

Symptoms of a leaky gut include:

- ☐ Anxiety, depression, ADHD
- ☐ Fatigue, headaches, brain fog, memory loss
- ☐ Immune deficiencies
- ☐ Nutritional deficiencies
- ☐ Skin rashes, eczema, rosacea, acne
- ☐ Sugar and carb cravings
- ☐ Diarrhoea, constipation, bloating

Ways to heal a leaky gut:

- ☐ Avoid wheat, gluten, baked goods
- ☐ Avoid processed meats, refined oils
- ☐ Avoid snack and junk food
- ☐ Avoid artificial sweeteners, dairy products
- ☐ Avoid alcohol, sodas and sugary drinks
- ☐ Improve overall vegetable variety
- ☐ Include ferments and sprouts
- ☐ Include healthy fats like avocado
- ☐ Include cultured dairy products like buttermilk and greek yogurt
- ☐ Include lots of bone broth

Legumes

Legumes are fruits or seeds from the Fabaceae family of plants. They include beans, peas and lentils and are full of fibre and micronutrients.

The high fibre content can interfere with thyroid hormone replacement so an excess of legumes can easily put you into this situation.

Legumes also contain a high content of lectins which is a type of protein that we can struggle to digest. Since thyroid people often have digestive issues, these may add a burden until the gut microbiome and digestive process has been restored to good health.

Lemon Balm

The lemon balm bush smells like nothing else. So fresh and uplifting. For thyroid disease it is a TSH antagonist so must only be used in hyperthyroidism and Graves Disease.

Studies have indicated it can stop antibodies attaching to the thyroid receptor in Graves Disease so it would be a useful herb to try to lower antibodies and improve TSH levels.

It is also a carminative, mild sedative and spasmolytic so addresses many symptoms of hyperthyroidism by helping to calm them.

Lemon Myrtle

Lemon Myrtle is a native Australian Tree that thrives in the subtropical rainforests of south east QLD (Australia) and its leaves, when crushed, have the most amazing lemon/lime fragrance.

Not only does it smell ridiculously divine, the oils emitted by the crushing of the leaves have the most incredible benefits.

Lemon Myrtle is said to be:

- ☐ Anti-inflammatory
- ☐ Anti-bacterial
- ☐ Antispasmodic
- ☐ Anti-fungal
- ☐ Germicidal
- ☐ Sedative qualities

- ☐ Reduces infections
- ☐ Clears the mind
- ☐ Promotes Happiness
- ☐ Gives a sense of rejuvenation
- ☐ Uplifting in depression
- ☐ Calming influence
- ☐ Potent antioxidant

Lemon Water

Lemon Water is one of the simplest yet positively impacting things we can do for our bodies.

Many people think that lemon is acidifying but it actually forms what is called an Alkaline Ash in our body once metabolised. So don't be afraid of it.

Here are some of the benefits of a glass of warm water with a lemon squeezed into it:

- ☐ Alkalises the body
- ☐ Cleanses the Liver
- ☐ Improves digestion
- ☐ Flushes out toxins
- ☐ Improves our electrolyte balance
- ☐ Reduce pain
- ☐ Reduces inflammation
- ☐ Regulate the bowel
- ☐ Regulate the immune system
- ☐ Improve anxiety and depression
- ☐ Reduce blood pressure
- ☐ Improve skin health
- ☐ Improve gout symptoms
- ☐ Dissolve calcium build up
- ☐ Dissolve kidney stones
- ☐ Improve heart health
- ☐ Improve nerve function
- ☐ Relieve bloating and indigestion
- ☐ Detoxifies the blood
- ☐ Improves Energy
- ☐ Is antiviral

To make life easy for me, we have about 6 Lemon Bushes (not trees) which here in Australia are from Bunnings and called "Lots a Lemons" because they produce sooooo many lemons and are designed to grow in a pot.

They live up to their name and produce an abundance of lemons year round, which get juiced up and frozen into ice cubes, and placed in the deep freeze.

I then get out one container at a time and it is easy to add one cube to either cold water or hot water depending on the weather. EASY!

LaPorte, Danielle

Danielle is the author of The Desire Map and I mention her often to clients and friends alike because of what she does.

You see The Desire Map is about deciding what you want to feel in life instead of "what you want to be when you grow up" so to speak.

Some people need the feeling of security, others the feeling of joy. For me I need the feeling of freedom. Not just physically and geographically but I hate feeling boxed into something. I crave the freedom to change my mind, change my location, change my beliefs.

After reading Danielle's Desire Map and figuring out my core desired feelings, it was such an easy step after that to make my future dreams align with Freedom.

For example, I started learning kinesiology but realised as much as I loved it, I would need a clinic room to be able to practice it. My core desire of freedom sees me travelling with a laptop, so it was easy to see that kinesiology did not play a part in my bigger picture.

Get her book and figure out your core desired feelings. It will be worth it for your health and stress levels alone.

Leptin

A hormone made by our fat cells to regulate our hunger. It tells us when we are full.

For the full science version of understanding this hormone I recommend Dr Jack Kruse and his book.

Leucine

An essential amino acid, our body needs to get leucine from food, as we cannot make it from other ingredients.

Needed for all things protein and sugar related, leucine helps our bodies with:

- Improves endurance and reduces fatigue
- Diabetes and regulates blood sugar
- Low blood sugar symptoms (fatigue, headaches, dizziness)
- Promotes wound healing
- Encourages insulin release
- Improves burning of visceral fat
- Improves muscle weakness
- Improves chronic pain

Food sources of leucine include:

- Almonds and cashews
- Beans, lentils, legumes and soybeans
- Beef, chicken, eggs, fish and seafood
- Whey protein
- Whole wheat

Levothyroxine

The synthetic version of thyroxine used for thyroid replacement in hypothyroidism.

Libido

I always know when my thyroid is not optimal, and I encourage you to know your body that well too.

If my thyroid is low, I lose my libido (sex drive).

It is particularly obvious for me, because if hubby comes home after being away at work and I don't want to jump his bones, then something is wrong.

It may not be the same for you, but low libido is a common thyroid symptom.

Herbs to help enhance the libido include: Damiana, Korean Ginseng, and Tribulus Leaf.

Licorice

As I have written this book, I have been surprised at just how often Licorice has popped up for so many different reasons.

Specifically useful for adrenal support it is also helpful for gastritis, GERD, PCOS, androgen excess, recurrent cystitis, bronchitis, asthma, constipation and peptic ulcers.

Just be aware we are talking real liquorice here as in a root, not the lovely black aniseed strips we find in candy shops. They don't generally contain any liquorice anymore.

Try it in tea (very very sweet) or as a tincture, it is a mainstay in many of the herbal mixtures I make up.

Lipedema

Not long ago I found myself sitting in the clinic of a Lipedema / Lymphedema massage specialist. She looked at my legs and said "Oh, so you are a Lippy lady then"

I looked at her confused and went about telling her I had thyroid disease and was looking for lymphatic drainage massage to help with all things thyroid including fluid retention.

"Yes!" she said

"You are a classic case of Lipedema! A Lippy lady!"

As she went about the process of measuring the "clogged" spots, such as under my knees, my elbows and ankles my mind started to whirl in both fear and excitement at another possible piece of my thyroid puzzle being handed to me.

My masseuse explained that it was likely my lymphatic vessels were small and therefore clogged easily, and I would have always had thicker legs, all my life as a result (true). Once the lymphatic vessels are clogged, fluid pushes out into the tissues causing swelling and lipedema.

If not addressed this becomes permanent with the skin thickening and hardening, turning into Lymphedema, which is also called elephantiasis.

After going home and researching this some more and finding photos online, I realised that my legs very definitely looked exactly like a "Lippy Lady".

At this stage of the process, the main goal is to clear the lymphatics so that fluid can run through them and not be pushed out into the tissues.

This is what can be done:

- □ Drink plenty of warm water. Lymphatic fluid is like butter, colder will make it harder, warmer will make it more fluid and able to move.
- □ Get regular exercise. Again, warming up the body helps to make the fluid moveable.

- ☐ Use a rebounder. If you have followed me long enough you will know I love mine. They used to be called a lymphasiser as the action of jumping up and down moves the lymphatic fluid.
- ☐ Regular lymphatic Drainage massage
- ☐ Herbs for lymphatics such as Baptisia, Blue Flag, Calendula, Clivers, Echinacea Root, Myrrh & Poke Root
- ☐ Herbs for fluid retention such as: Bilberry, Butcher's Broom & Horsechestnut
- ☐ Being upside down or on an inversion machine helps the lymphatics drain
- ☐ Extremely low fat diet. Fat gets to where it needs to be through our lymphatics. If they are already clogged, more fat consumption makes it worse. I have always felt better on a low fat diet and the times I actually lost weight were always when I was eating little to no fat (even good fats).

Liquid Crystal Oracle Cards

These are my favourite Oracle Cards. Each card is a crystal from Atlantean Times and is great for people who love crystals but don't have the room or the finances for lots of them.

In fact, I am going to stop typing right now and draw a card for fun..... let's see what comes up!

First I always shuffle the cards till one falls out. I have always done it that way, because I don't want to choose.

...and the card I pulled is Imperial Topaz

- ☐ Confident Manifestation (selling lots of this book?)
- ☐ confidence, clarity, self love
- ☐ focus, order, understanding
- ☐ physically helps with digestion, nervous exhaustion and stress (book writing)
- ☐ Imagination is the only limit
- ☐ Affirmation "I confidently create my world"

Very woo woo I know, but I loooovvve them and they are just so fun!!!

List Writing

Let's face it.... Thyroid brain fog completely sucks!

For years I got around this issue by writing lists and even though my memory is sooo much better, it is a habit I continue to this day.

I keep most of my lists on my phone, simply because I always have it with me. But I also have many exercise books in my office for work lists.

The types of lists on my phone include:

- ☐ Groceries
- ☐ Gifts for upcoming birthdays
- ☐ Printer Ink order numbers
- ☐ Hair & makeup colour numbers
- ☐ Holiday dates
- ☐ My husbands roster
- ☐ blog post ideas

So, stop trying to remember everything, only to feel bad about yourself and inducing more stress when you forget! Use lists and give your poor thyroid brain a little break.

Lithium

Lithium is a Serotonin Transporter, so it gets our happy hormones to where they need to be.

We only need small amounts of it and generally we get it from our water. However, more and more people (including me) are using heavy filtration units to remove the fluoride, chloride and other hormonal disruptors in our tap water including the lithium.

It has made me suspect there is a huge correlation with the rise in purchased water in the last 2 decades and the rise in mental health issues, particularly depression and anxiety and the general lack of happiness. Are we all missing lithium now? (By the way you can test lithium in your body via a Hair Mineral Analysis)

I'm not suggesting we run out and get lithium prescribed, nor do we have to choose between lithium and fluoride in our water.

It means we have to look for other sources of it, and lucky for us many algae's and spirulinas are full of it, so we can have our cake and eat it too (just a metaphor, put down the cake).

Liver

I can never say enough about the liver, in fact it is one of the most common things I talk about in Thyroid School.

The first thing we must always know is that 70% of our thyroid hormone is converted in the liver. If our liver is sluggish then we will not be converting our hormone well at all, meaning most of us are probably taking far more medication than we actually need.

Anything we can do to clean up our liver is non-negotiable to my thinking so here are the main things I want you to know about liver health:

- ☐ Liver damage can occur from excess fat stores. You don't have to drink lots of alcohol to develop liver damage, simply being overweight can cause damage over time.
- ☐ Waking regularly between 1-3am can be a sign of a struggling liver.
- ☐ Not wanting breakfast can be a sign of a sluggish liver. Although this can also be an Adrenal sign, quite often it is the liver letting you know that it is still dealing with yesterday's toxins so please don't add to them by eating just yet (Well, at least I'm sure that's how your liver would talk if it could). The more you clean up your liver the more you will find you wake with an appetite!
- ☐ Glutathione is our Chief Antioxidant and is made in the liver. It is the first one in line to hose down the free radicals like toxins, chemicals and cancer when things get out of balance. If we don't have enough Glutathione, the job is then passed to Vitamin C (which has a smaller capacity for the job), if there is not enough of that the job then passes to Vitamin E (which has a smaller capacity again). If you don't have any of those, you will be struggling to protect your body against the nasties. Clean your liver so that it can make LOTS of glutathione.
- ☐ One of the primary jobs of the liver is to metabolise excess hormones such as oestrogen. If the liver is struggling that's when you will notice hormonal symptoms such as hot flushes in menopause and severe PMS or an intolerance to hormone replacement therapy.
- ☐ Good quality protein, regardless of it being from vegetable or animal sources will help the liver to do what it needs to do when it comes to detoxification.
- ☐ Flushing of the face can be a sign of poor liver health
- ☐ Beets & globe artichoke can help with liver drainage. I'm not talking about canned beets (which is full of sugar) or canned artichokes. The liver needs the specific antioxidants in these fresh foods. Try the beets in a juice or grate them into salads. You can also bake them (no oil) nice and slowly in the oven to retain their nutrients. WARNING: suddenly eating beets will cause pink urine!! Don't be alarmed and think something is bleeding!
- ☐ Grapefruit is a natural Liver detoxifier and is a superfood in my personal world! It is high in antioxidants, Vitamin C, Lycopene (in the pink variety), the pith is great for reducing plaque build up, and it is so effective at reducing cholesterol

that people on Statins are told not to eat it as it will increase the outcome to an unhealthy level. (Meaning too much of a good thing is never good) It is also great at helping to remove excess oestrogen which is why there are so many "cellulite diets" with grapefruit in them.

- What colour are the whites (sclera) of your eyes? Are they indeed white? Or more of a yellow colour? Do they have any blotches or strange marks in them? These are all signs in iridology of a compromised liver.
- The plough pose in Yoga restores outflow to the liver.
- Rosemary protects the liver. Many people focus on the Brassica Family for liver protection and health, which becomes problematic for thyroid people. As they contain goitrogens (which are somewhat destroyed when cooked) many people avoid them for the most part. Rosemary can do the same job without the goitrogen problem? Many liver herbs and supplements are now starting to use rosemary, so if you would prefer avoiding the brassica's as a detox method have a look around for one that has this amazing herb instead.

Lobectomy

The surgical removal of one half of the thyroid (it has two lobes) and is generally performed in cases of thyroid cancer or goiters.

Low Appetite

This is a common issue with overweight, hypothyroid patients. And it's so frustrating right? People look at you and just assume you eat too much when in reality you often forget to eat.

Lack of appetite can be caused by many things, so let's address the most common when it comes to thyroid disease.

- Low zinc - we need zinc for thyroid health and often we are low in it. Zinc is involved with taste, smell and appetite.
- Digestive conditions - IBS and Crohn's disease
- High calcium levels in the blood.
- Medications - some can cause nausea and a lack of appetite, particularly for hyperthyroid cases.
- Mental health issues - depression and anxiety can both cause a lack of appetite.
- Stress - if there is major trauma going on (which could simply be that you have a chronic disease).

It is important to remember, particularly if we carry extra weight, consuming very low calorie diets (so not eating much) will only slow down our metabolism further and can contribute to further issues with the thyroid.

Low Blood Pressure

See Blood Pressure

Low Fat Diet

The original low fat diet is The Starch Solution by Dr John McDougall and focuses on high starches (mostly vegetable starches such as potatoes) coupled with vegetables and little fat.

Anyone with lymphatic issues or gallbladder issues may consider this a diet worth trying.

If you check him out (Dr McDougall is full of amazing information) and are interested in following his protocol, check out Chef AJ too as she has a book based around her incredible weight loss using his method and has a Youtube channel showing you how to cook and eat this way.

Lupus

A systemic autoimmune disease also known as Systemic Lupus Erythematosus, it causes skin rashes (notably a butterfly shaped rash across the face and onto the cheeks), ulcers in the mouth and nose, joint pain and arthritis, inflammation of the heart and lungs, seizures, sensitivity to light, and low blood cell count.

It is common to find autoimmune thyroid disease in lupus patients, but more hypo than hyper. Generally the lupus comes first.

Lyme Disease

Growing at an alarming rate is the incidence of people with the tick borne illness Lyme Disease.

Characterised by a bullseye looking bite site, the poison can spread through the body causing damage to the brain, heart, severe inflammation of the joints leaving the victim with long term neurological issues and also can trigger autoimmune hypothyroidism.

Lymphatic

An agent used to flush out the lymphatic system.

Examples Include: Baptisia, Blue Flag, calendula, Clivers, Echinacea, Myrrh, Poke root

Lymphatic Health

Our lymphatic system has three main jobs:

- Remove excess fluid from our tissues (a big issue for thyroid ppl)
- Absorb fatty acids and transport fats
- Produce immune cells

Unlike our blood that has a heart to pump it around the body, our lymphatic system only has a series of one-way valves. No pump.

So to get these valves to open, and get the fluid inside moving we need to be either upside down (not always convenient quite frankly) or we move, you know.... like... exercise and stuff.

Lumps and Bumps

Tumors, lumps, bumps and cysts are related to lymphatic congestion. - Have you ever heard of nasty lumps and bumps referred to as garbage bags?? The analogy is that when we have an overload of toxins in our body, the lymphatics need to do something with it to keep us safe. So they build little garbage bags around the toxins to stop them from seeping into our cells. Clever huh?

But then, in our human wisdom, we have them removed! Now this is absolutely fine to do - however - if you continue to eat or live in the same manner that got you those little garbage bags in the first place then your lymphatics freak out. It goes searching for it's garbage bags and when it can't find them, it decides it better make more - many many more - just in case some of these go missing too! It is not a coincidence in any cancer that the surgeons look at the lymph nodes to see how far it has spread.

So I love this analogy (which, I can't be sure of where it came from but have a feeling it may have been Don Toleman) as it makes perfect sense to me as to why tumours tend to grow back after the doctor says "Yep, got em all!"

Your lymphatics take away any substance it doesn't recognise - So we have established that the lymphatics are our waste disposal system, but what exactly does it look to remove? Essentially anything it doesn't recognise. So that might be processed foods, pesticides, insecticides, food additives, food flavours, chemicals from skin care, hair care, dyes, makeup and cleaning products.

Now let's look at this scenario: If you are not exercising in any way because the thyroid fatigue has completely beaten you, then there is no way of moving the lymph fluid through the body. Add to that if you are eating a lot of processed,"easy" foods, then we have a recipe for disaster that is setting you up for complications to your already growing list of symptoms from thyroid disease.

So what do we do? I get thyroid fatigue! I do! I have been there! So all we can do here, is to try to stop as much of the bad stuff coming in as we can. Try upgrading a little at a time like buying organic processed foods or organic lipstick. A rebounder is awesome for fatigue, you can sit on the matt and have someone behind you bouncing up & down and it will allow your lymphatic to start flowing.

Inversion (being upside down) will open lymphatic valves - Remember our one-way valves that open when we move to let the stagnant lymphatic fluid through? Well being upside down will do it too! So you could go for one of those pieces of inversion equipment or make your own. At the very least, you can put your butt up against a wall and put your legs and feet up the wall which will open the lymphatic valves in your legs.

Tight clothes can block lymphatic flow - It is not just underwire bras that can block the flow. Tight jeans, shoes that leave a mark, and any of those undergarments that are designed to suck you in and make you smaller is going to cause stagnation in different areas.

Muscle contraction pumps lymph fluid - Any muscle contraction and relaxation will help to move the lymph in that area. So making fists while you are sitting down or going up and down on your tiptoes while you are waiting for the kettle to boil are all going to help move that fluid and any toxins it contains along.

Other ways to improve lymphatic health:

- ☐ We need HCL (good gut acid) & potassium for effective lymphatic flow
- ☐ Skin Brushing
- ☐ Lymphatic drainage massage weekly
- ☐ Floor exercises specific to moving clogged lymph (generally involves lots of bending joint type movements)
- ☐ Low fats and oils
- ☐ Lots of warm water (never cold, lymph fluid is like butter, when it is hot it will flow like a liquid but when it is cold it will be hard and solid)

- Fresh veggie juices, particularly carrot, cucumber and beets
- Don't sit too long, get up every hour and maybe swap your chair out for a fit ball.
- Liquid herbals from a qualified herbalist can help move lymphatics out

Lymphedema

A case of swelling in either arms or legs caused by a blocked lymphatic system in that extremity.

Often the cause is from having a lymph node removed during the treatment of cancer but can also happen due to ageing, excess weight, rheumatoid arthritis and infections.

Lymphedema is thought to not be curable, but specialised massage therapists, compression stockings and exercises that pump or bend the afflicted limb may help to manage the condition.

Herbs to help include: Butcher's Broom, Dandelion Leaf, and Horsechestnut.

Lymph Nodes

Throughout our lymphatic system we have from 500-700 lymph nodes connecting the vessels together.

They are the cleaning stations of the lymphatic vessels. All waste, viruses, pathogens and other toxins end up in the nodes for cleaning and then the clean lymphatic fluid is sent out the other end and on its way.

When we have enlarged lymph nodes it generally indicates a pathogen of some kind is being battled. Like when the nodes in our neck become enlarged when fighting a cold or virus.

In the case of cancer, it can break away from the tumour site and travel through the body via the blood or lymphatic system. That is why often when tumours are cut out, the nearby lymph nodes are checked for cancer also, and if necessary, they are removed.

Herbs that may help enlarged lymph nodes: Baptisia, Blue flag, Calendula, Clivers, Echinacea Root, and Poke root.

Lysine

An essential amino acid we need lysine for:

- antiviral activity
- absorption of calcium

- ☐ maintaining a lean body
- ☐ bone growth
- ☐ hormone production
- ☐ collagen synthesis
- ☐ muscle protein synthesis

Deficiency symptoms may include:

- ☐ dizziness, fatigue & stress
- ☐ bone loss, osteoporosis
- ☐ lack of concentration
- ☐ infertility, low sperm motility
- ☐ irritability
- ☐ loss of appetite and body weight
- ☐ low immune function
- ☐ Meniere's Disease
- ☐ Shingles
- ☐ female hair loss
- ☐ cold sores
- ☐ angina, Bell's Palsy

Reasons we may need more lysine:

- ☐ hypothyroidism
- ☐ excessive exercise
- ☐ herpes infection
- ☐ low protein diet
- ☐ macrobiotic diet
- ☐ surgery recovery

Food sources include:

- ☐ Chicken, fish, lamb
- ☐ Dairy products, whey protein
- ☐ Oats, watercress, mung bean sprouts
- ☐ Brewers yeast

Daily Adult dosage:

- ☐ 32mg/kg body weight

M

Mindset

When I set my mind on something, it takes a lot for me to let go of it. Right or wrong. So when I make important choices I need to be really sure it is what I want, because even if I decide down the track that maybe it wasn't the best choice, it takes a shift in the tectonic plates for me to give in.

That's just who I am.

To make a change in thyroid health, you need a similar mindset I'm sorry to say.

You need to be sure with absolute unwavering conviction that you can heal. And by healing I mean

- ☐ Feeling healthy and happy even while taking medication
- ☐ Feeling on top of the world even though you no longer have a thyroid
- ☐ Reversing your antibodies but still taking medication and feeling great
- ☐ Reversing all need for medication
- ☐ Reversing antibodies, medication and symptoms

It can mean so many things. It could be as simple as forgiving yourself for thinking thyroid disease was your punishment to bare in this life.

My mindset around thyroid disease is that I will never stop improving it. If I can reverse it completely along with all the symptoms and medication, that's awesome. If I spend the rest of my life still on medication, but happy and healthy and teaching others what I know then that's just as awesome.

It is because of my mindset that I am able to keep going when things aren't going my way. I know it's just a blip.

I would love for you, right this minute, to decide you are going to take on the mindset of healing and be like a dog with a bone. Never let go of that mindset.

MACA Root

A native plant of Peru the Maca root is used to improve hormones. With high levels of potassium, Vitamin B6, iron and Vitamin C it is used for the following:

- ☐ increase sex drive in both men and women
- ☐ increase male fertility by improving sperm quality and quantity
- ☐ improve menopausal symptoms
- ☐ improve energy and boost mood
- ☐ improve memory and learning

It comes in powder form and many people add it to their smoothies. If you do try it (it is readily available in health food shops) then you may want to have a regular thyroid test in case it affects your thyroid hormone levels.

Macadamia Nuts

I grew up in Queensland, Australia and lived for many years just down the road from the Big Pineapple and The Macadamia Nut Farm. Very tropical sounding I know. Part of that time was spent in the garage using Dad's vice to crack open the hulls of macadamia nuts that grew all around the area. I still love doing that with hubby, only now we have a fancy cracker so we don't have to go out to the shed.

I love macadamia nuts, and they have 6 times more omega 3s than 6s, which is better for us since most of us get far too many omega 6s.

100g of these little nuts give us:

- ☐ 16% DV in Protein (thyroid pathway)
- ☐ 34% DV in Dietary Fibre (hormones, gut health)
- ☐ 2% DV in Vitamin C (thyroid pathway, adrenal health)
- ☐ 3% DV in Vitamin E (thyroid pathway, antioxidant)
- ☐ 80% DV in Vitamin B1 (thyroid, hair, hyperthyroidism)
- ☐ 10% DV in Vitamin B2 (thyroid pathway)
- ☐ 12% DV in Vitamin B3 (mental health)
- ☐ 14% DV in Vitamin B6 (mental health, progesterone)
- ☐ 3% DV in Folate (MTHFR & liver)
- ☐ 9% DV in Calcium (bone health)
- ☐ 20% DV in Iron (thyroid, gut acid, fatigue)
- ☐ 33% DV in Magnesium (Sugar & Stress)

- □ 19% DV in Phosphorus (liver, bones)
- □ 11% DV in Potassium (thyroid, fatigue, fluid)
- □ 9% DV in Zinc (immunity, thyroid, mental health, wound healing)
- □ 38% DV in Copper (skin, collagen, nerves)
- □ 207% DV in Manganese (thyroid pathway)
- □ 5% DV in Selenium (thyroid pathway)

That's a pretty awesome list for less than a cup of macadamia nuts.

I try not to have too many fats cause they just don't agree with me (but that's my unique presentation) but if I am going to make one of those raw desserts or a raw sour cream (recipe under Sour Cream), then I always use macadamia nuts instead of cashews. As a bonus the flavour works better too as it is more of a non-flavour where as cashews have a very distinct flavour.

Macrophage

Immune cells that wrap themselves around an invader (pathogen) and force an immune response in the body.

Magnesium

Magnesium is required in our body for so many processes that a long term deficiency in it can have pretty major affects.

Magnesium is required for:

- □ Regulating calcium, sodium & Potassium
- □ DNA replication
- □ Regulation of body temperature
- □ Muscle contraction
- □ Heart muscle health
- □ Fatty acid oxidation
- □ Immune health
- □ Insulin sensitivity

Deficiency Symptoms of Magnesium include:

- □ Addictions

- ☐ Heart Palpitations
- ☐ Cold Hands/feet
- ☐ Fluid Retention
- ☐ Difficulty Swallowing
- ☐ Constipation
- ☐ Anxiety, Irritability, Agitation, Depression
- ☐ Tinnitus & vertigo
- ☐ Chronic pain, arthritic and joints
- ☐ Carpal Tunnel Syndrome
- ☐ Fatigue
- ☐ Low Temperature
- ☐ Unstable blood sugar
- ☐ Muscle pain, twitching, cramps, weakness
- ☐ Blurred vision
- ☐ Insomnia
- ☐ Unstable or high Blood Pressure
- ☐ Kidney & gallstones
- ☐ Cravings for sugary foods

Factors that contribute to Magnesium deficiency:

- ☐ Sweating
- ☐ Increased Urine output
- ☐ Alcohol & coffee
- ☐ Stress
- ☐ Oral Contraceptive Pill
- ☐ Hormone Replacement Therapy
- ☐ Pregnancy
- ☐ Diuretics
- ☐ ACE inhibitors
- ☐ Beta Blockers
- ☐ Blocked by Cadmium
- ☐ Blocked by Excess Copper

Food sources of Magnesium include:

- ☐ Almonds, cashews & seeds
- ☐ Cocoa

- Molasses
- Wholegrain
- Eggs
- Parsnips

Daily Requirements of Magnesium:

- Adults - 350 mg
- Toxicity Dose - >15 g

Malic Acid

An acid found in apples, currants and other tart fruits, it helps our Krebs Cycle (energy production) to function optimally.

A deficiency in this may present as fibromyalgia, muscular pain and just sheer physical exhaustion.

Malignant Thyroid Nodule

A thyroid nodule that has turned cancerous (malignant). Only 5% of thyroid nodules are malignant and the outcome is usually positive.

Maltose

Malt sugar that is comprised of two glucose units and is the sugar found in beer.

Mammograms

A test to look for lumps in the breast which involves plates pressing down on either side of the breast to take an X-ray. The goal is for women to have these regularly after the age of 50 for early detection of breast cancer.

Manganese

Manganese is required for:

- Co-factor in the making of thyroid hormone
- Critical for T3 production

- ☐ Carbohydrate metabolism
- ☐ Smooth muscle relaxation
- ☐ Dopamine & neurotransmitter function
- ☐ Mitochondrial integrity

Deficiency Symptoms of Manganese include:

- ☐ Hypothyroidism
- ☐ Poor balance & dizziness
- ☐ Poor cognitive function and concentration
- ☐ Lowered metabolism
- ☐ Fatigue
- ☐ Reduced Hair & Nail growth
- ☐ Loss of hearing / tinnitus
- ☐ Osteoporosis
- ☐ Pancreatic damage

Factors that contribute to Manganese deficiency:

- ☐ Diabetes
- ☐ Pregnancy
- ☐ Calcium supplementation
- ☐ Vegetarianism
- ☐ Blocked by lead
- ☐ Blocked by excess copper

Food sources of Manganese include:

- ☐ Almonds, pecans, walnuts, sunflower seeds
- ☐ Avocado, corn, olives, carrots
- ☐ Legumes, buckwheat, wholegrain
- ☐ Pineapple juice
- ☐ Kelp

Daily Requirements of Manganese:

- ☐ Adults - 2.5 - 7mg
- ☐ Toxicity levels - >1000mg

Mango

My love of mangoes is another giveaway of my Queensland upbringing. And they are just pure Thyroid Goodness in a glass!!

When I was pregnant with our son, for awhile that was all I could eat due to morning sickness. It then accidentally was the first food he ever tried, and now as a teenager, it is one of the few fruits he actually loves. Funny that.

So let's get to the list!! Why should we eat Mango???

1 average mango gives us:

- ☐ 2% of DV in Protein (thyroid pathway)
- ☐ 15% of DV in Fibre (oestrogen & hormone clearance, gut health)
- ☐ 32% of DV in Vitamin A (thyroid pathway)
- ☐ 96% of DV in Vitamin C (thyroid pathway, adrenal health, antioxidants)
- ☐ 12% of DV in Vitamin E (thyroid pathway, antioxidant)
- ☐ 11% of DV in Vitamin K (blood & bone health)
- ☐ 8% of DV in Vitamin B1 (thyroid, hair, hyperthyroidism)
- ☐ 7% of DV in Vitamin B2 (thyroid pathway)
- ☐ 6% of DV in Vitamin B3 (mental health)
- ☐ 14% of DV in Vitamin B6 (mental health, progesterone)
- ☐ 7% of DV in Folate (Liver health & MTHFR)
- ☐ 2% of DV in Calcium (bones)
- ☐ 5% of DV in Magnesium (stress & Sugar)
- ☐ 9% of DV in Potassium (thyroid, fatigue, fluid)
- ☐ 2% of DV in Selenium (thyroid pathway)
- ☐ 1% of DV in Zinc (immunity, thyroid, mental health, wound healing)
- ☐ 3% of DV in Manganese (thyroid pathway)
- ☐ 2% of DV in Phosphorus (liver, bones)
- ☐ 1% of DV in Iron (thyroid, fatigue, gut acid)
- ☐ Glycemic Load of 10

This all adds up to:

- ☐ Improves sleep & insomnia
- ☐ Calms the nervous system
- ☐ Are an anti-cancer food
- ☐ Can help in prevention Cardiovascular diseases

- ☐ Can help in prevention of kidney disease
- ☐ Alkalizes the body
- ☐ Flushes out toxins
- ☐ Prebiotic (food for good probiotics)
- ☐ Improve Eye health
- ☐ Improve skin health
- ☐ Improves fluid balance

And they are just such a happy fruit to smell and eat too!

Margarine

Also called Oleo, margarine is a spread made from polyunsaturated oils and water.

As thyroid people we don't need to get into the pros and cons of butter vs margarine because there is an overriding thyroid issue with margarine. It contains PUFAs which inhibit thyroid hormone from getting to our cells.

See PUFAs

Marshmallow

Marshmallow root is amazing for gut health. Particularly if there is an upset stomach or irritated gut lining involved.

Another herb that no longer exists in the ingredients that make up our current day little fluffy sugary delights, it is a demulcent and emollient which means it soothes and lines the gut.

This makes marshmallow valuable in GERD, peptic ulcers, gastritis, IBS, constipation, ulcerative colitis and general improvement of the gut lining.

It also has the same action in the lungs so is helpful with asthma, bronchitis, and coughs.

Due to its ability to line the stomach, it is best to take other medications away from it as it may inhibit absorption.

Massage

Who doesn't love a good massage?

Some don't but the majority of us adore the pampering and feeling of well being it brings us afterwards.

There are many varieties of massage available to us and it's always good to choose one that is specific to our symptoms at the time. Here are some of my favourite kinds:

- Lymphatic Drainage Massage - soft stroking movements to help move lymphatic fluid.
- Remedial Massage - for an issue or pain in a certain joint or muscle.
- Aromatherapy Massage - the use of specific essential oils used for issues are massaged into the body. Used for stress, anxiety, depression, tension and pain.
- Swedish Massage - gentle full body relaxing massage great for the first timer. Used for tension and relaxation.
- Hot Stone Massage - the use of large smooth stones that have been heated to a comfortably hot temperature are used as tools, mainly over the back, neck and shoulders (Incredible feeling!) Used for pain relief, relaxation, stress and tension.
- Shiatsu Massage - a Japanese massage to promote relaxation, stress, anxiety, depression and tension.
- Trigger Point Massage - the focus is on areas of muscle tension in the body and the broad flowing strokes are used to reduce pain.
- Deep Tissue Massage - not for the sensitive among us, this one involves finger pressure into the deep layers of our muscles and tissues to relieve tension and pain.

I regularly have lymphatic drainage and Hot stone massages when I am at home which helps with the many hours I spend sitting and writing.

When I head to Bali then I get any massage they have on offer, because it's so cheap, but I do find myself having to ask them to be ultra gentle with me.

Meadowsweet

A fantastic natural antacid, meadowsweet is also anti-inflammatory, mucoprotective (protects the mucous lining of our gut) and astringent.

Useful for peptic ulcers, gastritis, GERD, diarrhoea, IBS, gut inflammation, cystitis, myalgia and the common cold.

Medical History

Knowing our medical history is one of the most important things we can do for our health.

If we don't know where we have come from we cannot even begin to figure out where we are heading right?

It is a simple process of dividing a piece of paper into 2 sides, one for the mother, one for the father and then write down all the diseases and deaths for each side of the family.

Often the patterns emerge and it becomes really obvious what genetics you are facing if you don't look after yourself.

The other reason this is a great exercise to do, is that every time you go to a new doctor or practitioner you can simply take a copy for them.

Medical Medium

Anthony William is a Medical Medium from the US and is behind the best selling book: Thyroid Healing.

For those not in the know, a medical medium is somebody who diagnoses or pinpoints medical issues through clairvoyant abilities.

Told by his angels at aged 4 that his grandmother had breast cancer Anthony sat on her knee and told her, after which it was confirmed medically.

Anthony believes (via his angels guidance) that most thyroid disease is caused by the Epstein Barr Virus. The virus likes to hide in the thyroid gland, and our autoimmune system goes after it to kill it, with the thyroid being collateral damage.

He explains in his book the 4 stages of Epstein Barr virus, with its ultimate goal being feeding off the nervous system.

Even if you are not a believer in medium's or angels, much of his information is medically backed and makes perfect sense.

Meditation

You would have to be living under a rock to have not come across information that tell us the 1001 benefits of meditating. But in case you have been under a rock, I'll tell you again ok?

- ☐ Reduces stress, anxiety
- ☐ Promotes self awareness, self love, emotional health
- ☐ Improves attention span, memory, clarity
- ☐ Helps fight addictions
- ☐ Rewires the brain
- ☐ Reduces the risk of heart attack and stroke
- ☐ Reduces blood pressure

- Reduces inflammation at cellular level
- Promotes kindness, compassion, empathy

Don't know where to start? Try one of the many guided meditations on Youtube, or if you want a specific thyroid meditation, a long time friend of mine, Gemma who is an amazing meditation teacher, has a thyroid meditation on her site.

You can find her at https://gemmacolqhoun.com

Mediterrenean Diet

A heart healthy diet based on the eating habits of Italy, Greece and Spain.

- Whole grains
- Herbs and Spices
- Fruits and vegetables
- Beans, nuts and olive oil
- Fish and seafood twice a week
- Moderate to small amounts of diary, eggs and poultry.

Like many diets, half of the value in them is all of the processed junk and sugars that are not in there to start with. Although I do love a good Greek Salad.

Medium Chain Fatty Acids

MCT's are fats like coconut oil, and palm kernel oil.

They are said too:

- increase lean muscle mass
- increase fat burning
- decrease body fat
- reduce cholesterol
- improve brain function
- improve memory
- increase energy and endurance
- decrease blood sugar

Although coconut oil particularly is the star right now, keep in mind it is still saturated fat and too much of anything is never good.

Medullary thyroid cancer

A rare and aggressive type of thyroid cancer that forms in the parafollicular cells. If caught early and is still contained within the thyroid survival rates are nearly 90%.

Melatonin

Our sleep hormone that is regulated by the pineal gland. It can be purchased in supplement form to help fall asleep and also for shift workers whose body clock struggles to make melatonin any more due to lack of sunlight.

Meniere's Disease

A condition of the inner ear that affects the Vestibular and auditory systems. Meniere's Disease affects balance, movement and hearing due to a buildup of fluid clogging the inner ear.

Since thyroid disease is completely tied up with fluid retention, this is a common issue with thyroid people.

Signs & Symptoms:

- ☐ Vertigo - spinning room sensation, dizziness, lightheaded, loss of balance
- ☐ Tinnitus
- ☐ Loss of Hearing
- ☐ Fullness / pressure in the ear.
- ☐ Headaches

What contributes to Meniere's Disease:

- ☐ Acetaminophen - causes water retention and upsets the body's balance of electrolytes
- ☐ Antacids - high in sodium
- ☐ Aspirin - increases tinnitus
- ☐ NSAIDS - ibuprofen
- ☐ Nicotine - constricts blood flow to the inner ear.

Diet to improve Meniere's Disease:

- ☐ Fluid reducing diet
- ☐ Drink fluids throughout the day to flush out excess fluid

- ☐ Reduce Salt to less than 1500mg daily
- ☐ Avoid MSG due to the high sodium content
- ☐ Reduce sugar as it causes an insulin response which then causes the body to retain sodium which retains water.
- ☐ Caffeine contributes to tinnitus and fluid regulation
- ☐ Alcohol contributes to fluid imbalance

Nutritional supplements to improve Meniere's Disease: Ginger, Lipoflavonoids, Magnesium, Potassium, Vitamin B6

Herbs to support Meniere's Disease: Gingko, Horsechestnut, Wood Betony, Horsetail, Dandelion Leaf, Parsley,

Memory

Memory can be an issue in thyroid people, particularly hypothyroid. This is simply due to the enormous numbers of T3 receptors in the brain. If they are not getting hormone, then it will manifest into lowered cognitive function of all kinds.

One of the best brain herbs out there is bacopa, and it has the added bonus of being a thyroid stimulant.

Other herbs to improve memory include: Gingko, Korean ginseng, paeonia, Rhodiola, rosemary, Sage, Schisandra, and Siberian Ginseng

Menopause

The end of reproduction in a woman's life, menopause is a natural part of life that is marked by 12 months since the last period.

At this time the adrenal glands take over the helm of making hormones from the ovaries, but the estrogen it makes is not as strong so adrenal health is now the focus for a smooth, symptom free transition.

Herbs to support menopause include: alfalfa, black cohosh, Kava, Korean Ginseng, Ladies Mantle, Sage, Shatavari, St John's Wort, Tribulus Leaf, and Wild Yam

Mental Health

It is said in many health circles that there are many people out there with mental health issues such as depression and anxiety that are actually undiagnosed thyroid patients.

We have a huge concentration of thyroid hormone receptors in our brain, so if we are not getting enough hormone it will show up in the form of mental health issues. Conversely, if we are getting too much hormone, and everything is going to fast, it will also manifest in the brain.

Although I am a fan of trying to use food and nutrition instead of supplements where possible, when it comes to mental health sometimes we need the extra help before we can even get our heads around the idea of changing our food.

The two supplements that I have found work the best and makes the most obvious impact in a really short time are:

- Algotene - an algae that grows in Western Australia and is a natural source of lithium. I have spoken at length with the makers of this supplement and it does not interfere with any anti-depressants and is classed as a "functional food" much like spirulina or chlorella.
- Complex B Vitamins - activated is better, because thyroid people already have compromised systems, so let's just make this job a little easier for it shall we?

Depression

I only suffered depression when I tried natural thyroid medication strangely enough. After 3 months or so on it, I was suddenly getting through my days simply because my husband was telling me what to do next.

"Now you are going to have a shower"

"Now we are going to go for a walk"

"Now you are going to .... etc

It was during a walk along the beach that some little voice deep down inside said: "it's the medication".

I went back to thyroxine the very next day and within a week or so I was back to my usual self. Remember, not everything works for everyone.

I remember what a hideous, lost, dark time it was and I feel for others that go through it on a regular basis.

So don't discount medication influences if you are going through this awful experience.

Herbs to help depression: Damiana, Lavender, Lemon Balm, Siberian Ginseng, St John's Wort

Anxiety

I find that I suffer with chronic anxiety if my thyroid medication is not right.

This manifests for me as constant worry. You probably know the kind, did I leave the iron on, did I shut the garage door when I left home this morning, what if I have a crash on the freeway and nobody is there to pick up my son from school. Constant little nagging thoughts that took up my day.

It was not until my thyroid improved and I got my conversion working that one day when researching and writing something about it for Thyroid School that I realised I no longer had those fears and that constant nagging anxiety.

Again, it comes down to optimising the thyroid pathway, improving conversion and getting hormone in the right amounts to the brain.

Panic Attacks

Yes I will put my hand up here and say that I have experienced these awful, scary things.

But, because I keep a thyroid diary of all my symptoms, foods and feelings I finally figured out that it was a coffee and diary related issue.

Once again, that was many years ago, and since I have cleaned everything up, I can drink coffee again (even once a day if I want too, but I don't) and if I want to treat myself to dairy I can do that too with no fears of attacks. I just don't do it often, and am always working on my pathway.

One tip I learned along the way is throwing cold water on your face during a panic attack which affects the vagus nerve. This kicks in the parasympathetic nervous system which is our rest & digest system. It takes us out of the "fight or flight" sympathetic nervous system.

Mercury

This is a hideous toxic metal that loves to head straight for the thyroid and make its home there.

Exposure can come from lots of sources and industries including:

- ☐ body talcs and powders, cosmetics
- ☐ silver fillings, vaccines, haemorrhoid suppositories
- ☐ fungicides, herbicides, pesticides
- ☐ wood preservatives, paint, batteries
- ☐ large fish
- ☐ mercurochrome, thermometers, inside fluorescent light bulbs
- ☐ lamp makers, boilermakers, dentists, electroplaters, mirror makers, textile printers

What mercury does in the body:

- ☐ increase the production of free radicals
- ☐ decrease the production of glutathione
- ☐ increases inflammation
- ☐ inhibits insulin production
- ☐ increases food intolerance to wheat and milk proteins
- ☐ blocks selenium, iron, vitamin B12, melatonin, zinc, sulphur, vitamin E, Molybdenum and carnitine in the body

How to chelate (excrete) it from the body:

- ☐ Increase zinc, selenium, iron, magnesium and sulphur either from food sources or supplements
- ☐ Chlorella helps detoxify mercury
- ☐ Cilantro eaten daily (2 tablespoons over 3 months)
- ☐ Dr Mercola has a really specific mercury detoxification protocol at https://www.mercola.com

Metabolic Syndrome

This is the collective term given to somebody who has the following:

- ☐ High Blood Pressure
- ☐ High Cholesterol
- ☐ High Blood sugar
- ☐ Increased body fat around the middle

Since we are already at risk of all of these issues with thyroid disease then having all three wouldn't be hard. This then leads us down the road of further complications for developing more serious diseases such as:

- ☐ Increases risk of kidney disease by 200-400%
- ☐ Increases risk of Cardiovascular disease
- ☐ Increased risk of Stroke
- ☐ Increased risk of Fatty Liver Disease
- ☐ Increased risk of Heart Attack
- ☐ Increased risk of Hardening of the Arteries
- ☐ Increased risk of Diabetes
- ☐ Increased risk of Nerve Damage

To reverse Metabolic Syndrome is a lifestyle choice and will mean in most cases completely changing the current diet and habits. Examples are:

- Getting daily exercise
- Losing weight
- Giving up smoking, alcohol, caffeine
- Vegetarian diet full of vegetables and limiting fat, salt & sugar.
- Use herbs such as Cinnamon, Coleus, Gymnema & St Mary's Thistle.

This will not happen quickly, however if early death is not in the diary, then working with a specialist in this field, that will help keep things going in the right direction would be money well spent.

Metabolism

The rate at which our "inner furnace" is burning. The thyroid regulates our metabolism.

Methionine

An essential amino acid that helps us with:

- making adrenaline, antibodies, and carnitine
- methylation reactions, methylation pathway
- free radical scavenger, antioxidant
- normal cell function
- precursor to cysteine, which build proteins in the body
- prevent liver damage particularly when taking acetaminophen

Used therapeutically for the following conditions:

- alcoholism, heroin addiction
- allergies, chemical sensitivities, pesticide exposure
- atherosclerosis, high cholesterol, gallstones, liver disease, kidney failure, Parkinson's Disease
- burns, fatigue, surgery

Food sources of methionine include:

- Beans, beef, dairy, eggs
- Fish, sardines, whey protein
- Onions, garlic, liver

Michaels, Jillian

The star of the original series "The Biggest Loser" Jillian Michaels has hypothyroidism.

Microbiome

The new term used for our gut bacteria. There are more bacteria in our gut than cells in our body, so it is right they should have a fancy name.

Migraines

Migraine sufferers are at 41% higher risk of becoming hypothyroid.

Another study states that hypothyroid sufferers are at a much higher risk of getting migraines.

I think what we can safely assume there is a connection right?

On further investigation, I found theories around it being connected with temperature, more specifically low temperature which is a symptom of hypothyroidism. It is suggested that when temperatures dip too low, this brings about fluid leakage in the brain tissues causing the migraine pain.

My thought process here is for those who suffer is to track temperatures and migraines to see if you have a correlation and look into Wilson's Temperature Syndrome a little more thoroughly.

Millicurie

A unit of measure for radioactive iodine.

Mint

What's not to love about mint right? It's just so fresh and, well, minty!

To show you the value of what's inside mint I'm going to use the measurement of 100 grams which is a lot of mint, however all the other measurements were in 2 tablespoons and I would like to think we could all manage a few more leaves than that for the sake of our health!

So 100g of peppermint has:

- ☐ 32% of DV in Dietary fibre (hormonal clearance, gut health)
- ☐ 7% of DV in protein (who knew?)

- ☐ 85% of DV in Vitamin A (Thyroid Pathway)
- ☐ 53% of DV in Vitamin C (thyroid pathway, adrenals)
- ☐ 5% of DV in Vitamin B1 (Thyroid Health)
- ☐ 16% of DV in Vitamin B2 (Thyroid Pathway)
- ☐ 9% of DV in Vitamin B3 (Mental Health)
- ☐ 6% of DV in Vitamin B6 (Mental Health, progesterone)
- ☐ 29% of DV in Folate (MTHFR & Liver)
- ☐ 24% of DV in Calcium (thyroid & bones)
- ☐ 28% of DV in Iron (thyroid, fatigue, gut acid)
- ☐ 20% of DV in Magnesium (sugar & stress)
- ☐ 7% of DV in Phosphorus (Liver, bones)
- ☐ 16% of DV in Potassium (thyroid, fatigue, fluid)
- ☐ 59% of DV in Manganese (thyroid pathway)

Wow!! who knew common old mint contained pretty much a bit of everything? So while we may not sit down to 100g of it at once (unless you make it the base of a Moroccan salad perhaps instead of lettuce) clearly anywhere we can throw this little gem will give us a boost!

I have a client who has used mint to signal to herself it is the end of the meal. In an effort to stop eating dessert with her family, she started eating a couple of mint leaves after eating her meal and kept telling herself, the meal was finished now. Well it worked for her! Never again did she crave dessert after having her mint leaves! Genius!!

Miscarriage

In both hypothyroidism and hyperthyroidism there is a greater risk of miscarriage in the first trimester.

If this is something you have or are experiencing, I'm here with you, and when you are ready to take action, then give it your best as I know you will.

- ☐ The first step here is to get your thyroid levels optimal.
- ☐ Have a salivary hormone test to see where your estrogen and progesterone are at. Progesterone is the hormone that holds the baby in the womb, so if it is low that will struggle to happen.
- ☐ If you are hyperthyroid, working with a specialist to be on the lowest amount of antithyroid drugs possible to keep you stable will help.
- ☐ Be kind to yourself and know that you are doing your best in every minute of every day.

Herbs for repeated miscarriage: Black Haw, Chaste Tree, Cramp Bark

Herbs to support threatened miscarriage include: Black Haw, chaste Tree, Cramp Bark, Squaw Fine, True Unicorn Root, Wild Yam

Modality

A word used to describe a type of treatment.

Acupuncture, Chiropractic, Bowen Therapy are all different "modalities".

Molecular Mimicry

This occurs when 2 different substances look so similar that the body treats them the same.

An example is that gluten and thyroid cells look chemically similar and therefore often removing gluten from the diet brings down antibodies.

Mold

Mold can have a negative effect on the pituitary gland, and since that is involved in telling our thyroid what to do, we may have problems if the mold is not removed from the environment.

Molybdenum

Molybdenum is required for:

- Lipid metabolism
- Iron metabolism
- Copper metabolism (Wilson's Disease)
- Purine metabolism
- Sulfation Pathway metabolism

Deficiency Symptoms of Molybdenum include:

- Anaemia
- Anxiety
- Fatigue
- Weight Gain
- Zinc Deficiency

- Joint Issues
- Gout
- Infertility
- Irritability
- Perfume Intolerance
- Sulphite allergies
- Tachycardia
- Tooth Decay
- Weight Gain

Factors that contribute to Molybdenum deficiency:

- High Protein Diets
- Blocked by excess Copper
- Low Zinc levels
- Fluoride
- Blocked by Lead

Food sources of Molybdenum include:

- Beans & Peas
- Legumes & Lentils
- Lamb, pork, liver & kidney
- Oats
- Oysters
- Sunflower Seeds,

Daily Requirements of Molybdenum:

- Adults - 75 - 250 ug
- Toxicity level - >2000 ug

Mono Meals

Mono meals is like food combining on steroids.

This is a diet where only one type of food is eaten at each meal which allows the body easier digestion.

For example you may have a bowl of apples for breakfast, a plate of melon for lunch or a handful of blueberries as a snack. Generally it is the raw food eaters or fruitarians that might follow this type of framework, however I have on many occasions only eaten roast chicken for lunch or dry roasted potatoes and nothing else.

It always leaves me feeling energised and nourished as opposed to eating those two things together which can sometimes leave me bloated.

Morbid Obesity

This is a term for someone whose BMI is over 40 or is 100 pounds over their ideal weight for height.

Motherwort

This is an herb for hyperthyroidism only as it has an antithyroid action.

It also helps with many of the symptoms of hyperthyroidism such as nervous fast heart beat, anxiety and to calm racing nerves.

It is to be used with caution in pregnancy, so work with a qualified herbalist.

MSG

Did you know that scientists often use MSG (monosodium glutamate) to fatten mice when they want to study anything to do with weight? If that does not put into perspective how little MSG we should be eating, I'm not entirely sure what will.

Apart from weight gain, MSG contributes to:

- inflammation
- is a neurotoxin
- Migraines
- Liver Disease
- Endocrine Disorders, Diabetes, Fibromyalgia, Chronic Fatigue Syndrome
- Lymphoma
- Epstein Barr Virus
- Confusion, Memory loss, Depression, Insomnia

If that isn't a list of thyroidy things I don't know what is!!

MSG is hidden in so many things, so here is a list of not so obvious as well as obvious sources of where it may be lurking. It is not always in these products, but it would be wise to check the ingredients.

Other names for MSG:

- ☐ Plant Protein Extract
- ☐ Hydrolyzed Vegetable protein
- ☐ Hydrolyzed Plant protein
- ☐ Calcium & Sodium caseinate
- ☐ Yeast Extract (vegemite / marmite etc)
- ☐ Textured Protein (meat substitutes)
- ☐ Autolyzed Yeast
- ☐ Hydrolyzed Oat flour
- ☐ Malt Extract
- ☐ Malt Flavouring
- ☐ Bouillon Broth
- ☐ Stock Flavouring
- ☐ Natural Flavouring
- ☐ Natural Beef or Chicken Flavouring
- ☐ Seasoning & Spices
- ☐ Soy Protein Concentrate
- ☐ Soy Protein Isolate
- ☐ Whey protein Concentrate

So the take home message here is to check everything we consume. Particularly the vegetarians who live off a lot of the meat substitutes. Or make everything from scratch (80% of the time - balance!) so you know what is going into your body.

MTHFR

More and more people are having DNA type testing done that tells them if they have any gene irregularities so to speak.

MTHFR which stands for Methylene-TetraHydroFolate Reductase is becoming a common gene variation, and with the people who have that variation, they cannot convert folate into its active form to be able to use the nutrients.

Kind of like in thyroid disease, if you are not converting T4 to T3 properly, you cannot fully utilise the thyroid hormone, with MTHFR mutation you cannot get folate as you don't convert it.

What this means is that those people will always need to take "activated folate" that has already been converted into 5-Methyltetrahydrofolate (the active form).

You can find out if you have this mutation, plus others, if you are nosey like that through 23 and me.

https://www.23andme.com/

Multiple Endocrine Neoplasia

Multiple Endocrine Neoplasia (MEN) is a rare inherited syndrome presenting as tumors growing on several endocrine organs at the same time.

Multiple Endocrine Neoplasia type 2 (MEN2) is when the tumors are specifically: medullary thyroid cancer, parathyroid tumors and pheochromocytoma (tumors on the adrenals)

Multiple Sclerosis

Many autoimmune diseases are associated with Multiple Sclerosis (MS) a nasty disease where nerve damage causes problems with vision, balance, muscle control and coordination along with experiencing pain and fatigue.

It appears most sufferers of MS have low tyrosine levels which is the amino acid required (with iodine) to make thyroid hormone.

Anthony William (Medical Medium) says that it is a stage of Epstein Barr Virus (seriously, get his thyroid book!).

One thing for sure, is that MS symptoms can mimic thyroid symptoms, or is it the other way around? If you have MS, get your thyroid checked regularly.

Muscle Weakness

see Myasthenia gravis

Mushrooms

Love them or loathe them, they pack a nutritional punch.

Don Toleman has reported that people have regrown their thyroid after surgical removal by eating 2 cup of mushrooms everyday. Not sure of the validity but I trust Don so why not? Because of that, let's look at what 2 cups of whole button mushrooms contain:

- 8% of DV in Dietary Fibre (hormonal clearance, gut health)
- 12% of DV in Protein (thyroid pathway)

- ☐ 6% of DV of Vitamin C (thyroid pathway, adrenals)
- ☐ 8% of DV of Vitamin D (hormone health)
- ☐ 10% of DV of Vitamin B1 (thyroid, hair, hyperthyroidism)
- ☐ 46% of DV of Vitamin B2 (thyroid pathway)
- ☐ 34% of DV of Vitamin B3 (Mental Health)
- ☐ 10% of DV of Vitamin B6 (mental health, progesterone)
- ☐ 8% of DV of Folate (Liver Pathway & MTHFR)
- ☐ 2% of DV of Vitamin B12 (Energy & MTHFR)
- ☐ 6% of DV of Iron (thyroid pathway, fatigue, gut acid)
- ☐ 4% of DV of Magnesium (sugar & Stress)
- ☐ 8% of DV of Phosphorus (Liver, bones)
- ☐ 18% of DV of Potassium (Thyroid, fluid, fatigue)
- ☐ 6% of DV of Zinc (immunity, thyroid, mental health, wound healing)
- ☐ 30% of DV of Copper (skin, nerves, collagen)
- ☐ 4% of DV in Manganese (thyroid pathway)
- ☐ 26% of DV in Selenium (thyroid pathway)
- ☐ Glycemic Load of 2
- ☐ Contains Tyrosine (thyroid pathway & mental health)
- ☐ Contains Tryptophan (mental health)
- ☐ Contains Iodine - although I could not find definitive amount
- ☐ Regulates the immune system
- ☐ Help protect against Breast Cancer

I can see why they are great thyroid food with all that selenium and potassium, let alone all the other goodies.

Myasthenia Gravis

A chronic autoimmune disease, Myasthenia gravis (MG) causes muscle weakness in the skeletal muscles.

Symptoms include:

- ☐ weak arms and legs
- ☐ difficulty breathing, swallowing, chewing
- ☐ hoarse voice and difficulty talking
- ☐ double vision, drooping eyelids, facial paralysis

As this is an autoimmune disease it is not uncommon to also have thyroid disease. I know of at least one person on Thyroid School that has both, but that is because she is brave enough to talk about it. Hi Gloria!

MG is treated with immunosuppressants and corticosteroids and in really serious cases, the thymus is removed (the immune systems white blood cell maker).

Myotherapy

A type of physical therapy focusing on musculoskeletal pain. It is a specialised form of massage that helps to release muscles. You do not see a massage therapist for this, you would find a trained Myotherapist.

Myxedema

A severe or advanced form of hypothyroidism that comes from being under treated or untreated.

Symptoms include:

- ☐ swollen face
- ☐ swollen body, especially the legs
- ☐ thickened skin
- ☐ decreased breathing
- ☐ extremely low body temperature
- ☐ confusion, mental slowness, shock, seizures
- ☐ low blood oxygen levels coupled with high carbon dioxide levels (due to the decreased respiration)
- ☐ myxedema coma - medical emergency

This can happen if someone stops taking thyroid medication which is common in the elderly if they forget to take it. It can also occur due to trauma, infection, severe stress or sudden illness.

N

Negotiable

Have you got a list of what's negotiable and non-negotiable in your healing journey? By this I mean, what won't you budge on?

I won't budge on buying organic carrots. But other organic veg is negotiable depending on the price. Why? Because I found out that many farmers plant carrots in their fields when they become too hard after many crops have been grown and fertilised.

They plant carrots which draw out all the fertilisers, pesticides and insecticides from the soil making them soft and plantable again.

Now I'm not entirely sure how true that is, but the source was pretty reliable in my eyes, so because of that, organic carrots are non-negotiable.

The food protocol I follow is negotiable. It has to be because as my body changes it needs different things so I have to be open to change on that level.

My exercise program is negotiable but doing exercise in general is non-negotiable.

Drinking alcohol is negotiable, drinking green juice everyday and lemon water every morning is non-negotiable.

So I ask again, do you have a list of what is negotiable and non-negotiable? Often having this list makes life feel less rigid and a little more flexible.

NAC

N-Acetylcysteine is a nutrient that can "resuscitate" mitochondria (energy) in long term hypothyroidism.

It increases the production of glutathione (our master antioxidant) and enhances excretion of mercury and lead.

It is also used therapeutically for:

- Acetaminophen overdose
- AIDS
- Cancer treatment
- Heavy metal poisoning
- Ethanol poisoning
- Infertility
- Motor Neuron Disease
- Sjogren's syndrome

Nails

Our nails can tell us a lot about the health of our body by giving us physical signs.

- Moons - when the half moons at the base of our nails are missing it can indicate a thyroid disorder. On my hand they are missing on the outer fingers of my left hand which leads me to believe that it is my left thyroid lobe that is still not doing so well. Just a theory though.
- White spots - zinc deficiency
- Split, peeling & cracked - deficiency in biotin, thyroid hormone, low stomach acid and low essential fatty acids
- Spoon shaped nails - iron deficiency
- Flat on top but squared edges - iron deficiency
- Ridges running vertically - silica deficiency
- Split nails vertically - silica deficiency
- Brittle nails - Vitamin A deficiency

Nutrients needed for nail health include: Biotin, Vitamin A, manganese, silica
Herbs to help nail health include: Gotu Kola, Horsetail, and Nettle Leaf

Nail Varnish

I love painting my nails. It makes me feel very girly and feminine even if my nails don't grow very long.

However much of the nail varnishes on the market are filled with endocrine disruptors that would have my medication heading in the wrong direction really quickly if I used them all the time.

The nail varnish industry is starting to catch on though and now we can find a variety of paints that boast "5 free" "7 Free" "10 Free" meaning they do not contain those top endocrine disrupting chemicals.

- 5 Free - they have removed formaldehyde, dibutyl phthalate, toluene, camphor, formaldehyde resin
- 7 Free - the first 5 removed plus ethyl tosylamide, xylene
- 10 Free - the first 7 removed plus fragrances, parabens, animal products.

Some great brands are:

- Sienna Byron Bay (a personal favourite as they are Aussie like me)
- Kester
- Butter - London
- Nailberry - Paris-London

Naltrexone

Low Dose Naltrexone is a medication generally used for alcohol and opioid addiction, and works on balancing the immune system.

Now it is more commonly used in the following disorders:

- Hashimoto's
- Multiple sclerosis
- Fibromyalgia
- Fatigue and Pain
- Chronic Fatigue Syndrome

Natural thyroid hormone Replacement

See Armour

Nature-Throid

A medication for hypothyroidism made from animal thyroid glands (usually pigs) containing T4, T3, plus cofactors T1, T2, calcitonin and iodine.

See Armour

Neonatal Hypothyroidism

See congenital hypothyroidism

Nerve impingement

This is simply when our skeletal body is out of alignment and impinges or puts pressure on our nerves causing pain.

This actually puts the body into flight or fight which means it has activated the sympathetic nervous system which then causes the adrenals to release cortisol.

A chiropractor, physiotherapist or Bowen Therapy can all help with this.

Nervine

An agent that tones and strengthens the nervous system.

Examples Include: Bacon, Damiana, Gotu Kola, Green Oats, Motherwort, Oats Seed, Polygonum multiform, Schisandra, Skullcap, St John's Wort, Vervain

Nettle Leaf

The leaves of the nettle are useful specifically for Osteoarthritis, rheumatism, rheumatoid arthritis, Hay fever, dermatitis & urticaria. But when we look at the breakdown of nutrients and what it can do it is clearly a friend to the thyroid also!

If you were to eat nettle - (many use it in soups) I suppose it is a bit like an earthy spinach flavour. I put mine in herb tea and just make sure I drink 1-2 cups everyday, so I am getting a hit of nettle goodness, without the handling issues.

If you were to get your hands on Nettle for soup then this is what is in 100g:

- ☐ 28% of DV in Fibre (hormonal clearance, gut health)
- ☐ 5% of DV in Protein (thyroid pathway)
- ☐ 40% of DV in Vitamin A (thyroid pathway)

- □ 623% of DV in Vitamin K (blood, bones)
- □ 1% of DV in Vitamin B1 (thyroid, hair, hyperthyroidism)
- □ 9% of DV in Vitamin B2 (thyroid pathway)
- □ 2% of DV in Vitamin B3 (mental health)
- □ 5% of DV in Vitamin B6 (mental health, progesterone)
- □ 48% of DV in calcium (bones)
- □ 9% of DV in Iron (fatigue & thyroid)
- □ 14% of DV in magnesium (sugar, stress)
- □ 39% of DV in manganese (thyroid)
- □ 7% of DV in Phosphorus (bones, liver)
- □ 7% of DV in Potassium (thyroid, fluid, fatigue)
- □ 2% of DV in Zinc (thyroid, mental health, immunity, wound healing)

That all adds up to:

- □ Reduces joint pain
- □ Reduces Arthritis pain
- □ Is anti-inflammatory
- □ Has antihistamine properties
- □ Stimulates hair growth
- □ Helps control blood pressure
- □ Helps with urinary tract health
- □ Reduces fluid retention
- □ Is a diuretic
- □ Is a wound healer
- □ Helps with kidney health

Neuroprotective

An agent used to protect neural (brain) pathways.

Example: Gingko

Nightshades

Nightshades are foods from the Solanaceae plant family.

Vegetables from the nightshade family can exacerbate arthritis and autoimmune conditions due to their high content of lectins, a protein that can bind cells together.

Cooking can reduce the amount of lectins however if arthritis and inflammation are a major issue then an elimination diet would be helpful to see if these foods are making your issue worse.

They include:

- White potatoes
- Tomatoes,
- Tomatillos
- Sweet bell peppers
- Eggplant
- Chilli
- Goji berries
- tobacco.

Night Sweats

Can be both menopause related and thyroid/adrenal related.

The adrenals take over the making of hormones after menopause, but a smooth transition requires healthy adrenals, so night sweats would be a sign to focus on adrenal health.

NKC

The shortening for Natural Killer Cells which are immune cells sent to destroy an invader.

NLP

The shortening for Neuro-linguistic Programming which is a tool used by psychologists or trained practitioners to help people with disorders, mental health issues and post traumatic stress.

The process involves the practitioner helping you to arrive at your own answers as they believe all the knowledge you need is between your ears.

NSAIDS

Nonsteroidal anti-inflammatory drugs (NSAIDs) are pain relievers, reduce fevers and inflammation and prevent clots and come under the names of Aspirin, Ibuprofen, Advil, Naproxen, and Celebrex.

They might be magic at relieving our pain however they come with an increased risk of stomach ulcers, heart attacks and kidney disease.

Safer options include Turmeric and Boswellia.

Nuclear Receptor Proteins

Proteins in our cells that sense steroid hormones and thyroid hormones

O

Oprah's Life

One of the many celebrities in our world that has thyroid disease is Oprah. I say this just to remind us that we can absolutely still have a fulfilling life with this crappy disease.

Yep ok she may have a lot of help that we may not be able to afford, but she still shows up and changes the world.

Another notable celebrity that I admire with thyroid disease is Jillian Michaels from Biggest Loser fame. Honestly, she turned her weakness into her strength!

Hillary Clinton managed to be the first female to run for the presidency. I can only imagine the physical workload she endured during her campaign. But she showed up and didn't let thyroid disease be the reason she couldn't do it.

Sofia Vergara has curves for days. I have no doubt she has to be extremely careful with what she eats and how she manages to learn her lines with thyroid brain is a wonder to me! But she shows up and gets the job done so we can laugh at her characters antics every week.

Obstructive Goitres

A goitre that grows and begins to press on the trachea. Noticeable wheezing, and coughing is a symptom of this issue.

It may be a slow progression or sudden painful enlargement, but generally occurs in patients who have had goitres for a lengthy period.

Obstructive Sleep Apnea

An issue that occurs when the throat closes over during sleep, causing loud snoring and a cessation of breathing for up to a minute at a time.

This can occur in any age group or gender and can be caused by:

- Enlarged tonsils and adenoids
- Being overweight
- Excess tummy fat (less room for lungs)
- Narrow throat or other structural abnormalities such as a deviated septum.

The dangers of leaving this untreated are:

- Extreme fatigue
- Lack of oxygen in the body
- Poor concentration
- High anxiety, depression, low mood and stress
- Increased risk of high BP, heart attack and stroke
- Higher risk of diabetes

How to help it?

- Reduce or remove alcohol and smoking
- Increase exercise and aerobic fitness
- Sleep with a wedge
- Your doctor may recommend a CPAP machine to wear at night which keeps the airways open and oxygen flowing

Oil Pulling

The act of "pulling" oil through your teeth and swishing it around your mouth for 15 mins first thing in the morning.

It removes toxins and bacteria from the mouth which stops it entering the body. Many people have reported enhanced health and wellbeing when practicing this daily, particularly with any oral diseases.

You can use coconut oil or sesame oil, but make sure when you are finished you spit the white solid residue that you end up with into a tissue and dispose in the bin or you will clog up your drains.

Omega 3

When we think of Omega 3 fatty acids we mostly think of foods from the ocean, although there are many plant and land animal foods that contain this nutrient.

We need Omega 3s help for:

- ☐ Reduce inflammation
- ☐ Fight Autoimmune Disease (inc lupus, rheumatoid arthritis, Crohn's Disease, Diabetes, MS)
- ☐ Reduces Non-alcoholic Fatty Liver Disease
- ☐ Improves Joint Health
- ☐ Improves Skin Health
- ☐ Mental health (depression, mood swings and anxiety)
- ☐ Brain Health (cognition, memory, dementia, alzheimers)
- ☐ Metabolic Syndrome (high BP, Sugars, Cholesterol)

I was listening to a talk by Jon Gabriel a while back and he says it takes 6 months to coat your cells completely with Omega 3 which causes cells to regain sensitivity to insulin.

Insulin Resistance is so common in thyroid issues, so Omega 3 daily for a minimum of 6 months may help to reduce it.

We find Omega 3s in the following foods:

- ☐ 2 Tbsp Flax Seeds contain 133% of DV
- ☐ ¼ cup of Walnuts contain 113% of DV
- ☐ 3.2 oz Sardines contain 61% of DV
- ☐ 4 oz Salmon contain 55% of DV
- ☐ 4 oz of Beef contain 46% of DV
- ☐ 4 oz Shrimp contain 14% of DV
- ☐ 2 cups of Romaine Lettuce contain 5% of DV

Omega 6

We actually get too many Omega 6s in our diet, that is the whole reason I have added an entry for them. While the healthy body requires them as they help inflammation during healing, as thyroid people we are always inflamed so do not need any extra help.

Our ideal ratio of Omega 3:Omega 6 should be 1:1 but no more than 1:5. In reality most of us get a ratio of 1:20 which is alarming.

Sources of Omega 6s include:

- ☐ Safflower, grapeseed, and sunflower oils
- ☐ Nut oils
- ☐ Wheat germ
- ☐ Salad dressings & mayonnaise
- ☐ Shortening

While there are other high sources in the fruit and vegetable world such as avocados, olives and berries, it appears most of our imbalance comes from the oils, dressings and shortenings (particularly in cooking). Just removing or cutting those items way down would mean we could eat the vegetables with no change to our ratio.

Omega 9

Mostly found in animal protein and vegetables, omega 9s cannot be produced by us, which Omega 3 and 6 can be.

Generally though if we are eating a well rounded diet, then we should be getting what we need of this fatty acid.

We need Omega 9 for:

- ☐ Increased energy
- ☐ Improve mood
- ☐ Improve cognitive function
- ☐ Reduce the risk of Cardiovascular Disease
- ☐ Reduce the risk of Stroke

Omega 9 foods include:

- ☐ Hazelnuts
- ☐ Macadamia Nuts
- ☐ Almond butter
- ☐ Avocado oil
- ☐ Olive oil

Onions

Onions are amazing little vegetables. They can be put into so many dishes and helps us in a million ways.

One cup (210g) of onion gives us:

- ☐ 11% of DV in Dietary Fibre (hormone clearance, gut health)
- ☐ 6% of DV in Protein (thyroid pathway)
- ☐ 8% of DV in Vitamin B1 (thyroid, hair, hyperthyroidism)
- ☐ 4% of DV in Vitamin B2 (thyroid pathway)
- ☐ 16% of DV in Vitamin B6 (mental health, progesterone)
- ☐ 27% of DV in Biotin (hair, skin, nails)
- ☐ 8% of DV in Folate (MTHFR, liver)
- ☐ 15% of DV in Vitamin C (thyroid pathway, adrenals, antioxidant)
- ☐ 5% of DV in Calcium (bones)
- ☐ 16% of DV in Copper (nerves, skin, collagen)
- ☐ 3% of DV in Iodine (thyroid pathway)
- ☐ 3% of DV in Iron (thyroid pathway, fatigue, gut acid)
- ☐ 6% of DV in Magnesium (stress, sugar)
- ☐ 14% of DV in Manganese (thyroid pathway)
- ☐ 11% of DV in Phosphorus (bones, liver)
- ☐ 7% of DV in Potassium (thyroid, fatigue, fluid)
- ☐ 2% of DV in Selenium (thyroid pathway)
- ☐ 4% of DV in Zinc (thyroid, mental health, wound healing, immunity)
- ☐ Glycemic Load of 5
- ☐ They are anti-inflammatory
- ☐ They help support bone & connective tissue
- ☐ They improve cardiovascular health

And did you notice this one has iodine in it!! Talk about a thyroid superfood!

Opioids

A class of drugs including heroin, oxycodone, codeine and morphine.

This class of drugs have an effect on the nervous system which brings about pain relief and a feeling of pleasure.

Some opioids can increase TSH and therefore affect thyroid function.

Oral Contraceptive Pill

Generally an estrogen based medication, the OCP can affect your thyroid with an increased level of T4 being produced.

Although they have proven to be extremely convenient and life changing for women in general, there are many downsides to it that remain unknown to the general population taking them.

They include:

- Deplete the body of good gut flora
- Increase the risk of breast and ovarian cancers
- Contribute to osteoporosis
- Increase the risk of blood clots and stroke
- Increases the bodies load of estrogen which interferes with the thyroid transport leading to lower amounts of thyroid hormone getting into our cells
- Lowers folate, Vitamin B12 and Vitamin B6 levels
- Lowers our muscle building ability, resulting in weaker muscles
- Can cause a low libido
- Causes autoimmune issues

Many women take Chaste tree to try and help their hormones however it is important to note that this herb will have no effect while taking the OCP.

Orbital Decompression Surgery

This is a surgery carried out that removes bones and fat in the eye socket mostly in Grave's eye disease.

Generally this 3-4 hour surgery is performed endoscopically (through the nose) and is considered safe and effective and improves quality of life.

Oregano

This lovely aromatic herb found in all our favourite Italian and Greek recipes is amazing at killing the bad guys.

It is anti fungal, antibacterial and an antioxidant so is extremely helpful for restoring bowel and gut flora. It can also be of use when healing from peptic ulcers caused by Helicobacter.

Useful also for bronchial issues, so be sure to throw it into your food liberally at all times.

Ornish, Dean

Dr Ornish was one of the original physicians to treat heart disease and other chronic diseases with a whole foods, plant based diet.

He was the physician to President Bill Clinton after his bypass and continues to advocate good health through this way of eating.

Author of many books including "Eat More, Weigh Less", "UnDo It" and his original book "Dr Dean Ornish's Program for Reversing Heart Disease" he offers many programs on his website to help with changing to a healthy lifestyle. www.ornish.com

Orthomolecular Medicine

Medicine, where the Doctor specialises in using nutritional supplements in treating and correcting diseases.

Often supplements are prescribed but are made up specifically for each patient.

Osteoarthritis

A form of arthritis that occurs mostly in the knees, hips and hands, osteoarthritis is the most common form of arthritis.

Originally thought to be caused by wear and tear it is now believed to be a condition brought about by the joint working to repair itself causing inflammation.

Being overweight, doing repetitive movements such as kneeling, and squatting can contribute to this condition.

Topical Herbs to help with the inflammation are: Arnica, Cayenne, Comfrey, peppermint

Herbs to take internally to help with the inflammation are: Boswellia, Cat's Claw, Celery, Devil's Claw, Ginger, Juniper, Nettle Leaf, Polygonum, Prickly Ash, Rosehip, Turmeric, Willow Bark and Withania

Osteoporosis

An increasingly common condition that causes low bone density, due to a loss of minerals. This then causes fractures which can cause further issues down the line.

Although most people fully get that our bones are losing calcium in this disease it is an easy assumption to jump to “replace the calcium”.

However I am going to say something that can be controversial, however it is true.

The countries with the highest rates of osteoporosis are also the countries with the highest intake of dairy foods.

Hmmmm, so what now?

My understanding from research over the years is simply that osteoporosis develops when our bodies become too acidic. Since our body is a smart cookie, it then looks for something to quickly alkalise it. The most abundant alkaliser we have in our body is calcium from our bones. Was that as big of a shock to you as it was to me when I first discovered it?

So what do we do?

- Remember that bones are made of more than just calcium for a start and we need a lot of other minerals for bone health such as molybdenum, Boron, phosphorous, magnesium, potassium, Vitamin D, and yes, calcium.
- Look for plant based foods that are high in calcium such as sesame seeds, swiss chard, bok choy, beet greens, mustard greens, spinach, and collard greens.
- Engage in weight bearing exercise regularly. The stress on the bones is what helps them to grow.

Also use common sense here. If you have been diagnosed with osteoporosis and you have always eaten dairy foods, perhaps eating more of them is not the answer?

Ovarian Cysts

Cysts that form in the ovaries are extremely common and appear to be caused by excess estrogen.

Generally they are non-cancerous and not painful so often go undiagnosed until they cause an issue.

Ovarian cysts can secrete hormones which cause weight gain and other metabolic issues, so it can be the missing piece of the puzzle for some women.

Anything to do with estrogen and hormones such as endometriosis, fibroids and cysts should all be treated in a way to lower estrogen levels, by removing *xen-estrogenic* foods and balancing hormones.

Herbs that may help to reduce ovarian cysts include: Chaste Tree, False Unicorn Root

Oxalates

A substance found in some foods that when combined with calcium form salts and can crystallise and become stones lodging in our organs.

There are some studies that suggest that people with thyroid disease are unable to process the calcium oxalate compounds and so we have a higher risk of developing stones which may lodge in our thyroid.

Symptoms of excess oxalates include:

- ☐ Joint pain
- ☐ Cystitis (burning with urination)
- ☐ Burning sensation with bowel movements
- ☐ Kidney stones
- ☐ Leaky gut
- ☐ Depression

High oxalate foods include:

- ☐ Dried Fruit, rhubarb, raspberries, oranges, pineapple, dates, figs
- ☐ Buckwheat, wheat berries, rice bran, wheat bran, brown rice, millet, cornmeal
- ☐ Potato, yams, corn, beets, pumpkin, spinach, swiss chard, turnips, parsnips, carrots, celery, green peppers, avocado
- ☐ Legumes, nuts and seeds, soy foods
- ☐ Cocoa (chocolate), black tea, stevia
- ☐ grapefruit juice, carrot juice, rice milk
- ☐ Processed meats

As you can see that is a really large amount of healthy foods so I would only be concerned if you were always exhibiting the burning sensations.

Otherwise, if you are consuming these in a balanced way with other foods, and not having constant burning then continue as you were.

Oxygen

I know we all know what oxygen is, but I have added this because there is an important aspect I want you to know about it.

Diseases such as cancer cannot grow in our body if the cells are well oxygenated. They just can't. Cancer needs a sickly, stale suffocating environment (much like the disease itself right?) to thrive.

So if losing weight or getting fit is not enough of a reason to work up a sweat, maybe avoiding the Big C is?

Here are some ways to oxygenate your body:

- Get plenty of fresh air (a no-brainer I know, but we still need reminding)
- Exercise, particularly aerobic exercise that leaves us puffing and panting thinking we are dying. You know the kind right?
- Walk an hour a day on top of your puffing and panting exercise routine
- Indoor plants help to oxygenate our environment and therefore us.
- Alkalise your body
- Diaphragmatic or Yogic Breathing
- Hydration is important here
- A recent study suggests that a ketogenic diet increases oxygen uptake
- Intermittent fasting

Ozone Therapy

Ozone is a type of oxygen therapy that helps to stop the growth of harmful pathogens such as viruses, bacteria, fungi and yeast. It is an oxygen gas called O3 (Pure oxygen is O2) and it is administered to the body intravenously.

The benefits of ozone therapy include:

- Stimulate the immune system
- Reduce oxidative stress in the body
- Reduce some breathing disorders
- May prevent some types of cancer
- Possibly anti-ageing

For unusual therapies like these, particularly when needles are involved, always research the practitioner thoroughly.

P

Pleasure

I forgot about pleasure as the years went by.

I forgot about dresses that make me feel girly.

I forgot about a hairstyle that made me feel flirty.

Everything I purchased from the clothing store needed two functions only.

Did it fit?

Dit it make me look smaller?

Where is the pleasure in that?

But I also forgot about the pleasure in dancing.

I forgot about the pleasure in laughing.

Many times over the years my husband would force me to dance or sing on the spot and wouldn't let me go about my day until I had. He has always saved me from myself, even when I couldn't see it.

Now I actively search for the pleasure.

I actively look for the moments that make me feel good.

Because when I feel good, when I feel pleasure, I can feel my stress levels lowering, which always makes for better thyroid health.

Paeonia

The root of this plant with the divine flowers is useful for PCOS, endometriosis, fibroids, androgen excess, estrogen excess, memory, concentration and mental performance.

It is a mild skeletal muscle relaxant, anti-inflammatory, cognition enhancer, and estrogen modulator.

Paleo Diet

A way of eating based on our ancestral diet. Foods consumed on this diet include:

- Meats including beef, chicken, lamb etc
- Fish and seafood
- Eggs - free range
- Fruits and vegetables
- Tubers - potatoes, sweet potatoes, yams
- Nuts and seeds
- Healthy fats such as EVOO, Coconut oil
- Salt, herbs and spices

All grains, dairy, legumes and processed and sweet foods are removed from the diet.

Pete Evans is a huge advocate of this lifestyle and has written many books about it, and produced a television series about how to eat this way.

Panaxea

A brand of supplements developed by Daniel Webber, that is based on Traditional Chinese Medicine and other western herbs.

I particularly like the Thyrocaps and Zlim Trim. You will need to see a practitioner to order these though.

Panic Attacks

See Anxiety

Papaya

Papaya or Paw Paw depending on where you are from is an unusual fruit which people generally either love or hate.

Often though the people who say it tastes weird have not had the experience of eating a tree ripened pawpaw.

1 medium papaya will give you:

- ☐ 313% of DVI in Vitamin C (thyroid pathway, adrenals)
- ☐ 29% of DVI in Folate (MTHFR, mental health)
- ☐ 67% of DVI in Vitamin A (thyroid pathway, skin)
- ☐ 8% of DVI in magnesium (stress, sugar)
- ☐ 22% of DVI in potassium (thyroid, fatigue, fluid)
- ☐ 22% of DVI in fibre (hormones, gut health)
- ☐ 11% of DVI in Vitamin E (thyroid pathway, antioxidant)
- ☐ 10% of DVI in Vitamin K (bones, blood)
- ☐ 7% of DVI in Calcium (bones)
- ☐ 2% of DVI in Iron (thyroid pathway)
- ☐ 2% of DVI in Manganese (thyroid pathway)
- ☐ 3% of DVI in Selenium (thyroid pathway)
- ☐ 1% of DVI in Zinc (thyroid, mental health, immunity, wound healing)
- ☐ 5% of DVI in Vitamin B1 (thyroid, hair)
- ☐ 6% of DVI in Vitamin B2 (thyroid pathway)
- ☐ 5% of DVI in Vitamin B3 (mental health)
- ☐ 3% of DVI in Vitamin B6 (mental health, progesterone)
- ☐ Trace amounts of almost all the Amino Acids

Papaya also is said to:

- ☐ Prevent cholesterol oxidation
- ☐ Lower cholesterol levels
- ☐ Dry up mucus
- ☐ Helps heal skin issues such as eczema and psoriasis
- ☐ Soothes the gut
- ☐ Anti-viral and anti-inflammatory
- ☐ The seeds are anti-parasitic

So, who's ready to try some pawpaw with a drizzle of passionfruit or lime juice?? I can highly recommend both ways!

Papillary Carcinomas

The most common form of cancer of the thyroid

Parafollicular Cells

One of two cells in the thyroid gland. Parafollicular cells secrete calcitonin which help balance calcium levels.

Parathyroid Gland

Four very small glands located on the thyroid (2 on each lobe) that produce parathyroid hormone (PTH).

Their job is to measure calcium in the blood and secrete the appropriate amount of PTH to keep calcium balanced.

Partial Thyroidectomy

See lobectomy

Passionflower

An herb useful for sleep or insomnia issues along with anxiety, irritability, nervousness, tension headaches, tachycardia and palpitations.

It is a mild sedative, anxiolytic, hypnotic and spasmolytic.

Pau D'Arco

This is the first herb I researched at length when I suffered from candida. It is actually a bark and has incredible antibacterial, anti parasitic, anti fungal, anti tumour and immune enhancing properties.

Used mostly for candida and parasites it is also often used as a side therapy for cancer.

Avoid in pregnancy and when taking blood thinners such as warfarin.

PCOS

Polycystic Ovary Syndrome (PCOS) is one of the most common female hormonal disorders

It presents as

- ☐ elevated insulin
- ☐ menstrual irregularity
- ☐ excess hair growth
- ☐ acne
- ☐ obesity
- ☐ elevated testosterone
- ☐ multiple ovarian cysts

Treatment includes:

- ☐ Low sugar diet
- ☐ Diabetes medication
- ☐ Birth control pills

Herbs that may help include: Black Cohosh, Chaste Tree, Gymnema, Licorice, Paeonia, Thuja, and tribulus Leaf

Pears

This ordinary, often left out fruit has a tonne of goodness for our thyroid health.

1 medium Pear contains:

- ☐ 10% of DV in Vitamin C
- ☐ 9% of DV in Vitamin K
- ☐ 22% of DV in Fibre
- ☐ 4% of DV in Vitamin B2 (thyroid pathway)
- ☐ 3% of DV in Vitamin B6 (mental health)
- ☐ 3% of DV in Folate (MTHFR & Liver)
- ☐ 1% of DV in Vitamin E (thyroid pathway)
- ☐ 2% of DV in Calcium (thyroid & bones)
- ☐ 3% of DV in Magnesium (stress & sugar)
- ☐ 5% of DV in Manganese (thyroid pathway)
- ☐ 6% of DV in Potassium (thyroid health)
- ☐ 2% of DV in Zinc (immune & Healing)
- ☐ 17% of DV in Copper
- ☐ Promote cardiovascular health
- ☐ Promote Colon health

- Is hypoallergenic, so great for people with sensitivities
- Settle an upset tummy
- Quenches Thirst
- Decrease risk of Diabetes Type 2
- Are anti-inflammatory
- Improve Insulin Resistance
- Helps the body retain calcium, so helps prevent osteoporosis

I love pears with porridge (oats have a different gliadin molecule to other glutinous grains so some people like me are fine with it)

I also love it stewed and of course fresh dipped in peanut butter.

Pedal Edema

Fluid retention (edema) in the lower legs and feet.

Pendred Syndrome

A condition characterised by a large goiter and being deaf/mute.

Caused by insufficient thyroid hormone production combined with inner ear dysfunction.

Pepsin

The main digestive enzyme in the stomach. It breaks down protein.

Peppermint

This wonderfully scented common herb is one we should just automatically throw into any food or drink we can think of.

It has an amazing list of actions such as spasmolytic (calms spasms), carminative (calming to the nervous system), cholagogue (helps release bile from the gallbladder), antiemetic (stop vomiting), antitussive (calm coughs), antimicrobial (kills bugs), mild sedative, topical analgesic (pain relief), topical antipruritic (stops itching).

With this array of actions it is useful in IBS, Gall bladder dysfunction, nausea, tummy bugs, cough's cold's and flu's, and also nice and mild flavour for little ones with colic.

Why wouldn't you want to get used to drinking peppermint tea or growing it in your garden with all of those actions??

Perfume

I love perfume!

BUT... where do we spray it? Usually straight onto our neck where it soaks directly into our thyroids.

The problem with that is most perfumes contain endocrine disruptors which can harm our thyroid and interfere with its hormone production.

As an alternative, try pure essential oils as a perfume.

Or if you must spray your favourite Channel or Miss Dior then spray it onto your clothing instead of your skin.

Perimenopause

The transition period to menopause.

Pernicious Anemia

Caused by a lack of Intrinsic Factor in the gut which is required to make Vitamin B12.

People without Intrinsic Factor need Vitamin B12 injections for life.

Phosphorous

Phosphorus is required ink the body for:

- bone growth and mineralisation
- calcium balance
- energy metabolism
- energy production
- activates B-Vitamins
- muscle contraction

Deficiency Symptoms of Phosphorus include:

- anxiety, irritability, apprehension, chronic fatigue, nervous disorders, general malaise

- vertigo, rickets, cardiac arrhythmias
- muscle weakness, shallow breathing,

Factors that contribute to Phosphorus deficiency:

- excess calcium, excess coffee, excess antacids
- malabsorption, gluten sensitivity
- pregnancy, growth, lactation, premature birth

Food sources of Phosphorus include:

- almonds, cashews, sesame seeds
- beef, chicken, eggs, offal, salmon, sardines, tuna
- cheese, milk, chickpeas

Daily Requirements of Phosphorus:

- Adults 800 mg

Pineal gland

A tiny gland in the brain that regulates melatonin, the sleep hormone.

Pineapple

Pineapple is loaded with manganese which is a cofactor in the making of thyroxine.

Manganese also facilitates bone formation, carbohydrate metabolism, blood clotting, lipid metabolism, smooth muscle relaxation, and improves the integrity of the mitochondria which is our energy centres.

1 cup of Pineapple contains:

- 11% of DV in Vitamin B1 (thyroid, hair)
- 4% of DV in Vitamin B2 (thyroid pathway)
- 5% of DV in Vitamin B3 (mental health)
- 11% of DV in Vitamin B6 (blood & bones)
- 7% of DV in Folate (MTHFR, mental health)
- 105% of DV in Vitamin C (adrenal Health)
- 2% of DV in Calcium (bones)

- ☐ 20% of DV in Copper (skin, collagen, nerves)
- ☐ 3% of DV in Iron (thyroid pathway)
- ☐ 5% of DV in Magnesium (stress, sugar)
- ☐ 77% of DV in Manganese (thyroid pathway)
- ☐ 2% of DV in Phosphorus (liver, bones)
- ☐ 5% of DV in Potassium (thyroid, fatigue, fluid)
- ☐ 2% of DV in Zinc (immunity, thyroid, wound healing, mental health)
- ☐ 9% of DV in Fibre (hormones, gut health)
- ☐ 2% of DV in Protein (thyroid pathway)

This makes pineapple

- ☐ Anti-inflammatory
- ☐ Anti-viral
- ☐ Antioxidant
- ☐ May protect against macular degeneration
- ☐ Helpful in reducing joint & muscle pain

So have you ever tried a pineapple smoothie?? Literally just cut up an entire pineapple and whack it into a high-speed blender. Don't add anything to it, except maybe some mint and you have a thyroid winner!! Be careful though if you have blood sugar issues with this one.

Pituitary Gland

The gland in the brain that directs the thyroid to make hormones by producing Thyroid Stimulating Hormone (TSH). It is also involved in breast growth, milk production, skin pigmentation, body growth and metabolism.

Plantar Fasciitis

Inflammation in the soles of the feet, often worse in the morning causing pain to walk.

PNS

Parasympathetic Nervous System.

When this kicks in we are in Rest & Digest mode.

Pollution

Liver disease is so common now and it is easy to see why. As the central processor of all our toxins, chemicals & hormones, our liver has quite a job to keep on top of it all.

Not only do we all eat food full of chemicals, fruit and vegetables that have been sprayed with chemicals, but all we have to do is go outside and breathe and our poor liver has to deal with pollution as well.

So the people and clients that have said to me over the years "I eat very cleanly, my liver is fine" I have always asked this "So, do you breathe?"

Let's take a really simple example.

We (mostly) all live somewhere near at least one car, tractor, truck or vehicle with wheels right? Well, every time someone hits the brakes in that vehicle the substance Cadmium is released into the air and we breathe it in. you can read more about cadmium under that entry, but let's just say it has a huge affect on our hormones.

And that is just one example.

I am a realist though. I understand it's not possible to move house or change jobs or go live on an uninhabited island somewhere. More power to you if you can!

So what do we do? We change what we physically and financially can, and try not to stress about the rest.

Need examples:

- ☐ Use plants to clean the air inside our home
- ☐ Buy a fancy air filtration unit for home
- ☐ Don't use chemicals for cleaning
- ☐ Don't use fly sprays or fragrance sprays
- ☐ Remove shoes before entering the house
- ☐ Eat unsprayed or organic foods where possible
- ☐ Detox regularly
- ☐ Get back into nature on holidays and weekends

If we don't already do any of these things then changing just one of them will have a huge impact on our health.

Polygonum Cuspidatum

An anti ageing rhizome... have I got your attention?

This little beauty (see what I did there?) is an antioxidant, anti inflammatory, antitumor and anti ageing.

It helps with osteoarthritis and rheumatoid arthritis, metabolic syndrome and preventing cardiovascular disease as well as slowing down the ageing process due to its high levels of resveratrol.

Polygonum Multiflorum

Like its sister rhizome, this processed root also slows the ageing process and I have found is a common ingredient in hair products to reverse greying.

It helps to calm the nerves, improves fatigue, is an antioxidant, reduces high cholesterol, strengthens connective tissue, and is used also with tinnitus and dizziness.

Pomegranate

Whilst they are quite messy to get into, they are so worth it. They are a little bit sweet and a little bit tart and go perfectly sprinkled on top of salads (which will make you look like a chef).

1 medium 4"pomegranate contains:

- ☐ 48% of DV in Vitamin C (thyroid pathway, adrenals)
- ☐ 8% of DV in Vitamin E (thyroid pathway, antioxidant)
- ☐ 58% of DV in Vitamin K (blood, bones)
- ☐ 13% of DV in Vitamin B1 (thyroid, hair)
- ☐ 9% of DV in Vitamin B2 (thyroid pathway)
- ☐ 4% of DV in Vitamin B3 (mental health)
- ☐ 11% of DV in Vitamin B6 (mental health, progesterone)
- ☐ 27% of DV in folate (mental health, liver)
- ☐ 3% of DV in Calcium (bones)
- ☐ 5% of DV in Iron (thyroid, fatigue, gut acid)
- ☐ 8% of DV in Magnesium (stress, sugar)
- ☐ 10% of DV in Phosphorus (bones, liver)
- ☐ 19% of DV in Potassium (thyroid, fluid, fatigue)
- ☐ 7% of DV in Zinc (immunity, thyroid, wound healing, mental health)
- ☐ 22% of DV in Copper (skin, nerves, collagen)
- ☐ 17% of DV in Manganese (thyroid pathway)
- ☐ 2% of DV in Selenium (thyroid pathway)
- ☐ 45% of DV in Fibre (hormonal clearance, gut health)
- ☐ 7% of DV in Protein (thyroid pathway)

This all adds up to:

- ☐ Fight Cancer
- ☐ Reduce Arthritis
- ☐ Improve heart health
- ☐ Reduce Joint Pain
- ☐ Improve Memory
- ☐ Improve gut flora
- ☐ Lower bacterial infections
- ☐ Extremely high in antioxidants
- ☐ Improves weight management
- ☐ Lower cholesterol
- ☐ Reduce the risk of stroke
- ☐ Immune support
- ☐ Prevents constipation
- ☐ Improves Digestion
- ☐ Improves fatigue

Postpartum Thyroiditis

A presentation of hyperthyroidism followed by hypothyroidism and then returns to normal or stays at hypothyroid after the birth of a child.

Potassium

It is estimated that over 30% of the population are deficient in potassium. While it is not required directly in the thyroid pathway, it is required for great thyroid health and wellbeing.

Potassium is required for:

- ☐ Blood pressure control & regulation
- ☐ Smooth muscle function
- ☐ Muscle contraction
- ☐ Nerve & heart function
- ☐ Hydration
- ☐ Regulation of pH
- ☐ Fluid balance

Deficiency Symptoms of Potassium include:

- ☐ Acid pH
- ☐ Bone & joint pain
- ☐ Oedema (fluid retention in cells)
- ☐ Cognitive issues
- ☐ Constipation
- ☐ Continuous thirst
- ☐ Depression
- ☐ Dry skin
- ☐ Fatigue
- ☐ Headaches
- ☐ High Blood Pressure (caused by salt)
- ☐ Insomnia
- ☐ Irregular heart beat
- ☐ Irritability
- ☐ Muscle weakness
- ☐ Rheumatoid arthritis
- ☐ Stroke
- ☐ Tachycardia

Factors that contribute to Potassium deficiency:

- ☐ Adrenal tumours, stress
- ☐ Cortisone Therapy
- ☐ Diabetes
- ☐ Diuretics
- ☐ Excess salt, coffee, tea, alcohol & sugar
- ☐ High Blood Pressure
- ☐ Liver Disease
- ☐ Malnutrition

Food sources of Potassium include:

- ☐ 1 cup beet greens = 37% DV
- ☐ 1 cup swiss chard = 27% DV
- ☐ 1 cup beetroot = 15% DV
- ☐ 1 cup sweet potato = 27% DV

- ☐ 1 cup white potato = 26% DV
- ☐ 1 cup lentils = 21% DV
- ☐ 1 cup avocado = 21% DV
- ☐ 1 medium banana = 12%DV
- ☐ 1 cup green peas = 11% DV
- ☐ 1 cup onions = 10% DV
- ☐ 1 cup kidney beans = 20% DV
- ☐ 1 cup carrots = 11% DV
- ☐ 1 cup tomatoes = 12% DV
- ☐ 1 cup asparagus = 12% DV
- ☐ 1 cup Romaine/Cos = 7% DV
- ☐ 1 medium Papaya = 14% DV

Daily Requirements of Potassium:

- ☐ Adults - 2-5 g

Prebiotics

Prebiotics are the food source of probiotics.

Many years ago I watched a program on the BBC where they were testing which had better results on gut flora: taking probiotics or feeding the existing gut probiotics with prebiotic food.

They took a group of cowboys who were all in the same environment (breathing the same microbes etc) and gave half a daily dose of probiotics and fed the other half a diet rich in the prebiotic fibre called Inulin.

Foods rich in Inulin include:

- ☐ Jerusalem Artichoke
- ☐ Garlic
- ☐ Onions & Leeks
- ☐ Asparagus
- ☐ Dandelion Greens
- ☐ Chicory Root
- ☐ Apples & Apple Cider Vinegar
- ☐ Seaweed
- ☐ Flaxseeds

Can you guess which group came out with the highest count of good guys in their poop at the end of the trial???

Yep, prebiotics, which shows that food is more powerful than supplements if you are consistent.

Probiotics

Probiotics is an umbrella term for the many strains of bacteria we need in our gut for healthy gut function.

As discussed under prebiotics, it is far more beneficial to feed our existing good bacteria than it is to add probiotics in on top.

However there are some specific strains that are useful for specific purposes.

- ☐ L.Rhamnosus - Gut support, eczema
- ☐ L.Plantarum - Inflammation
- ☐ L.Casei - Brain function, diarrhoea
- ☐ L. Acidophilus - vaginal health, diarrhoea, acne
- ☐ B. Lactis - obesity, immunity
- ☐ B.Breve - skin, weight loss, allergies
- ☐ B.Bifidum - stress, infections, gut health
- ☐ B.Longum - immunity, liver, cholesterol
- ☐ B.Infantis - immunity, Gut health
- ☐ B.Animalis - obesity, immunity

Working with a naturopath the specialises in gut health would be beneficial if you are needing specific strains of probiotics.

Processed Foods

It doesn't take a genius to know that we should not be eating the likes of takeaway food daily. A treat? Sure! But even weekly would be a stretch unless your thyroid symptoms are completely under control.

Processed foods however are a grey area, because most of us don't understand exactly what they are.

Reading the section on gluten will help you further understand why we must always know what a processed food is.

Here are some examples:

- ☐ Baked Potato = Whole Food
- ☐ Mashed Potato = Processed Food
- ☐ Corn Cob = Whole Food
- ☐ 100% Corn Tortilla = Processed Food
- ☐ Juicy Apple = Whole Food
- ☐ Apple Juice = Processed Food
- ☐ Brown Rice = Whole Food
- ☐ Rice Noodles = Processed Food

Do you see what I mean? It doesn't have to be unhealthy to still be processed, and while most of these healthy processed foods our body knows what to do with, obviously it is much more efficient at dealing with the whole food.

Because our body is already compromised, the more we can eat whole foods, the more energy our body has on healing what needs to be healed.

I would love to say these are the only kinds of processed foods we all eat, but the fact is they are not. It's so easy now to pick up a fully prepared Indian meal in the supermarket and heat it at home, or grab half price Lean Cuisine's for the week at work, but these meals are full of numbers and additives and are more types of processed meals we are consuming now.

Our thyroid is a magnet to chemicals and toxins, so any harmful numbers or additives in those meals could be damaging our health further, making it that much harder to feel better which is the goal right?

Of course we will always use processed foods in some way. It is our lifestyle now after all, and we are all busy and looking for what is quick and easy. But if we can cook from scratch 80% of the time then our body and thyroid will thank us for it.

Progesterogenic

An agent used to improve progesterone levels.

Example: Chaste Tree

Progesterone

Progesterone is an anti-cancer hormone

If we have high oestrogen levels, you can safely assume you have low progesterone levels, as it is the progesterone in the second half of your cycle (after ovulation) that kicks out the oestrogen. Progesterone opposes oestrogen

When we are in overdrive the body diverts progesterone to the adrenals to help support cortisol production. This leads to excess estrogen and low progesterone for the reproductive cycle.

For healthy progesterone levels (particularly after menopause) you need healthy adrenals which are usually out of balance if you have a thyroid problem. I know it seems like everything is working against you, but look at it in the way that everything is linked, so by improving one thing we will improve another and so on. I have always seen my health as a set of domino's, once I get one thing sorted it will have a domino effect on the rest, and that is essentially how it is going to date. Everything seems to be improving together rather than one thing at a time.

Also don't forget that Oestrogen is stronger than progesterone, so working on liver health (which is what processes and eliminates bad oestrogen) needs to be a day after day battle. It takes a long time, so don't think 1 bottle of supplements will do the job. Your liver has to deal with all toxins, chemicals, hormones etc so needs daily help.

Progesterone boosting nutrients:

- [ ] Vitamin C
- [ ] Vitamin B6
- [ ] Vitamin E
- [ ] Zinc
- [ ] Magnesium
- [ ] Coconut oil
- [ ] Indole-3-carbinol
- [ ] B vitamins
- [ ] Omega 3s

Prozac

Prozac is also called Fluoxetine. And the FLUO is the big alarm bell for us thyroid people. The Fluo means it is a fluoride based medication.

Regardless of the need for it (I'm not disputing some need this medication) it will have an affect on the thyroid due to it's fluoride content which blocks iodine in the thyroid.

Add to that, any synthetic medication builds up in the liver, which we need to activate 70% of our thyroid hormone then we are clearly in trouble if we are taking prozac regularly.

Now, I'm not sure what the answer is to those that need it, however, one thing is for certain, anyone on this, MUST keep a close eye on their thyroid health and do everything possible to counteract the medication by detoxing the liver.

Here is a warning though. It is NEVER wise to go cold turkey on removing medication of any kind, without supervision. And it is NEVER wise to detox from such medication without supervision. There are 2 reasons for this.

- It may have serious consequences on the mind or body if we are without the medication.
- Detoxing suddenly from a medication may send the store we have of it in our liver gushing into our bloodstream which can cause an overdose.

I guess the moral of this story is that we must always know the ingredients of our medications and what the effects may be on us and our thyroid health, and go in with our eyes open.

We don't have to disagree with our doctor, but if something is NEEDED for our own health and wellbeing , then a conversation should be had as to how this can be done with the least possible harm to our thyroid and liver.

PUFAS

PUFAs which are polyunsaturated oils is hijack the thyroid hormone transport protein which means there is no room for thyroid hormone to get on board. Resulting in lowered thyroid hormone actually getting into our cells where it is needed.

These oils include:

- canola, safflower, hydrogenated vegetable, vegetable, rapeseed, margarine, corn, sunflower, soybean, cottonseed, rice bran, grapeseed, peanut, wheatgerm, linseed, flaxseed, vegetable shortening, trans fats

Pulmonary Edema

Fluid in the spaces of the lungs. It is a symptom of congestive heart failure.

Pump Soap

Commercial pump soap (so I am not talking about organic here) contains lots of ingredients that the thyroid doesn't like - particularly Triclosan.

Triclosan is a known endocrine disruptor and our thyroid is part of the endocrine system. So not only does this ingredient harm the thyroid and suppress it, but it also does harm to the other endocrine organs which are the Adrenals, Parathyroids, Reproductive organs, Hypothalamus, Pituitary, Pineal Gland and the Pancreas.

So this is just a simple way of removing some excess load on your thyroid and endocrine system. Remember that, little things we do every day add up - both the good and the bad. So while washing our hands once in a while at a public bathroom won't hurt, if we are washing them many times a day at home, day in and day out, then that can be a problem.

Purgative

A substance that causes an evacuation of the bowel.

Q

Quitter

I am not a quitter.

There may be times in my life where I decide that whatever protocol I am following or strategy I am using to improve my thyroid health is not getting me anywhere, but I don't just quit.

First I make sure I have followed the strategy or program for at least 4-6 weeks to get a good sense of how it is affecting me. I diarise everything during this time.

If at the end of that time, I feel that I am honestly better suited to something different, and not just giving up because it is hard, then I make the choice to "Archive" that program or protocol for a possible later date.

Sometimes I never go back to it, other times I may rediscover it many years later only to find that it now is making a difference. Maybe my gut health or liver health has improved enough that the protocol is effective now where it wasn't before.

Everything I do is strategic with my thyroid health, so quitting is just not a part of it. Taking on that mentality serves no-one.

So my advice to you is to never quit. Take a break when you need to, archive as much as you have to, re-evaluate, re-strategize and go again. You are so worth it.

Quick Weight Loss

This is actually really dangerous which is why it needed its own section.

Our fat cells contain hormones, toxins, heavy metals and other pathogens because our body thinks it is a wise place to keep them. And it is.

But when we lose weight quickly those toxins get released into an already overburdened body and our liver has to cope with processing them.

Since our liver is also generally not doing as well as it should, this can cause a back up of toxins or a recycling of them.

Many times women have reported getting breast cancer after a massive weight loss. They say how happy they are that because they lost weight they were able to detect the lump, but the theory is out there that it was the weight loss that actually caused the cancer.

Now, I am not saying don't lose weight, what I am saying is, that quick weight loss in any way needs to be accompanied with a helping hand for the liver to process this huge burden.

QiGong

An holistic form of movement similar to Tai Chi that combines meditation, controlled breathing and certain movements to improve mind, body and soul pathways.

It has been around for over 2,000 years and helps the body and mind find its balance, but also increases flexibility and strength.

Quitting

Quitting something is a tough thing to do, but the most important start is to get your mindset right.

It doesn't matter if you are quitting smoking, sugar or a bad relationship, getting in the right mindset is the key to taking the first step, and is what will keep you getting back up when you stumble.

Because you will stumble. That is completely normal. Here are some tips:

- Knowing your "why" is a great start. Write it in big letters and plaster it anywhere you can see it.
- If it is a food item you are quitting find out the nutrients you need. For example if you are quitting sugar, you will need magnesium to help you through the cravings.
- Ask for help. You don't need to do this alone, so don't be scared to ask whomever you need to, family, friends, practitioners.

There is a kinesiology exercise that is great for quitting which helps break through blocks you didn't realise you had.

It is called 70 x 7 and this is what you do:

- ☐ Everyday write your issue 70 times followed by whatever comes to mind when you write it.
- ☐ Do this everyday for 7 days.

For example:

- ☐ I want to quit sugar
- ☐ But I love sugar
- ☐ I want to quit sugar
- ☐ But I don't think I can
- ☐ I want to quit sugar
- ☐ I love cake too much
- ☐ I want to quit sugar
- ☐ I could lose weight if I did

So you get the idea. It doesn't matter what comes up, good or bad, write it down. Often you will repeat things, that's ok, other times you may be stuck. I have found this process reveals things I didn't know I was resistant about.

Give it a go if you are quitting anything!

R

Routines

Most of us struggle with some kind of brain fog either in spurts or almost daily. When we are in the throws of complete confusion and brain fog, the way through it is having routines in place that your brain knows so well, that you can operate on auto pilot.

Have you ever driven home from work and then realise in horror as you pull into your driveway that you don't remember any detail of your trip home? That happened because your brain knows your routine and while you were zoning out thinking about the workmate that stole your lunch, it took you home.

Routines are different to habits though. Routines are a familiar way of doing things. So you may have a morning routine that involves 5 habits in a particular order.

Many successful people swear by having a morning routine, so can you imagine what you could get done if you had your own routine that kicked in regardless of what head space you are in?

Another advantage of routines are for the times when mental health issues are dragging us down. Due to the high number of T3 receptors in our brain, it is the first to suffer when there is not enough thyroid hormone to go around, leading to depression, anxiety, panic attacks and brain fog.

When these times hit, having a routine to follow can be the one thing that keeps our head above water.

Racing Heart

See Tachycardia

Radioactive Iodine

The thyroid soaks up iodine, so radioactive iodine was developed as a way to destroy the thyroid, kind of like a trojan horse. It is used for thyroid cancers and Graves Disease and is usually given in pill form.

Radioactive Thyroid Tests

Although it sounds like it has something to do with radioactive iodine, it is not, and is simply a type of test used to diagnose thyroid disease.

This involves the ingestion (swelling) of a radiotracer to give specific information about the thyroid including shape, size and function.

It is more often used for hyperthyroidism.

Raw Food Diet

The Raw Food Diet exploded into our lives about a decade ago, as an answer to every health issue or disease around.

It involves only eating raw fruits, vegetables, nuts and seeds.

Like any diet, often it is the removal of all the bad stuff that has the greatest effect on the outcome, but any diet that encourages a larger consumption of plant food has to be good.

One of the things I love about the Raw Food cuisine is their desserts. A raw "cheesecake" can be made from nuts and fruits and taken to a dinner party with no one suspecting it is a health food. They are so good!

Receding Gums

Due to the dry mouth issues that both kinds of thyroid disease can experience, receding gums can be an issue. It is a must for anyone with thyroid disease, to have regular dental checkups. Just say no the fluoride treatments ok?

Rebounding

The one exercise I have always enjoyed is rebounding.

It is also known as a mini-trampoline or in the 80s it was called a lymphasizer, because that is what it does - moves our lymph around our body.

It is easy on the joints and you can plonk it down in front of the television, bouncing away while you watch your favourite show.

Favoured by NASA, rebounding has a remarkable ability to strengthen all cells and organs in the body due to the force of gravity. Many people who have lost weight with no excess skin, say that it was due to the rebounding they did daily.

I personally use a Bellicon Rebounder which is known as the Rolls Royce of rebounders, but for 20 years I used cheap ones so start with what you can afford.

Referred Pain

Pain that is originated in one part of the body, but presents itself in another part of the body.

Examples:

- Lung and diaphragm - left side of the shoulder and neck
- Liver and gallbladder - right side of the shoulder and neck
- Heart - left side of the chest and down the underside of the left arm, also between the shoulder blades in the middle of the back
- Kidney - lower half of the trunk front and back to half way down the thighs

I find this fascinating and a whole new way of looking at pain, and hearing what our body is trying to tell us.

There are a lot of images on Google that will show you diagrams of this.

Reflexology

I did a semester of this when I was studying naturopathy and it is amazing. It involves massaging different zones on the feet and the benefits are felt in corresponding organs.

A really experienced reflexologist can even pick up on diseases developing before you know about them.

The spot for the thyroid is on the inside edge of the big toes. So if you just massage your hole big toe and down a little bit, you will stimulate it.

Reflux

Acid reflux is essentially gut acid coming back up the esophagus where it does not belong. It causes pain, burning, discomfort and anxiety.

See GERD

Rehmannia

The root of a plant useful for adrenal fatigue, autoimmune disease, rheumatoid arthritis, asthma, urticaria, chronic nephritis and constipation.

It is an adrenal tonic, anti-inflammatory, antihemorrhagic and antipyretic.

Reiki

A modality that involves hands on healing (although usually the hands are hovering not so much touching) and transferring energy from the practitioner to the patient.

It is said to promote peace, balance, harmony, dissolve emotional blocks and release stress and tension in the body.

Reishi

This mushroom is often used as a side therapy with treating cancer due to its immune modulating qualities.

Useful during chemotherapy, radiotherapy, immune deficiency, chronic infections, chronic fatigue, fibromyalgia, convalescence, and autoimmune disease.

For those with Hashimoto's or Graves, it might be a good one to use fresh in food on a regular basis, if you can get a hold of it.

Restless Leg Syndrome

The first time I experienced this sensation I was at a comedy show with friends. We were sitting right in the middle of a large row in the theatre and all I can remember is the incredibly uncomfortable feeling of just needing to get up and run and move.

Its official name is Willis-Ekbom Disease and while symptoms tend to be in the early evening, they can become extremely severe at night.

It is related to the following:

- ☐ Levothyroxine (yes our medication may be the cause)
- ☐ iron deficiency (common in thyroid conditions)
- ☐ medications such as antidepressants, antipsychotics, antihistamines, and antinausea drugs
- ☐ nerve damage
- ☐ alcohol, cigarettes and coffee
- ☐ end stage kidney failure

Herbs that can help include: Butcher's Broom, Ginkgo, Gotu Kola, Horsechestnut, Kava, Mexican Valerian, Prickly Ash, Valerian

Other treatments to consider may be Acupuncture, TENS (transcutaneous electrical nerve stimulation), addressing any of the above possibilities and making sure magnesium and potassium levels are optimal.

Resveratrol

The anti-ageing nutrient, resveratrol helps with:

- ☐ inflammation
- ☐ lipid oxidation (LDL Cholesterol)
- ☐ improves liver detoxification
- ☐ protects the heart
- ☐ induces cell death in some cancers

It is used therapeutically for:

- ☐ Ageing, high fat diets,
- ☐ Alzheimers
- ☐ atherosclerosis, metabolic syndrome, cardiac hypertrophy
- ☐ prevention of colon, liver, pancreas, prostate, stomach and thyroid cancer
- ☐ nephrotic syndrome

Reverse T3

Reverse T3 (RT3) is a form of thyroid hormone the body cannot use, but acts as a T3 blocker.

Since T3 is our active hormone and for us to use it and feel well it has to be inside our cells (not just floating around in the blood where tests can detect it) then it needs an easy entry into our cells.

When we are stressed in any way, physically, mentally, emotionally, then our body produces RT3 to act as a guard outside our cells.

RTs's job is to stop T3 entering the cell. Why would it want to do that? In our body's attempt at keeping us safe while we are under stress, it slows down all the systems our thyroid runs such as the metabolic system so that we will essentially go back to bed and hibernate until the danger passes.

Since we all live with some form of stress (if you don't, please call me so I can learn how you do it) this can have a huge effect on thyroid function.

Selenium has the ability to downgrade RT3, so it is something we need to be either taking or consuming in foods rich in this mineral on a permanent basis.

Rhodiola

An herb that is useful for immune deficiency, emaciation, physical stress, fatigue, mental performance, concentration and memory, chronic fatigue syndrome, fibromyalgia and post virals.

It is an adaptogenic, antioxidant and antitumor.

Riedel's Thyroiditis

Chronic inflammation and scarring of the thyroid causing fibrosis. It can spread to surrounding tissues.

It is a rare inflammatory disease and only about 30% of people end up with thyroid disease. It is treated with prednisolone and may require surgery.

Rolfing

A complementary modality that uses soft tissue manipulation to ease pain and stress. It is aimed at realigning the body and improving its function. If you can imagine it looks like a massage, but with more specific movements that help release the fascia around our muscles .

Romaine Lettuce

Romaine Lettuce is also known as Cos Lettuce and is the most nutrient dense of all the lettuces and the darker the green leaves the more goodies inside.

2 cups of Romaine Lettuce contains:

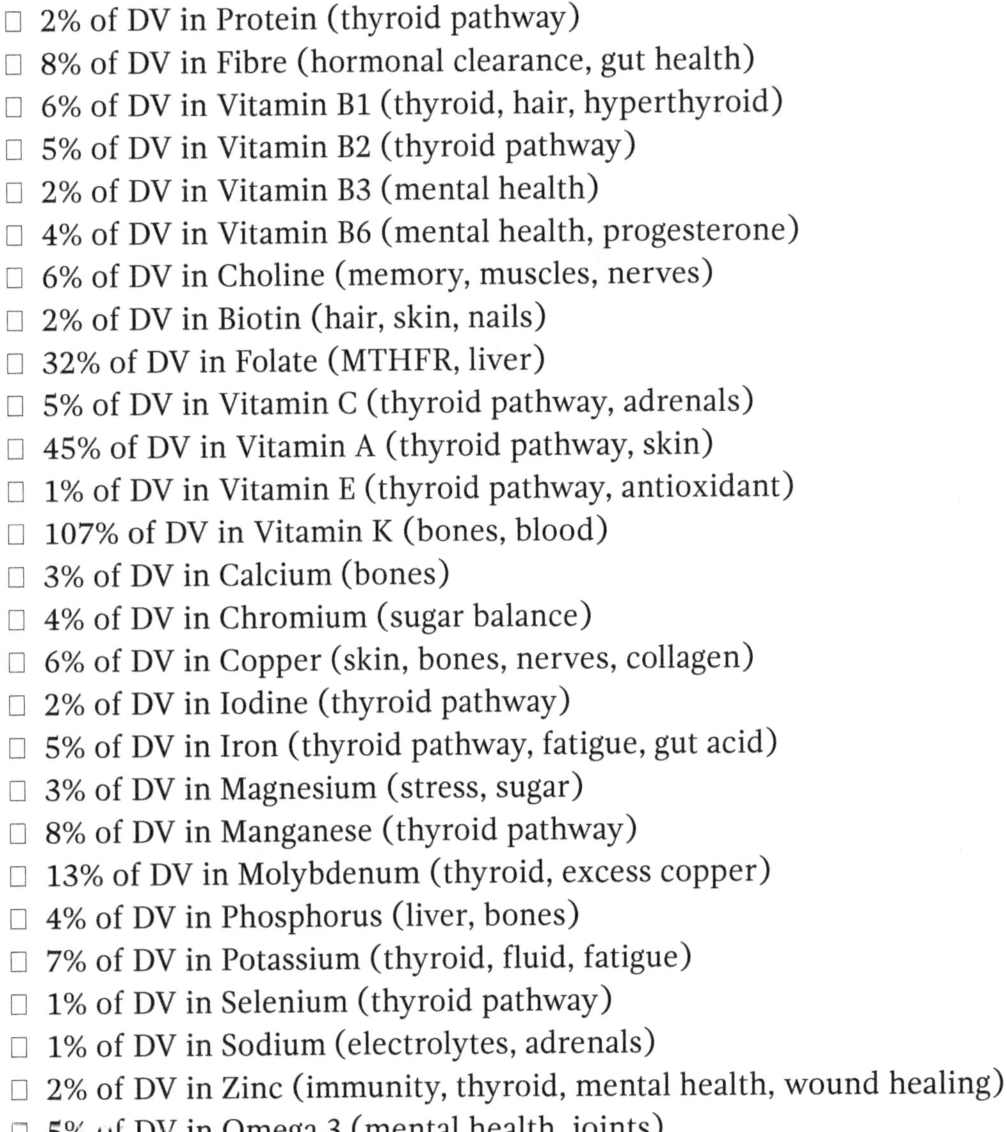

- ☐ 2% of DV in Protein (thyroid pathway)
- ☐ 8% of DV in Fibre (hormonal clearance, gut health)
- ☐ 6% of DV in Vitamin B1 (thyroid, hair, hyperthyroid)
- ☐ 5% of DV in Vitamin B2 (thyroid pathway)
- ☐ 2% of DV in Vitamin B3 (mental health)
- ☐ 4% of DV in Vitamin B6 (mental health, progesterone)
- ☐ 6% of DV in Choline (memory, muscles, nerves)
- ☐ 2% of DV in Biotin (hair, skin, nails)
- ☐ 32% of DV in Folate (MTHFR, liver)
- ☐ 5% of DV in Vitamin C (thyroid pathway, adrenals)
- ☐ 45% of DV in Vitamin A (thyroid pathway, skin)
- ☐ 1% of DV in Vitamin E (thyroid pathway, antioxidant)
- ☐ 107% of DV in Vitamin K (bones, blood)
- ☐ 3% of DV in Calcium (bones)
- ☐ 4% of DV in Chromium (sugar balance)
- ☐ 6% of DV in Copper (skin, bones, nerves, collagen)
- ☐ 2% of DV in Iodine (thyroid pathway)
- ☐ 5% of DV in Iron (thyroid pathway, fatigue, gut acid)
- ☐ 3% of DV in Magnesium (stress, sugar)
- ☐ 8% of DV in Manganese (thyroid pathway)
- ☐ 13% of DV in Molybdenum (thyroid, excess copper)
- ☐ 4% of DV in Phosphorus (liver, bones)
- ☐ 7% of DV in Potassium (thyroid, fluid, fatigue)
- ☐ 1% of DV in Selenium (thyroid pathway)
- ☐ 1% of DV in Sodium (electrolytes, adrenals)
- ☐ 2% of DV in Zinc (immunity, thyroid, mental health, wound healing)
- ☐ 5% of DV in Omega 3 (mental health, joints)

Who would have thought there was so much in lettuce? Even Omega 3, iron and iodine?

Romaine also has astringent qualities to it, which means it helps dry up water and excess fluid in our body, perfect for thyroid conditions.

This is one that should be added to our daily diet, and if looking for a kale swap out, then this is the one for you!

Rosehip

A berry that is useful for vitamin C deficiency, osteoarthritis, gastritis, diarrhoea, thyroid disease, irregular heartbeat and Urinary Tract Infections,

It is anti-inflammatory, antioxidant and an astringent.

Rosemary

A common household herb with so many useful indications and tastes so good with potatoes.

Rosemary is amazing for mental health and hormone health and also contains a good smattering of vitamins and minerals and Essential Fatty Acids.

The attributes of Rosemary include:

- Carminative, Spasmolytic, Antioxidant
- Anti-microbial, Circulatory Stimulant, Hepatoprotective (liver protector)
- Improves memory, concentration, mental performance
- enhances Liver detoxification (the hormone pathway)
- Helps prevent CVD, improves tension headaches
- improves hair loss symptoms
- Has a similar effect as cruciferous vegetables in the liver (indole-3-carbinol) with no goitrogenic effects.

An extremely hardy plant, it grows well in a pot or the garden so you can grab some and add it to potatoes or roast veg, or even just keep some sprigs on the desk to smell!!

Round Up

Roundup is the brand name for Glyphosate, an herbicide used readily since the 70s.

Theory has it that this herbicide, that is sprayed onto many crops, is actually the real cause of gluten issues and intolerances, not so much the grain itself. It is also implicated in many diseases including thyroid cancers.

There is a growing evidence of its dangers, and I noticed in the last year or so that the council workers that drive around spraying verges with this herbicide actually now have a warning on the back of their trucks stating they are using it.

If you have it in your garden shed, it might be time to get rid of it.

S

Social Media

This is a blessing and a curse.

I didn't jump on the whole Facebook bandwagon until I decided to have an online business, and to be honest, if I thought I could be successful without it I would be the first to hit "Deactivate".

Having said that, the connections I have made and people I have met and become close friends with even though we have never met face to face is heart warming and mind boggling.

The big problem for us as thyroid patients though is that there can be a lot of differing information. One person says this, another says that. It becomes so confusing.

Another downside of social media can be finding yourself in a downward spiral of despair, and complaining and typing "...why me, it isn't fair, nobody understands..." in any thyroid thread you can find. And that really gets you nowhere sorry.

I am very careful on Thyroid School to keep things upbeat and, while having a little moan is encouraged, so is picking yourself up, brushing yourself off and finding a solution.

Staying stuck in "Why Me" is just a distraction from doing the real work (wink wink).... so maybe social media is not your best friend or a great research tool when it comes to thyroid health.

Sacral Chakra

Located in the centre of the trunk just above the navel.

- ☐ Governing color - orange
- ☐ Key Issues - Relationships, addictions
- ☐ Body System - Genitourinary
- ☐ Endocrine Gland - Adrenals
- ☐ Crystals - Fire opal, carnelian, emerald, moonstone, aquamarine
- ☐ Aromatherapy - Sandalwood, Jasmine, Rose Oil, Ylang-Ylang, Champaca

Salicylates

A group of chemicals found in foods and products that people often have a sensitive too.

Anything we eat or use on our body that our body disagrees with will cause inflammation and an immune response. It is part of our thyroid responsibility to figure out what our body likes or doesn't like.

Salicylate sensitivity symptoms may look like:

- ☐ Headaches
- ☐ Anxiety, Panic Attacks, Behavioural issues
- ☐ Joint Pain, Muscle cramps and tremors
- ☐ Inflammation
- ☐ Fluid retention
- ☐ Digestive issues
- ☐ Mouth ulcers

Salicylates are found in A LOT of food so if we think we have a sensitivity, then trying an elimination diet would be worthwhile. Remove the group of foods for a minimum of 4 weeks, and then introduce them back in, while recording any reactions.

This is not an extensive list but it is the main offenders.

- ☐ Aspirin
- ☐ Peppermint tea
- ☐ All forms of black tea
- ☐ Wine & Champagne (sorry)
- ☐ Commercial toothpastes & soaps
- ☐ Peppermints & Chewing gum
- ☐ Almost all herbs & spices

- ☐ Almonds & Peanuts
- ☐ Apricots & plums
- ☐ Rockmelon, Pineapple, Oranges, Berries, Dates
- ☐ Tomatoes, Peppers, Zucchini (courgette) & mushrooms
- ☐ Chips & crackers
- ☐ Worcestershire sauce

Salivary Hormone Test

A test done by spitting into a vial, often up to 4 times a day to test cortisol levels and other hormones that fluctuate.

More accurate than blood testing as it gives an overall picture or pattern.

Many integrative doctors and naturopaths offer them

Salt

Craving salty foods is part of adrenal issues and Adrenal issues are part of thyroid problems.

So we need salt. Over the years, though we have been bombarded with the messages that we must avoid salt, which then upsets our electrolyte balance and adrenal health.

The problem has not been salt, but the kind of salt.

White Table Salt & Iodised salt

These are really of no help to us nutritionally or for our thyroid. Anything synthetic like this is going to eventually cause imbalances as our body requires a host of minerals and nutrients to be able to be absorbed.

Pink Salt

Pink salt - also known as Himalayan Salt contains almost 90 individual micronutrients. Sodium is just a portion of those nutrients. When we use pink salt, the micronutrients in it help us to absorb and use the sodium the way our bodies need to.

This is the salt I use and will continue to use.

Sea Salt

Another option for hypothyroid people, but perhaps not so much for the hyperthyroid people depending how much salt you tend to eat.

Sea salt (make sure you buy the dirty unprocessed one) is packed with iodine, but also full of other nutrients to help us absorb it.

However, due to the iodine content, it is wise to go gently gently, remember not enough can do the same as too much.

Salute the Sun

When I studied Naturopathy, one of my lecturers was a gorgeous Indian woman with a great figure!

I asked her one day what she did in the way of exercise and she said that she did Salutes to the Sun.

I knew about this yoga sequence but was confused as to how she used it for exercise.

She told me she did 6 sequences slowly followed by 6 sequences fast every single morning.

I gave it a go and wow it knocks it out of you! There are many videos on Youtube showing how to do this sequence and it is achievable for any size or fitness level.

Apart from the exercise component, this sequence also:

- Improves digestion
- Improves kidney function
- Boosts Immunity
- Improves flexibility
- Improves blood circulation and heart health
- Promotes weight loss
- Encourages emotional stability
- Tones muscles

SAMe

S-adenosyl-methionine (that's why it is called SAMe) is a nutrient that plays a part in Methylation and therefore mental health. It is only found in supplement form and facilitates:

- synthesis of adrenaline, creatine, Coenzyme Q10 and glutathione
- methylates DNA
- protects, enhances and regulates cell growth

It is used therapeutically in the following:

- □ alcohol toxicity,
- □ ageing, arthritis, depression, anxiety
- □ Parkinson's Disease, Down's Syndrome, fibromyalgia
- □ fatty liver, liver cancer, hepatitis, cirrhosis

Schilling Test

A test to determine a person's ability to absorb Vitamin B12. It is used in patients with chronic Vitamin B12 deficiency.

Schisandra

An herb used to help with liver detoxification, liver damage, fatigue, physical stress and to help improve physical and mental performance.

It has Hepatoprotective, antioxidant, adaptogenic, nervine, antitussive and antidepressant qualities.

Scleroderma

An autoimmune disease that causes the hardening of connective tissue in the body. Symptoms include hard thickened skin, cold fingers, small red spots on the face and chest, swollen joints, swelling, heartburn, diarrhoea, weight loss. A skin biopsy is required for diagnosis in most cases.

Sea Vegetables

Sea Vegetables include things like Kelp, Nori, Dulse, Wakame, and Agar.

While the thyroid absolutely needs iodine for health, the best way to get this is not through supplementation but through natural food sources.

The reason for this is that there are many other micronutrients in food that complement each other. When you just take a single mineral it is easy to have too much of it.

So if you ingest your iodine from a source like sea vegetables you will get the iodine but you will also get Vitamins A & C, manganese, Vitamins B1, B2, B3, B6, iron, zinc, protein, potassium, phosphorus and calcium. A much more well-rounded thyroid boost.

Homemade Sushi tonight?

Sedative

An agent used to calm the nervous system.

Examples Include: California Poppy, Chamomile, Hops, Kava, Lime Flowers, Passionflower, Peppermint, Valerian, Wild Cherry, Withania, Zizyphus

Selenium

Selenium is an extremely vital mineral that appears three times in the thyroid pathway.

Selenium is required for:

- ☐ Making T4 hormone
- ☐ Converting T4 to T3
- ☐ Down regulating RT3
- ☐ Joint Health
- ☐ Metabolism
- ☐ Autoimmune Disease
- ☐ Cancer
- ☐ Heart Disease
- ☐ Diabetes
- ☐ Increases Mercury excretion

Deficiency Symptoms of Selenium include:

- ☐ Arthritis
- ☐ Depression
- ☐ Hypothyroidism
- ☐ Infertility
- ☐ Liver damage
- ☐ Muscle pain and tenderness
- ☐ Early ageing
- ☐ Sleep apnoea
- ☐ Cognitive decline

Factors that contribute to Selenium deficiency:

- ☐ Alcohol
- ☐ Crohn's Disease
- ☐ High Cholesterol
- ☐ Pregnancy
- ☐ Smoking
- ☐ Vitamin C Deficiency
- ☐ Blocked by Mercury
- ☐ Blocked by Arsenic
- ☐ Blocked by Cadmium
- ☐ Blocked by Aluminium

Food sources of Selenium include:

- ☐ Alfalfa
- ☐ Brazil Nuts, Cashews & peanuts
- ☐ Crab, fish, tuna & oysters
- ☐ Eggs
- ☐ Celery, garlic, onions

Daily Requirements of Selenium:

- ☐ Adults - 50-200 ug
- ☐ Toxicity - <2 mg

Self Examination

There is a quick way of checking your thyroid for any lumps or bumps.

It is simply a matter of taking some water in your mouth and as you swallow it look in the mirror. The action will highlight anything unusual.

Do this regularly and you will always know what your thyroid looks like and be alerted straight away if something is not right.

Serotonin

An inhibitory brain neurotransmitter, serotonin is our happy hormone, but it does more than just make us happy.

It plays a vital role in appetite regulation, gut health, migraines, and pain perception.

To make serotonin our brain needs tryptophan which is an amino acid. But then we need to convert the tryptophan into 5-hydroxytryptophan for it to be useful. This step requires:

- Iron - Lentils, spinach, sesame seeds, swiss chard
- Vitamin B3 - Tuna, chicken, turkey, salmon, brown rice
- Calcium - sardines, sesame seeds, spinach, beet greens
- Folate - Lentils, asparagus, spinach, legumes

Then once we have converted the 5-hydroxytryptophan, we can convert that into serotonin. For this step we need:

- Magnesium - Pumpkin seeds, swiss chard, sesame seeds
- Zinc - Lamb, beef, pumpkin seeds, sesame seeds, lentils, quinoa
- Vitamin C - Papaya, bell peppers, kiwi fruit, pineapple, citrus
- Vitamin B6 - Tuna, turkey, sweet potato, sunflower seeds, bananas

Considering we thyroid people tend to have deficiencies in many of these, is it any wonder we also struggle with depression and anxiety??

Sesame Seeds

These tiny little seeds that usually come on the top of white fluffy bread (put the bread down) but they are also a powerhouse of nutrients.

Just 1 oz (28g) of these little seeds contain the following:

- 9% of DV in Protein (thyroid pathway)
- 16% of DV in Dietary fibre (hormonal clearance, gut health)
- 15% of DV in Vitamin B1 (thyroid, hair, hyperthyroidism)
- 4% of DV in Vitamin B2 (thyroid pathway)
- 6% of DV in Vitamin B3 (mental health)
- 11% of DV in Vitamin B6 (mental health, progesterone)
- 7% of DV in Folate (mental health, reproduction)
- 28% of DV in Calcium (bones)
- 23% of DV in Iron (thyroid, fatigue, gut acid)
- 25% of DV in Magnesium (stress, sugar)
- 18% of DV in Phosphorus (liver, bones)
- 4% of DV in Potassium (thyroid, fatigue, fluid)

- ☐ 13% of DV in Zinc (thyroid, mental health, immunity, wound healing)
- ☐ 35% of DV in Copper (skin, nerves, collagen)
- ☐ 35% of DV in Manganese (thyroid pathway)
- ☐ 2% of DV in Selenium (thyroid pathway)
- ☐ They also contain a substance called sesamin which protects the liver and increases Vitamin E supplies.

All of these factors make them helpful for

- ☐ Osteoporosis
- ☐ Rheumatoid Arthritis
- ☐ Asthma
- ☐ Lowering blood pressure
- ☐ Migraines
- ☐ Sleep patterns in menopause
- ☐ Reducing PMS
- ☐ Colon Cell Health
- ☐ Lowers cholesterol (high in phytosterols)

So, it's time to get fancy and start sprinkling these little beauties on everything! Salads, Vegetables and meat all look a little nicer with sesame seeds sprinkled on top!

Shitake

Like the Reishi mushroom, shiitake is an immune modulator and antitumor and is useful to help through chemotherapy and radiotherapy.

It is a great mushroom to purchase (this one is easier to get fresh) instead of regular mushrooms for autoimmune disease, fibromyalgia, virus recovery, chronic fatigue, and chronic infections.

Shomon, Mary

Mary Shomon would be the original Thyroid Patient Advocate as far as my memory serves me.

Mary has great solid information about feeling well with thyroid disease and has published over a dozen books. The New York Times Best Selling Author is found at https://www.mary-shomon.com

Shoulder Stands

No, I can't do one either, but shoulder stands are considered the queen of yoga moves while the headstand is the king.

They are particularly good for the thyroid due to the pressure it is placed under while in this position.

Shoulder Stands help with:

- ☐ Regulates thyroid & parathyroid hormone secretion
- ☐ Hormone balancing
- ☐ Heart health
- ☐ Respiratory health
- ☐ Constipation
- ☐ Improved flexibility
- ☐ Increased strength
- ☐ Stimulating the throat Chakra (speaking your truth)
- ☐ Insomnia
- ☐ Increases the metabolism
- ☐ Tones muscles

This will be an ongoing tussle between me and my body!

Siberian Ginseng

This herb is also called Eleutherococcus which is how many herbalists refer to it... I'm sure it's just so they can say the name!

It helps with physical stress, fatigue, mental performance, concentration, mild depression and chronic immune deficiency.

The herb has an immune modulating affect and is considered an adaptogenic.

SIBO

Small Intestinal Bacterial Overgrowth

Silent thyroiditis

An acute illness occurring mostly in women after childbirth the presents as becoming hyperthyroid followed by hypothyroid and then returning to normal function.

Silicon

Silicon is a mineral that is now rather lacking in our soils, so it is easy to become deficient in it. It is required for:

- bone calcification
- connective tissue resilience
- stops cholesterol becoming plaque
- muscle contraction
- nerve transmission
- collagen integrity
- synthesis, growth quality of hair, skin, nails, mucus membranes, bones, cartilage and connective tissue

Factors that contribute to Silicon deficiency include:

- Ageing, growth
- arthritis, musculoskeletal pain, bone fractures, osteoporosis, Paget's Disease
- atherosclerosis, hypertension
- weak nails, hair loss, low estrogen

Daily Requirements of Silicon:

- Adults - 9-14 mg

Silver Fillings

See Dental Health

Sitting

There is a saying "Sitting is the new smoking".

We are not designed for sitting on our backsides for endless hours a day, yet we are all doing it. Generally we have to because we are working. I am doing it endlessly as I write this book.

Sitting is inflammatory though. And thyroid disease is an inflammatory disease. Anything we can do to reduce inflammation is something we must try.

I have a 3 drawer filing cabinet which I put my laptop on and it is a good height for me to stand and type, which is great when I don't need to refer to textbooks.

The times when I need to be at my desk for the extra space I set an alarm (in another room) every hour. That way I must get up to turn it off. I then spend 10 minutes doing some form of exercise.

I can jump on the rebounder, or ride the exercise bike, or lift some weights in my husbands gym, or go up and down the steps a few times.

There are also some really amazing "standing desks" available now that may work for you. Any way that you can, reduce the amount of time you spend inflaming your body further by getting up out of your chair.

Sinusitis

Sinusitis is linked to poor lymph circulation and it is quite common in Thyroid Disease I am finding, to have a buildup of toxic lymph fluid trying desperately to get out any orifice it can find.

So employing several of the lymphatic techniques available, such as rebounding, exercise, deep breathing and using a neti pot would be a great way to start clearing the congestion.

Keep in mind that your thyroid lies right in the firing line if your head and nose passages are full of toxic garbage. Removing it will help your thyroid to breathe again.

Herbs for acute (flared up) sinusitis include: Andrographis, Echinacea Root, elder Flower, Eyebright, Garlic, Horseradish, Ribwort and Thuja.

Herbs for chronic long term sinusitis include: Andrographis, Echinacea Root, Elder flower, eyebright, Garlic, Golden Rod, Golden seal, Ground Ivy, Horseradish, Propolis, and ribwort.

Sjogren's Syndrome

An immune disorder which presents as dry mouth and dry eyes. The immune system in this case is going after the cells that produce saliva and tears.

A definite link or correlation, mostly with hypothyroidism.

Skin

Not only does it absorb 60% of anything we put on it, but it also does so in 26 seconds!!!!!

Now that can be a good thing if we are using lovely essential oils or magnesium oil, or soaking in an epsom salt bath, but if we are using petroleum based commercial body creams and soaking in chemical laden bubble baths, then it is not such a good thing.

This is just a gentle reminder that anything we put on our skin, is going to be in our blood stream and into our cells quicker than the time it takes to put it on our skin!!

PUT THE COMMERCIAL SKIN CREAM DOWN!!!!!!!!

We need to love ourselves enough to make this small change. We can all find an alternative, no matter what our budget and it's a simple thing that can improve our thyroid health everyday.

Skin Brushing

Skin Brushing is the act of running a body brush (generally made of natural bristles) over the body in short regular stroking movements towards the heart, which is the direction of our lymph vessels.

It is said that skin brushing:

- ☐ Improves lymphatic flow
- ☐ Removes toxins
- ☐ Improves dry skin
- ☐ Reduces Cellulite
- ☐ Improve elimination channels
- ☐ Naturally exfoliates skin
- ☐ Improves circulation
- ☐ Encourages cell renewal of the skin
- ☐ Deters ingrown hairs
- ☐ Eliminates clogged pores
- ☐ Improve Energy

It is a great wake-me-up in the mornings and makes you feel like you have been for a quick run even if you haven't, but the trick to getting results is daily action.

I know when I am good at skin brushing every day, I never have to worry about dry skin and I always see a noticeable smoothing of my bumpy thighs!

Skin Tags

I have read many times that skin tags on the body are a sign of sugar imbalance and glucose intolerance.

I have asked on Thyroid School and have had differing responses, but thought you may find the information curious and interesting.

If anyone out there wants to count their skin tags, go on a sugar free diet for 6 months and count them again, I would love to know the outcome!

Slippery Elm

An herb that helps soothe the digestive system helping with peptic ulcers, reflux, ulcerative colitis, IBS, constipation, diarrhoea, diverticulosis, haemorrhoids, cleanse the colon, lower gut inflammation and boost weight loss.

It has demulcent, emollient and laxative properties.

Slippery elm is known as a mucilage (something that is like a soothing thick gel) It can be purchased it at most health food stores.

Smoothies

Smoothies are whole foods that have been blended into a thick drink.

They are NOT a juice! In case you haven't read the juice entry yet, here is a reminder:

Smoothies are Food - Juice is Medicine

Is one better than the other? NO.

They both have different uses and are champions in their own right.

Smoothies are a food because they still retain all their fibre, which kicks in our digestive process the moment we start to drink them.

Great for detoxing if you are not one to cope with a juice fast, it makes you feel fuller and less like you are on a diet. Also great as a recovery food because the process of breaking the cell wall in the blender has helped to partially digest the food, making it easier on the gut to complete the job.

Green smoothies (mostly green vegetables) have been used with great success by some people to lose massive amounts of weight, by simply drinking them at every meal instead of eating. It is very easy to end up drinking too many sugars, fats and calories when living off smoothies.

Thinking we are doing right by our health, dates, syrups, nuts and fats can quickly become the main portion of the smoothie which does not contribute to good health if they are consumed daily.

For a really good smoothie detox diet check out Jason Vale's Super Blend Me. It is a great, thoroughly researched and balanced set of recipes using smoothies that will help you avoid the traps of just throwing something together until it tastes good. It comes in App form that is very easy to follow and even prints out a grocery list for you.

Otherwise if you want to keep making your own, try to keep to a ratio of 80:20. 80% Vegetables and 20% nuts, fruits or added goodies.

Having said that, another use for a "not so healthy smoothie" is if you are struggling to wean yourself of milkshakes and ice cream. The following recipe is for a Chocolate Smoothie and may help you to change your taste buds. It is full of magnesium which also helps with cravings. So use this for transitioning or treats only, the rest of the time stick with the 80:20 rule for good health.

Chocolate Nut Smoothie

- ½ cup mixed nuts (I use Macadamia, Hazelnuts & Brazil nuts)
- 2 tablespoons Raw Cacao
- 1 Tablespoon Maca Powder
- 2 cups cold filtered water
- 1 frozen banana (freeze with skin off in chunks)
- 3 Medjool dates, pips removed
- Place all ingredients into a blender and whizz until smooth
- Alter the amount of water depending on the consistency you prefer.
- Lasts in the fridge for 3 days but fresh is always best!

Snow Peas

Snow Peas are also called mangetout depending on where we live and are extremely versatile, they can be thrown into salads, steamed lightly, used as a crudite, sliced open and stuffed with, well, stuff!

100g (around 4 oz) of snow peas contain:

- 6% of DV in Protein (thyroid pathway)
- 10% of DV in Dietary Fibre (hormones, gut health)
- 22% of DV of Vitamin A (Thyroid Pathway)

- ☐ 100% of DV of Vitamin C (thyroid pathway, Adrenal Health)
- ☐ 2% of DV of Vitamin E (Thyroid Pathway, antioxidant)
- ☐ 31% of DV of Vitamin K (Bone & blood)
- ☐ 10% of DV of Vitamin B1 (thyroid, hair, hyperthyroidism)
- ☐ 5% of DV of Vitamin B2 (Thyroid Pathway)
- ☐ 3% of DV of Vitamin B3 (mental Health)
- ☐ 7% of DV in Vitamin B5 (food conversion, energy)
- ☐ 8% of DV of Vitamin B6 (mental health, progesterone)
- ☐ 10% of DV of Folate (MTHFR & Liver)
- ☐ 12% of DV of Iron (fatigue, thyroid pathway)
- ☐ 4% of DV of calcium
- ☐ 6% of DV of magnesium (sugar & stress)
- ☐ 5% of DV in phosphorus (liver health)
- ☐ 6% of DV in potassium (thyroid health)
- ☐ 2% of DV in Zinc (wound healing)
- ☐ 12% of DV in Manganese
- ☐ 1% of DV in Selenium (thyroid pathway)
- ☐ It has a glycemic load of 3
- ☐ They are antioxidant, anti-inflammatory, support sugar regulation, promote heart health, and another perfect thyroid superfood!

Solar Plexus Chakra

Located between the navel and the bottom of the breast bone (sternum) it is the place we get nervous or feel funny when something isn't right.

- ☐ Governing colour - yellow
- ☐ Key Issues - Fear, power, anxiety
- ☐ Body System - Digestive system
- ☐ Endocrine Gland - Islets of Langerhans
- ☐ Crystals - topaz, yellow tourmaline, emerald, sapphire, citrine
- ☐ Aromatherapy - Clary sage, juniper, geranium

Solfeggio Frequencies

Solfeggio frequencies are chants used by Gregorian monks. The different frequencies the chants are sung in are said to have different healing abilities, the ultimate being to connect mankind back to source (God, Universe or whatever you prefer to call it).

The entire planet is in a constant state of vibration, which has a frequency. As humans we are around 60-70 Megahertz. Meat is around 2 MHz

I meditate to these often as it helps me to feel like I am addressing something specific. Plus I can find them all on Spotify so I have a playlist ready to choose from if I am feeling I need the help in any of these areas at any time.

- ☐ 174 Hz - Natural pain relief
- ☐ 285 Hz - Influence energy fields
- ☐ 396 Hz - Liberation of guilt and fear
- ☐ 417 Hz - Becoming unstuck and facilitating change
- ☐ 432 Hz - Natural frequency of the universe
- ☐ 528 Hz - Transformation, miracles and DNA repair
- ☐ 639 Hz - Relationships and Connection
- ☐ 741 Hz - Problem solving & expression
- ☐ 852 Hz - Awakening intuition
- ☐ 963 Hz - Awaken to our perfect state

174 Hz. A reliever of both physical and emotional pain by giving our body and organs a feeling of security, safety and love. A type of natural anaesthetic it helps our body to function normally, overcoming the pain it is experiencing.

285 Hz. As humans we are made up of energy. This frequency encourages our damaged cells to return to their original form, helping them to remember how they should be. Listening to this vibration helps to energise and refresh our body.

396 Hz. Used for balancing the Root Chakra, this frequency will help you achieve goals by overcoming the fear and guilt attached to them. Even deep seated guilt and fear that your conscious mind is not aware of can be calmed and let go of allowing peace and joy to take their place.

417Hz. Balancing the Sacral Chakra, this frequency removes negative energy from a situation, trauma, the body or environment which can keep you stuck in a pattern and resistant to change. This is a good one to play as you sleep, but can be used at any time.

432 Hz. Rudolf Steiner stated that music based on this frequency will support humanity on its way to spiritual freedom. The frequency of nature, 432 Hz helps us to ground and become more in-tune with the earth. If you live somewhere surrounded by traffic or industrial noise, this would be a good one to play in the background.

528 Hz. This is the vibration for the Solar Chakra and Om. It restores balance in the earth and raises your heart vibration to be at one with the earth. The frequency of health it improves longevity by repairing DNA, improving energy and encouraging clarity of mind. Many musicians working in the spiritual field use this frequency.

639 Hz. The frequency of Love and the Heart Chakra, this vibration helps to repair relationships and create harmony by improving communication and understanding of each other. Meditating to this vibration will help to fill you with positivity, tolerance, compassion and love.

741 Hz. The vibration for the thyroid as it is the frequency of the throat chakra. The throat chakra is about self expression and speaking our truth and is often dormant or blocked by the untruths we speak, not just to the world but to ourselves. This vibration helps with letting go of that by repelling negative feelings such as jealousy and anger, and becomes a protective shield to anything like this coming in. The frequency cleans the cells of toxins (of which the thyroid is a magnet) and encourages change to a simpler, healthier lifestyle with less toxins by helping you to see solutions through your intuition.

852 Hz. The frequency of the Third Eye it encourages you to see past illusions, hidden agendas and untruths. It is about awakening our intuition so that we can remember the spiritual order and communicate with spirit.

963 Hz. The frequency of the Crown Chakra this vibration helps to remind you of your perfect original state of light and being one with spirit.

Soy

I'm not going to get into the whole argument about soy. That's not what this book is about. Some people swear by it for their hormones, others find over time their thyroids have gotten worse from it.

I don't consume it apart from the occasional drizzle of soy sauce if I am eating potstickers because let's face it, that whole meal is less than thyroid friendly (80% rule remember?).

There is growing evidence to suggest soy milk is partly responsible for our children being too estrogenic (boys having man-boobs and girls getting their periods as young as 6) the other responsible part being xeno-estrogens.

There is a book called "Soy is not a Health Food" by Dr Kaayla Daniel which is worth reading with an open mind.

She says that Soy contributes to:

- malnutrition
- digestive distress
- immune system breakdown
- thyroid dysfunction
- cognitive decline
- infertility
- breast cancer
- heart disease
- brain damage
- kidney stones
- food allergies

I have not read the science or studies behind these, but you can make up your own mind about it, however if you have been eating or drinking soy religiously for many years and you're reading my book because you still don't feel well, then I lovingly suggest you trial going without it for a month or two. But do have your blood levels checked while you do this.

Sour Cream

Sour cream is a dairy product which really is not ideal in thyroid disease along with gluten and soy. I found though that although I didn't miss most other dairy foods, I struggled with sour cream for entertaining, making dips and so on.

I discovered raw sour cream many years ago and it is such a saviour when it comes to making a creamy treat that doesn't taste like "health food" if you know what I mean?

Most raw sour cream recipes online are made from cashews, which is a great idea if you struggle with mental health as they have prozac like qualities, but otherwise I use macadamia nuts because they have a blander flavour in the finished product making it more like sour cream.

On top of that macadamia nuts have the highest ratio of Omega 3 to Omega 6 which we want. We all get far too many Omega 6s as it is.

Raw Sour Cream Recipe

Ingredients:

- 1 cup raw macadamia nuts
- ½ cup water
- ¼ cup no flavour oil of choice
- 2 tablespoons Apple Cider Vinegar or lemon juice
- 1 teaspoon Onion Powder
- 1 teaspoon Herb Salt

Method:

- Place all ingredients in a high powered blender and blend until smooth and creamy
- Stores in the refrigerator for 1 week

Trust me when I say, this will change your world!

Spaghetti Squash

If you have not seen spaghetti squash, it is like a butternut pumpkin but once cooked the flesh pulls apart and looks exactly like strands of spaghetti.

It is extremely low in carbohydrates and is a great alternative to pasta if you are trying to cut back or looking for a healthy gluten free version.

Specific Carbohydrate Diet

A grain free dietary protocol that also removes sugar and lactose. Originally created for celiac it is also low in gluten. This makes it a fairly good starting protocol for thyroid people. The book can be purchased on Amazon.

Splenda

An artificial sugar substitute made with Sucralose (sucrose + 3 chloride atoms).

The problem here lies in the chloride atoms. Chloride is a halide on the periodic table and is in the same family as Iodide, Bromide and Fluoride.

Because Iodide is the lightest of these halides it can be displaced by the others. This means that where we have chloride in our body, it will take precedence over Iodide in the cells.

Now, since we need iodide for thyroid hormone production, you can see how ingesting chloride bromide and fluoride will upset our thyroid levels and production.

Apart from that, it is an artificial sugar which is being studied more and more for the dangers they pose to our health.

Side effects of regular use may include:

- ☐ Migraines
- ☐ Dizziness
- ☐ Acne
- ☐ Bloating
- ☐ Chest Pain
- ☐ Laxative effect
- ☐ Disturbs gut flora
- ☐ Lowers absorption of some medication
- ☐ Can lead to allergies
- ☐ Blurred Vision
- ☐ Weight Gain (kinda defeats the point with this one)

Statins

Pharmaceutical drugs that help to lower cholesterol.

Stevia

A natural sugar replacement miracle made from a plant that tastes sweeter than sugar and also improves sugar metabolism in the body. Readily available now in grocery stores.

Stress

After speaking to many thyroid people over the years I have found in most hyperthyroid cases that diagnoses was always preceded by an extreme amount of stress. Sometimes up to 12 months before, but there was always something.

Stress is implicated in pretty much every disease in one way or another, and thyroid disease is no different.

Emotional, mental and physical stress of any kind can increase our levels of RT3 in the body, which block our thyroid hormone T3 getting into the cells where we need it to feel well.

We will all respond differently to ways of reducing our own personal stress, but we have to never stop searching until we find what works for us. Our lives may very well depend on our ability to lower our stress levels.

Proven stress lowering techniques include:

- ☐ Breathing techniques
- ☐ Yoga
- ☐ Aromatherapy
- ☐ Music
- ☐ Exercise
- ☐ Get a Massage
- ☐ Get creative (paint, draw, make)
- ☐ Hugs
- ☐ Kissing your honey

Stroke

Following on from our entry on stress, did you know it makes our blood sticky? And since we are pretty much all under stress even if it is just the physical stress of having a chronic disease then our blood is going to be stickier than others which puts us at a higher risk of other diseases.

I read in a text book on cardiovascular disease not long ago that people with thyroid disease are at a 70% higher risk of getting CVD and having a stroke.

That made me sit up straight let me tell you! 70%? That's massive!! But it may explain why life insurance is twice the cost of my husbands even though he works in a high risk industry.

Even though it seems like bad news, I liked reading it, because it reminds me why my daily meditation is important. It reminds me why I prefer a lighter diet and it reminds me to remove the stuff in my life that may be causing me unnecessary stress.

St John's Wort

An herb that is taken for it's antidepressant qualities and is purchased readily off the shelf.

However, it has many contraindications including the contraceptive pill, digoxin, anticoagulants, methadone, HIV drugs, and cyclosporin so always discuss this herb with a professional.

St John's Wort when taken correctly can help with depression, anxiety, irritability, emotional stress, autoimmune disease, menopause symptoms, PMS, shingles, viruses, and insomnia.

It can take 4 weeks to have an affect on mental health.

St Mary's Thistle

An herb also known as Milk thistle or Silymarin it is used for liver health, hepatitis, fatty liver, gallstones, nausea, constipation, flatulence, bloating, type 2 diabetes, metabolic syndrome and heavy metal reduction.

It is said to be hepatoprotective, hepatic trophorestorative, an antioxidant and choleretic.

Sucrose

A sugar made up of 50% glucose and 50% fructose, cane sugar is the common table sugar in most households.

Sudorific

An agent which induces sweating in the body. Lack of sweat is common in people with hypothyroidism, so finding ways to increase it, particularly when trying to detox is helpful.

Herbs that induce sweating include: Black Walnut & Elder berries.

Sugar

We all know we shouldn't eat it, I don't really need to go into why do I? The only thing you should know is that when buying pre-packaged foods try and keep the sugar content under 5g per 100g and your body, pancreas and thyroid will thank you.

How about just a list of all the other sneaky names sugar goes by?

- ☐ Cane Sugar
- ☐ Cane juice
- ☐ Evaporated Cane juice
- ☐ Cane juice solids
- ☐ Cane juice crystals
- ☐ Agave Nectar
- ☐ Corn Syrup
- ☐ High Fructose corn Syrup
- ☐ Crystalline Fructose
- ☐ Fruit Sugar
- ☐ Fruit Juice concentrate
- ☐ D-fructofuranose
- ☐ D-arabino-hexulose
- ☐ Malt syrup
- ☐ Molasses
- ☐ Barley Malt
- ☐ Caramel
- ☐ Beet sugar
- ☐ Brown Sugar
- ☐ Raw Sugar
- ☐ Honey
- ☐ Golden Syrup
- ☐ Turbinado
- ☐ Dextrin
- ☐ Dextran
- ☐ Maltodextrin

Sulfation Pathway

The liver has many pathways down which it processes and recycles or neutralises different ingredients or toxins.

It is the sulfation pathway that is responsible for conversion of our thyroid hormone. It is also responsible for dealing with:

- ☐ excess cortisol
- ☐ food additives

- ☐ aspartame
- ☐ acetaminophen (paracetamol)
- ☐ environmental toxins
- ☐ xeno-estrogens
- ☐ flavonoids
- ☐ estrogen, progesterone, androgens
- ☐ and again thyroid hormones

To help this pathway run smoothly we need:

- ☐ sulphur
- ☐ methionine
- ☐ cysteine
- ☐ taurine
- ☐ glutathione
- ☐ N-acetylcysteine (NAC)
- ☐ Molybdenum
- ☐ Vitamin B12, Vitamin B9 (folate)
- ☐ Magnesium
- ☐ MSM
- ☐ SAMe

Inhibitors of this pathway include:

- ☐ NSAIDs - Non Steroidal Inflammatory drugs such as Aspirin
- ☐ Tartrazine - yellow food dye
- ☐ Molybdenum deficiency

Sunshine

We need sunshine to make us happy. But it also helps us make Vitamin D, which is actually a hormone.

The best way to encourage this is to expose your trunk to the sun for 15-20 mins in the middle of the day. Do not wipe off any sweat that it produces but rather let it soak back into the body.

Sweet Potato

Sweet Potato is an orange vegetable, and all orange fruits and vegetables have higher anti-inflammatory qualities which makes the great for us thyroid people.

But let's have a closer look at what the experts say is in 1 cup of Sweet potato:

- ☐ 8% of DV in Protein (thyroid pathway)
- ☐ 26% of DV in Fibre (Hormone & Colon Health)
- ☐ 769% of DV in Vitamin A (Thyroid Pathway)
- ☐ 65% of DV in Vitamin C (Adrenal Health)
- ☐ 7% of DV in Vitamin E (Thyroid Pathway)
- ☐ 6% of DV in Vitamin K (Blood & bones)
- ☐ 14% of DV in Vitamin B1 (Thyroid Health)
- ☐ 12% of DV in Vitamin B2 (Thyroid Pathway)
- ☐ 15% of DV in Vitamin B3 (mental health)
- ☐ 18% of DV in Vitamin B5 (food conversion, energy)
- ☐ 29% of DV in Vitamin B6 (mental health, progesterone)
- ☐ 8% of DV in Calcium (bones)
- ☐ 8% of DV in Iron (thyroid, fatigue, gut acid)
- ☐ 14% of DV in Magnesium (stress & sugar)
- ☐ 11% of DV in Phosphorus (Liver & bones)
- ☐ 27% of DV in Potassium (Thyroid Health)
- ☐ 4% of DV in Zinc (Healing & Immunity)
- ☐ 50% of DV in Manganese (Thyroid Pathway)
- ☐ 4% of DV in Iodine (Thyroid Pathway)
- ☐ 1% of DV in Selenium (Thyroid Pathway)

Because of this mix of micronutrients, they are helpful with nerve health, blood sugar regulation, inflammation and are loaded with antioxidants, are antifungal and antibacterial.

Swiss Chard

Also called Silverbeet, this leafy green vegetable is so good as a thyroid staple.

Just 1 cup of this leafy green a day will give you:

- ☐ 7% of DV in Protein (thyroid pathway)

- ☐ 15% of DV in Dietary Fibre (hormones, gut health)
- ☐ 214% of DV in Vitamin A (thyroid pathway, skin)
- ☐ 53% of DV in Vitamin C (thyroid pathway, adrenals)
- ☐ 17% of DV in Vitamin E (thyroid pathway, antioxidant
- ☐ 716% of DV in Vitamin K (blood, bones)
- ☐ 4% of DV in Vitamin B1 (thyroid, hair, hyperthyroidism)
- ☐ 9% of DV in Vitamin B2 (thyroid pathway)
- ☐ 3% of DV in Vitamin B3 (mental health)
- ☐ 7% of DV in Vitamin B6 (mental health, progesterone)
- ☐ 4% of DV in folate (mental health, MTHFR)
- ☐ 10% of DV in Calcium (bones)
- ☐ 22% of DV in Iron (thyroid, fatigue, gut acid)
- ☐ 28% of DV in Magnesium (stress, sugar)
- ☐ 6% of DV in Phosphorus (bones, liver)
- ☐ 27% of DV in Potassium (fluid, fatigue, thyroid)
- ☐ 13% of DV in Sodium (adrenals, electrolytes)
- ☐ 4% of DV in Zinc (immunity, thyroid, mental health, wound healing)
- ☐ 14% of DV in Copper (skin, collagen, nerves)
- ☐ 29% of DV in Manganese (thyroid pathway)
- ☐ 2% of DV in Selenium (thyroid pathway)
- ☐ Glycemic Load of 4

You know I always forget just how incredible this leafy green veg is until I type it again. Surely we can add 1 cup of this superfood a day shredded into our salad?

Sympathetic Nervous System

Our Sympathetic Nervous System (SNS) is the one that sends us into panic and anxiety. It's involved whenever we go into fight or flight or any of those stressful situations that have our hearts beating a little bit harder.

Synthroid

The brand name for a synthetic thyroxine (T4) replacement.

Systemic Lupus Erythematosus

See Lupus

T

Thyroid School

I had been out of Naturopathic College for a couple of years. I was working under the name online of Make Healthy Simple because that is a super power of mine!

At the time I didn't know much about URLs and SEO and operating an online business, but I was just beginning to learn that nobody googles the words "How do I make healthy simple" (seems logical right).

I wasn't sure what to do about it, so tucked it away in the back of my thyroid brain and got on with life.

One day when driving around a really tight bend not far from our home, I heard the words "Thyroid School" spoken aloud from the back seat.

I know this is a little woo woo for some, but this has happened to me a couple of times over the years and I have learned to trust it. And no, there was nobody sitting in the back seat.

And so it began. I let myself fall into the one thing I didn't think I could help people with because I hadn't completely healed myself of it.

Since then I have learned that I didn't need to be healed to help people who weren't as far along in their journey as I was and now I get to see faces light up when they understand a little something more about their own disease.

I couldn't ask for a better way to spend my life than helping people take up the fight and realise they are worth spending the effort on.

T3

Triiodothyronine (T3) is the active thyroid hormone needed to get into our cells and make us feel good.

Only a very small amount is produced by our thyroid, the rest has to be converted from T4 in our liver and gut.

T4

Also called Thyroxin, the inactive hormone produced by the thyroid. It needs to be converted into T3 before we can use it

Tachycardia

A fast heart rate, classified as over 100 beats a minute.

Technetium

An isotope used for thyroid scans

Teflon

Although this awful coating is starting to get a name for being not that good for us, it still exists in some cheaper non-stick fry pans plus on the bases of irons.

Non-stick cookware and bakeware are coated with a chemical coating that once heated up imparts its vapour into the food.

Any chemicals are toxic to our thyroid, so this is something that we may be doing to harm our thyroid up to 3 times a day!!

I have switched to using baked enamel cookware which were very expensive and on layby for about a year (thanks to a very understanding kitchen store) but they are soooo worth it. They are going to be around forever - my son will get them!

Tendonitis

Tendonitis is simply an inflammation of a tendon. I was working as a cake decorator when I experienced tendonitis for the first time.

Shooting pains began running up and down my left arm making me believe I was having a heart attack. After a night in the ER, and a visit to my chiropractor I learned that the extremely repetitive nature of cake decorating coupled with inflammation inducing thyroid disease had given me this awful experience.

Also referred to as "Tennis Elbow" or "Swimmers shoulder" and it must be rested from any normal repetitive activities to heal.

I have learned as the years go by that whenever my body has become too inflamed, it will always result in those same shooting pains up my left arm and since that is a frightening thing I avoid it at all costs.

Curcumin is the active ingredient in Turmeric and is something that I take every day. If I am going to be doing anything that is harder on my joints, then I will take two a day. It keeps the pain away better than anything else I have ever tried.

Tertroxin

Artificial T3 made by Sigma Pharmaceuticals (Australia)

Taken with thyroxine Best taken 3 x daily

Testosterone

A hormone that produces male characteristics and is key in the development of male reproductive tissues.

Signs of low testosterone include

- low sex drive
- low muscle mass, increased body fat
- erectile dysfunction, smaller testes
- hair loss, fatigue
- memory problems

Testosterone is also found in women in smaller amounts.

Tetraiodothyronine 5'deiodinase

An enzyme that removes one molecule of iodine from T4

T Helper Cells

Immune cells that help direct immune activity and response. There are two kinds:

T-Helper 1 (TH1)

TH1 dominance - an immune imbalance in which the TH1 pathway is over abundant or over active. TH1 is involved when an immediate (or timely) response is required for a specific organ.

Examples of TH1 dominance diseases include:

- ☐ celiac disease
- ☐ crohn's disease
- ☐ Grave's Disease
- ☐ Hashimoto's Thyroiditis
- ☐ Multiple Sclerosis
- ☐ PCOS
- ☐ Rheumatoid Arthritis
- ☐ Sjogren's Syndrome
- ☐ Type 1 Diabetes
- ☐ Vitiligo

Support for TH1 dominance:

- ☐ Astragalus
- ☐ Echinacea
- ☐ Licorice root extract
- ☐ Melissa officinalis (lemon balm)
- ☐ Maitake mushroom
- ☐ Pomegranate

T-Helper 2 (TH2)

TH2 Dominance - an immune imbalance in which the TH2 pathway is over abundant or overactive. TH2 is involved with a delayed immune response.

Examples of TH2 Dominant diseases are:

- ☐ Allergies
- ☐ Asthma
- ☐ cancer
- ☐ Chronic Fatigue Syndrome
- ☐ Dermatitis
- ☐ Eczema
- ☐ Inflammatory Bowel Disease
- ☐ Lupus
- ☐ Sinusitis
- ☐ Ulcerative Colitis

Support for TH2 dominance:

- ☐ Pine Bark extract
- ☐ Grape seed Extract
- ☐ Green tea extract
- ☐ Resveratrol

T-Regulatory Cells

Immune cells that direct immune activity

T-Suppressor Cells

Immune cells that stop an immune reaction when necessary

The Good Goodbye

A book by Dr Gladys Ato that teaches how to let go of physical, mental and emotional traumas graciously and with love to allow for a new story.

Her words and teaching apply too many situations including saying goodbye to a loved one, a relationship, a habit or even a disease.

Stress has an enormous negative effect on the thyroid so navigating our way through such traumatic times in our life with grace and ease as an immediate impact on our thyroid health.

I also believe unless we are willing to let go of thyroid disease we will never be able to reverse our symptoms.

The Thyroid Secret

A great documentary/movie series by Izabella Wentz about reversing Hashimoto's Disease.

During the documentary Izabella interviews many experts about thyroid disease and shares her own journey.

Probably the best I have seen on Hashimoto's and hypothyroidism.

You can find more about the series at https://thyroidpharmacist.com

Throat Chakra

The throat chakra is located right where the thyroid is.

- Governing color - turquoise
- Key issues - self expression, speaking your truth
- Body system - Respiratory
- Endocrine Gland - thyroid and parathyroid
- Crystals - blue topaz, yellow topaz, sapphire, emerald, quartz, turquoise, chrysocolla
- Aromatherapy - lavender, chamomile, rosemary, thyme, sage

Thyme

Thyme is an acquired taste, like olives, avocado and coriander, but is worth the repeated effort.

The Medical Medium uses a thyme tea to help eradicate the virus in our body he says is the cause of thyroid disease.

It is not surprising it would be a virus killer as it is antibacterial, anti fungal, antimicrobial and an antioxidant. Because of these actions it is great for tummy bugs, diarrhoea, tonsillitis, gingivitis, bad breath, bronchitis, cold and flu.

Thyme is also an expectorant and spasmolytic so is useful in whooping cough, bronchial asthma, general coughs and stuffy noses.

Although I haven't tried it as a tea, I do add it to my steamed vegetables which I love and any salads I think it may match.

Thymus Gland

An endocrine gland located in the centre of the chest a few inches below the thyroid.

It is responsible for producing white blood cells to help the immune system fight off pathogens.

Thyroflex

A patented non-invasive testing method using reflexes, metabolic rate and symptoms to diagnose thyroid function.

Thyroglobulin

A protein involved in thyroid hormone production

Thyroidectomy

The removal of the thyroid gland.

Thyroid Antibodies

The soldiers that come out to fight when the thyroid is under attack.

Thyroid Binding Globulins

Proteins that transport thyroid hormones through the bloodstream to the cell receptor.

Thyroid Conversion

The process of converting inactive T4 into active T3 hormone.

- 70% of this happens in the livers sulfation pathway
- 20% happens in the gut
- 10% happens in other parts of the body

Thyroid Cysts

Lumps on the thyroid that are filled with fluid (nodules are filled with tissue).

Thyroid Dysgenesis

Congenital hypothyroidism can be caused by thyroid dysgenesis which results in a missing thyroid, an underdeveloped thyroid or ectopic thyroid.

Thyroid Eye Disease

Another name for Graves Orbitopathy

Thyroid Follicles

Small spheres of hormone producing cells within the thyroid gland.

Thyroid Hormone Resistance

Also called Refetoff Syndrome, this presents as elevated T4 and T3 levels but normal TSH.

Thyroid Lymphoma

A rare malignant tumour also called non-Hodgkin's lymphoma of the thyroid

Thyroid Remnant Ablation

The process of destroying leftover thyroid tissue after surgical removal.

Thyroglobulin Antibodies

(TGB Ab) Immune cells that indicate the immune system is attacking TGB in the thyroid gland

Thyroid Peroxidase

(TPO) An enzyme in the thyroid responsible for thyroid hormone production

Thyroid Peroxidase Antibodies

(TPO Ab) Immune cells that indicate the immune system is attacking TPO in the thyroid gland

Thyroid Receptors

The door that lets thyroid hormone into the cell. They can be found on almost every cell in the body.

Thyroid Stimulant

An agent used to increase the function of the thyroid for hypothyroidism.
Examples Include: Bacon, Bladderwrack

Thyroid Stimulating Hormone

TSH is Thyroid Stimulating Hormone. It is the messenger at the end of a feedback loop that tells our thyroid to either make more thyroid hormone or less.

Thyroid Stimulating Hormone Antagonist

An agent used to increase TSH levels, so works on the pituitary gland.
Example: Lemon Balm

Thyroid Storm

A life-threatening situation when hyperthyroidism is untreated or under-treated causing dangerous levels of blood pressure, temperature and heart rate.

Thyrotoxicosis

An excess of thyroid hormones flooding the body caused by nodules on the thyroid gland.

Thyrotropin Releasing Hormone

(TRH) A hormone sent from the hypothalamus to the pituitary gland to stimulate thyroid activity.

Thyroxine

The main thyroid hormone T4 (also the brand name of some synthetic T4 medications).

Tincture

A liquid herbal mixture generally made up by a qualified herbalist to drink at intervals throughout the day.

This type of natural remedy works quickly as the liquid goes directly into cells as opposed to tablets that go through the digestive process first.

The main issue with tinctures are the taste. I know myself that I don't get many clients who will stick to taking it as they generally taste awful! But they work well and quickly if you can manage the taste.

Tocotrienols

see Vitamin E

Toleman, Don

Referred to as the "Wholefood Medicine Man" Don has spent a lifetime researching whole foods and our connection to health. His light-hearted common sense approach to food and healing is easy and fun to listen to.

He is the author of The Farmacist Desk Reference books which are a must read.

You can find him at www.tolmanselfcare.com

Tonsils

Our tonsils are the lymphatic nodes that protect our thyroid.

Toothpaste

Changing my toothpaste was the first thing I ever did in my thyroid journey that made me realise I had a little control over my chronic disease.

I was 10 years or so into having hypothyroidism and had been on a dose of 250 mcg daily. It had never changed in all that time, and was what my body required to keep my TSH within range.

I was reading a health magazine one day when I saw an article about the possibility of fluoride causing thyroid problems. As I read on I decided that changing my toothpaste was really not that difficult so I went to the Health food store and purchased an herbal one.

I didn't think too much more about it until I had my blood tests and check up about 6-8 weeks after that. My doctor told me I had to lower my medication as I was taking too much.

So after 10 years of the same dose, 6 weeks of a non-fluoride toothpaste lowered my dose to 200 mcg daily for the first time.

Toxic Adenoma

A thyroid nodule that causes hyperthyroidism and produces extra hormone just from that nodule.

Toxic Multinodular Goitre

A goiter that causes hyperthyroidism and produces too much thyroid hormone.

Tremors

Hand tremors are a common symptom in hyperthyroidism and Graves Disease.

Triiodothyronine

The long name for T3 named for its Tyrosine and 3 molecules of iodine.

This is the active hormone that makes us feel well.

Truscott, Dana

The founder of the popular online blog Hypothyroid Mom, Dana shares in-depth articles and own personal story about thyroid disease and miscarriage and she doesn't shy away from the science and the controversy.

Tryptophan

An essential amino acid needed for:

- synthesis of Vitamin B3
- precursor of melatonin
- precursor of serotonin
- Reduces sweet cravings
- Reduces appetite

Symptoms of a deficiency include:

- anaemia, reduced plasma
- anxiety, depression, insomnia, poor concentration
- decreased serotonin & Vitamin B3
- pancreatic atrophy
- fatty liver, fibromyalgia

Therapeutically used for:

- aggression, anxiety, impulsiveness, depression, OCD, PMT, suicidal tendencies, violent behaviour,
- drug addiction, OCP use
- Down's Syndrome, fibromyalgia, IBD, Parkinson's Disease, ulcerative colitis
- hypertension, chronic pain relief
- appetite regulation, sugar cravings, stress

Food Sources of Tryptophan include:

- bananas, peanuts, legumes, lentils, oats
- pumpkin seeds, sunflower seeds, sesame seeds
- beef, dairy products, fish

Turmeric

This incredible rhizome will stain your fingers orange in a flash if using it fresh, but oh so worth it!

The studies about turmeric are growing rapidly and it seems to have so many applications that it is just worth learning how to make curry to be able to eat it every couple of days.

It is incredibly anti-inflammatory, which is amazing for osteoarthritis and rheumatoid arthritis, it lowers fat levels, is an antioxidant and is gaining traction for helping with digestion and gut issues such as Helicobacter.

Although it is excellent for helping detoxify both pathways in the liver, and is high in potassium which is great for the thyroid, I take it daily for my dodgy knee. As long as I take it, my knee will hold up under most exercises, walks, stairs or bike rides I choose to put it under.

The more it is studied, the more amazing things are being learned. Here is what we know about Turmeric so far:

- ☐ Anti-inflammatory
- ☐ Anti-oxidant
- ☐ Anti-depressant
- ☐ Anti - Stress
- ☐ Anti-microbial
- ☐ Anti-carcinogenic
- ☐ Improves peptic ulcers
- ☐ Improves osteoarthritis
- ☐ Improves arthritis
- ☐ Improves Liver detoxification
- ☐ Improves Asthma
- ☐ Cancer preventative
- ☐ Cardiovascular Disease preventative
- ☐ Alzheimer's Disease preventative
- ☐ Improves Cystic Fibrosis
- ☐ Improves high Cholesterol
- ☐ Improves Digestion
- ☐ Prevents Liver Disease
- ☐ Improves Allergies
- ☐ Improves Joint pain
- ☐ Reduces IBS symptoms
- ☐ Improves muscle regeneration
- ☐ Accelerates wound healing
- ☐ Prevents scar formation
- ☐ Improves psoriasis & scleroderma
- ☐ Improves dermatitis
- ☐ Reduces Blood Sugar in Type 2 Diabetes
- ☐ Extremely safe for long term use unless high potassium is an issue with any medications you are already taking.

From personal experience, my husband was having elbow pain from lifting weights, and curcumin (turmeric) completely took the pain away. If he stops taking it, the pain returns. The same for his mother who was having knee issues. The minute she stops it the pain comes back.

Tyrosine

Tyrosine is the T in all the T1-T2-T3-T4's
T = Tyrosine
3 or 4 = molecules of iodine

But we also need it in many other processes including:

- ☐ concentration, working memory, alertness (brain fatigue increases our demand for tyrosine)
- ☐ skin pigmentation
- ☐ synthesis of dopamine, noradrenaline, adrenaline
- ☐ regulate blood pressure

One really high source of Tyrosine is Peanuts. How many of us are addicted to Peanut Butter?

I have discovered the more I ask clients and people online the peanut butter thing is very common, so I personally think that tyrosine is the connection.

Good sources of tyrosine for thyroid people include:

- ☐ 100g Lean beef = 158% RDI
- ☐ 100g Pork chops = 140% RDI
- ☐ 100g Salmon = 132% RDI
- ☐ 100g Prawns = 84% RDI
- ☐ 100g Turkey Breast = 106% RDI
- ☐ 100g peanuts = 31% RDI
- ☐ 100g Pumpkin Seeds = 125% RDI
- ☐ 1 cup adzuki Beans = 59% RDI
- ☐ 1 cup lentils = 55% RDI
- ☐ 1 cup chickpeas = 41% RDI
- ☐ 1 cup raw oats = 102% RDI

So the interesting thing is that peanuts aren't really that high in comparison to others on the list.

Either way, it seems that if we are going through times of brain fatigue, brain fog or anything tough on our brains then upping our amounts of any of these foods (the ones that agree with us that is) is probably a great idea!

Most thyroid specific supplements also contain tyrosine.

U

Underestimate

I have a little sticky note on my computer screen as I write this. It says "NEVER UNDERESTIMATE YOURSELF KYLIE"

And yes it is in all caps like that too!

We forget what we are capable of sometimes. And even more so when we are struggling with chronic disease.

But let's give ourselves a pat on the back because often we are holding down jobs, running around after the kids, trying to have a social life when all we want to be doing is hiding under the covers and sleeping our lives away.

We achieve so much despite our fatigue, our confusion, our crappy memory, our extra weight, our racing hearts and our compiling fears.

If there is a dream you want to achieve, I believe you are better placed to do it then someone who doesn't have thyroid disease. Why? Because you already achieve so much despite your crappy symptoms!

So go get your sticky notes and write one for yourself. Stick it wherever you need to, and NEVER underestimate yourself ok?

Ulcers

Mouth ulcers are irritating and can be quite painful. They occur when a bit of tissue lining the inside of the mouth becomes damaged.

Generally harmless and quick to heal, if they are a common occurrence it may point to a deficiency in folate and/or choline.

Rinsing in saltwater (Himalayan or Sea Salt) or ionic silver may help to speed up recovery.

Ultrasound Scan

When I was first diagnosed with thyroid disease, I was sent for an ultrasound scan of my neck.

This was done to make sure there were no other abnormalities that may have been causing my lowered thyroid function such as cysts, nodules or tumors.

Ureas

Made from a combination of ammonia and carbonic acid, urea is a common ingredient in Pump soap.

It is also found in

- Hand and body lotions
- Hair products including shampoo, conditioner, styling products.
- Acne treatments
- Anti-ageing creams
- After Shave
- Some makeup such as foundation, mascara and lip balms
- Nail polishes

The reason we need to avoid this chemical is because it causes skin irritations such as dermatitis, joint pain, can interfere with heart regularity, reproductive problems, allergic reactions, weakens the immune system and it releases formaldehyde (a carcinogen).

It is listed in different ways on the ingredients panel so it may be called one of the following:

- Diazolidinyl urea
- DMDM hydantoin
- Imidazolidinyl urea
- Sodium hydroxymethylglycinate

Urinary Antiseptic

An agent used to inhibit a Urinary Tract Infection.

Examples include: Bearberry, Buchu, Juniper, Meadowsweet, Shepherd's Purse

Urinary Demulcent

An agent used to soothe & flush out the urinary tract during an infection.

Examples Include: Corn Silk, Couch Grass

Urinary Tract Infection

Urinary Tract Infections or UTIs seem to be a common issue with Thyroid People as they can be brought on by fluctuations in hormone levels.

I don't get them very often (every few years maybe) but there is a type of "First Aid" I use for myself and clients which has great success.

I don't think it would work as quickly if I didn't implement the whole strategy, so if you are a regular sufferer of these ghastly events then see an herbalist and always have the following on hand.

Here are the steps:

1. Alkalise! The first step is to flush your body with alkaline liquids to relieve the pain when going to the loo. That's what URAL does. But Lemon Water or even Green juice will do the job and give nutrients at the same time. For anyone that still thinks lemons are acid forming - that is only outside the body. Inside the body they form an alkaline ash and do the same thing as URAL does.
2. 1000mg Vitamin C every 2 hours
3. Zinc Tablet (30mg) once daily
4. Herbs! There is an herb called Barberry which actually dissolves the hook on the end of the particular strain of bacteria which is what causes the pain. Barberry mixed with a couple of other diuretic forming herbs such as corn silk and buchu taken 6 times a day, knocking it on its head pretty much the same day if you are vigilant about taking everything on the list the minute you suspect one is coming on.

The liquid herbs taste ghastly - not going to lie - BUT it is much nicer than dealing with the discomfort of a full blown UTI.

V

Vaccines

I am not going to go down the rabbit hole of this very controversial topic. However it is here to remind us that in all vaccines are ingredients that can harm the thyroid.

There is always a heavy metal (generally aluminium these days, but in the past mercury) to aggravate the immune system along with other interesting ingredients like formaldehyde.

We can't always avoid vaccines, but as long as we know what we are subjecting our bodies to we can make an informed decision about having it.

When I went to India last year, yes I had the suggested shots AND I took the Malaria tablets. It is totally down to personal choice here. Just know what you are having and perhaps implement the appropriate chelating agents afterwards.

Vaginal Dryness

The most common cause of vaginal dryness is a change in hormones, particularly a drop in estrogen levels which is the hormone that keeps the vaginal walls lubricated.

Other causes include:

- Douching (particularly if using a lot of chemicals)
- Medications (antidepressants, cold and flu medians and antihistamines)
- Sjögren's syndrome (an autoimmune disorder)
- Chlorine products, swimming pools etc

As it is generally around the estrogen levels, then estrogen creams or tablets may be prescribed.

Vaginitis

An inflammation of the vagina that causes bad odour, itching, pain, discharge and painful sex, vaginitis is often caused by bacteria (an infection), antibiotics, poor diet, chemical products such as lubricants, tight clothing but can also be caused by a change in hormones such as reduced estrogen.

A doctor would need to ascertain the cause and type so that the correct treatment can be used. Although I'm not a fan of cortisone creams and the like which is one of the methods of treatment, I know how uncomfortable this can be, so do whatever you need to make it end quickly, then address the underlying cause once you feel better.

Vagus Nerve

This important nerve is directly linked to our parasympathetic nervous system (the rest and reset part of our nervous system), so this is the nerve that we need to calm when we are feeling anxious or stressed. It also helps regulate our inflammation levels, immune response and hunger.

It is important that your conversion of T4 to T3 is optimal as it is the T3 that helps protect our myelin.

Ways to calm the Vagus Nerve include:

- ☐ Optimise thyroid conversion
- ☐ Splashing the face with cold water or even a cold shower. (why we feel refreshed after jumping into a cold pool or ocean)
- ☐ Breathing exercises
- ☐ Box Breathing (inhale for 4, hold for 4, exhale for 4, hold for 4 Repeat as long as necessary)
- ☐ Magnesium
- ☐ Improve Gut health
- ☐ Improve the myelin on your nerves by reducing sugar, alcohol and bad sleep and increasing good fats, vitamin C, iodine, zinc, and exercise.

Vale, Jason

Known as The Juice Master, Jason is an author, speaker and coach and has developed many programs around juicing and blending for weight loss and health.

An advocate of rebounding he has many videos online, along with his juicing videos.

Jason's apps are brilliant if you want to have a go at a juice fast as it even prints out shopping lists which makes it really easy.

If juicing seems a bit tough to start then his blending programs may help you as they have thousands of others.

Vanadium

A little known micronutrient, vanadium is required in our thyroid pathway for healthy function.

Deficiency symptoms in humans is not known.

Vanadium is required for:

- Iodine metabolism to make T4
- Balancing blood sugar
- Improves amino acid absorption in muscles

Food sources of Vanadium include:

- Black Pepper
- Chicken Fat
- Dill seeds & Linseeds
- Corn
- Mushrooms
- Parsley
- Shellfish & Seafood

Daily Requirements of Vanadium:

- Adults - 13 - 30 ug

Varicose Veins

Enlarged veins, mostly in the legs, caused by pressure on the legs such as obesity, extended periods of standing, constipation and pregnancy.

Although generally a cosmetic concern, if they become painful it is time to address the issue, particularly if they start to itch, change colour or begin to throb.

Although they can be common in hypothyroid patients due to inactivity and extra weight, they are not directly linked.

Ways to improve varicose veins include:

- Low impact exercise such as bicycling or swimming
- Losing weight (I know, this ones tough!)
- Not sitting or standing for long periods. Constant movement where possible
- Inversion tables or just putting your feet up regularly to improve circulation
- Skin Brushing to improve circulation
- Compression stockings if you must stand on your feet all day would be a good investment.

Vegan Diet

A vegan diet is one that removes all food that came from an animal. This includes:

- Dairy - milk, ice cream, cheese, sour cream etc
- Meats - lamb, beef, chicken, turkey, duck, offal etc
- Fish & Seafood - prawns, fish, crab, lobster, roe etc
- Honey - this is controversial but many vegans will not eat honey as it belongs to the bees
- Gelatine - as it comes from bones
- Protein Powder - made from whey
- Eggs - of any animal

When trying to decide if an eating regime is good for you it needs to be trialed for at least 4 weeks before making a decision.

This is because you will experience some form of detox and your body will need to adjust. If you only try it for a few days and then give up because you feel awful, you will never know if it really would have helped you.

Vegetarian Diet

Vegetarians will eat products from animals but not animals directly.

So for example they will eat:

- Eggs

- Dairy - milk, cheese, ice cream, yoghurt etc
- Honey

There are also different types of vegetarians:

- Pesco-vegetarians - will eat fish and seafood
- Lacto-vegetarians - will eat dairy, but not eggs
- Ovo-vegetarians - will eat eggs but not dairy
- Semi-vegetarians - will eat eggs, dairy and white meat from animals (no red meat)

Vertigo

The first time I experienced vertigo was the day after I had a colonoscopy. I sailed through the procedure, even with the surgeon bringing me out of the anaesthetic early (at my request) so that I could see the last part on the screen. I'm weird like that.

The next morning I woke up and stretched. I heard a strange click and then the whole room began to spin. It was so bad I ended up vomiting while trying to stay still as any movement made it worse.

My husband took me to the ER because we were concerned it was something to do with the previous days procedure.

As it happened, I was seen by a doctor who had just done a course on BPPV which is a type of vertigo caused by a crystal becoming loose in the ear canal upsetting equilibrium, and he knew that was what I was suffering from. He also knew how to fix it.

After an injection for the nausea and vomiting and giving me something called an Epley Manoeuvre, I was sent home.

I have had it about 3-4 times since then and I have now discovered for me personally it is a mechanical issue. By that I mean my neck is out of alignment.

If my neck is out of alignment and I am inflamed, those things will then set me off.

A possible cause of vertigo is Meneire's disease and is common in thyroid people, where there is a build up of mucous and pressure in the ear, nose and throat.

Possible other causes of Vertigo:

- Medical Medium says it is a symptom of the Epstein Barr Virus growing.
- Manganese deficiency
- Excess Copper

Very Low Calorie Diet

VLCD's are classified as less than 800 calories a day which are generally the Shake diets that are on the market.

Very low calorie diets are not the best option for thyroid sufferers because a very low calorie diet lowers the production of T3 thyroid hormone and increases the stress hormone RT3.

I spoke to a young lady on Instagram once as she had lost a lot of weight after having a gastric sleeve. She had hash tagged thyroid disease so I messaged her to ask if her thyroid had improved since having the operation. She told me that she didn't actually have thyroid issues until after she began losing weight. Since this kind of procedure automatically puts you on a VLCD, it is another example of it not being the best option if trying to reverse thyroid issues.

Vitiligo

A skin disease which presents as patches of white all over the body as skin colour is lost in those patches.

A common condition found in thyroid patients, patches generally start on the face around 20-30 years of age.

Although there is no known cure for vitiligo, since it is an autoimmune issue, working on calming down the immune system may be of help.

Visualisation

Visualisation is daydreaming on purpose.

It is digging deep into details and feeling how it would feel if you were actually doing the thing you are visualising.

Many athletes visualise their race or event many times over before hand and tests have shown that the areas in the brain that light up are the same whether it is actually happening or visualising with feeling.

Depending on your symptoms and where you are in your thyroid disease journey, visualising may be all you have available to you as a way to move forward.

Voice Hoarseness

This is a common symptom of thyroid disease because of the thyroid's proximity to the voice box. Any inflammation, or nodules will have a direct effect on the sound that is produced.

I remember when mine first changed, everybody would ask if I had a cold. When this went on for months eventually people realised this was my new voice.

Voice Therapy

There are a couple of ways to look at this.

Emotionally

Since the thyroid sits in the throat Chakra it is about speaking your truth, so any way of actually doing that is going to be beneficial.

It could be as simple as saying out loud what you are feeling. If you can say it out loud to someone you care about even better! It is said that saying an issue out loud to someone else lessens the stress around it by 50% even if no solution was reached.

Physically

Singing out loud at the top of your lungs is a great idea here... or even singing lessons! That is definitely on my to-do list.

The act of singing helps to tone and exercise our throat and vocal chords and as a knock on effect the thyroid.

Plus singing is just fun right? Anything fun improves the thyroid by reducing stress!

Vulnerary

Something used to hasten the healing of wounds.

Examples Include: calendula, Chamomile, Comfrey, Dan Shen, Echinacea Root, Golden Seal, Gotu Kola, Myrrh, Propolis, St John's Wort, Yarrow

W

Woman

During the process of thyroid disease and the 27 years I have had it, I slowly forgot how to be a woman.

Clothing was about what made me look slimmer.

No makeup because of the chemicals

High heels just hurt, so I said to everyone I was more of a sneaker girl.

My nails were brittle and broken.

I had no energy to do the things that girls love to do. Dance. Sing.

It was so easy to blame everything on thyroid disease.

Because frankly I just didn't have the energy to find solutions for these issues.

But I find myself now with a grown up son and reconnecting with my husband in a new way as so many empty nesters before me have done.

It started with an incredible lingerie shop that I was surprised to find stocked my size (Honey Birdette - You're Welcome - wink wink). Suddenly I felt sexy, and pretty and hope. Yes I felt hope that I could feel like a woman again.

That led to making the effort to have my nails done in low toxic varnish, and organic hair color to cover my greys.

And ... if you were to show up unannounced right now at my front door you would find me wearing my activewear (so that I can exercise in spurts to counteract long hours sitting here writing this book) and a pair of heels! Yup! While nobody is home, I am walking around in heels all day so that I can get used to them again. And I can't even tell you how feminine I feel just doing that small thing.

I am ready to be a woman again... and boy are you going to hear me roar...

Walker, Norman Dr

The original juicer, Dr Norman Walker lived to the age of 99 and advocated the use of juicing as medicine.

After retreating to a farm in France to recover from a breakdown in his early 50s he watched his host peel a carrot and noticing the juice that was on the peel he hypothesised about drinking the juice of a carrot, thereby taking the medicinal qualities straight into his cells.

He began by running the carrots through a feed grinder and squeezing the pulp in a tea towel to extract the juice.

Drinking the juice saw him return to vibrant health, at which time he went about developing, what is still considered the best juicer on the market today, Norwalk, and spending the rest of his life advocating a diet rich in juices, fruits and vegetables.

Dr Walker wrote many books which are a gold mine of information if you are interested in juicing (I have all of them!)

Walnuts

An incredible powerhouse of nutrition the walnut are a tree nut and are well known as brain food.

They can help with

- ☐ Reducing inflammation
- ☐ Boosts immunity
- ☐ Heart health
- ☐ Weight management and metabolism
- ☐ Brain and bone health
- ☐ Sugar regulation and diabetes
- ☐ Sleep regulation
- ☐ Mood stabiliser
- ☐ Astringent qualities to help dry up excess fluid

In 1 cup of chopped walnuts we get:

- ☐ 36% of DV in Protein (thyroid pathway)
- ☐ 452% of DV in Omega 3s (mental health, joint health)

- ☐ 3% of DV in Vitamin C (thyroid pathway, adrenal, antioxidant, immunity)
- ☐ 4% of DV in Vitamin E (thyroid pathway)
- ☐ 4% of DV in Vitamin K (blood, bones)
- ☐ 27% of DV in Vitamin B1(thyroid health, hair health, hyperthyroidism)
- ☐ 10% of DV in Vitamin B2 (thyroid pathway)
- ☐ 7% of DV in Vitamin B3 (mental health)
- ☐ 7% of DV in Vitamin B5 (food conversion, energy)
- ☐ 31% of DV in Vitamin B6 (mental health)
- ☐ 29% of DV in Folate (MTHFR conversion, liver health)
- ☐ 11% of DV in Calcium (bones)
- ☐ 19% of DV in Iron (thyroid pathway, fatigue)
- ☐ 46% of DV in Magnesium (stress, sugar)
- ☐ 40% of DV in Phosphorus (liver health, bone health)
- ☐ 15% of DV in Potassium (thyroid, fluid, fatigue)
- ☐ 24% of DV in Zinc (thyroid, healing, mental health)
- ☐ 93% of DV in Copper (skin, nerves, bones, collagen)
- ☐ 200% of DV in Manganese (thyroid pathway)
- ☐ 8% of DV in Selenium (thyroid pathway)

Like anything, too much of a good thing can become a bad thing, so while the nutrients may help with weight loss, if you overdo it, then it will help with weight gain instead. Balance in everything ok?

Water

We all know that we must drink water to survive right?

Thyroid people need it even more.

We need water to get our thyroid hormone to where it needs to be.

Proper hydration may allow many people to lower their medication needs because they are actually getting it into our cells.

If you never drink water, work with your practitioner, because you may need to track your levels and lower your medication needs when you increase your hydration.

Tap Water

Depending on where you live, you may need to filter your water, or it will add to your thyroid problems instead of improving them.

In some cities there is chlorine and fluoride added to the water supply, both of which block iodine. Plus it often comes through copper pipes which can cause an excess of copper in the body.

Find out what is happening to your water before deciding on what kind of filter you require.

Tank Water

I have heard many times people say they drink the cleanest water because they have tank water, so therefore rain water. I never disagreed.

Until I attended a seminar on hair analysis where I learned about what tank water actually contains.

Our rain water falls onto the roof, which is often covered in bird faeces, dust, pollutants from roads and factories nearby, it then runs down the roof collecting these as it goes and then into the gutters. Generally our gutters can be rusty and mouldy, so the water then collects little particles of heavy metals and mould as it continues into the tank where it can sit for long periods of time.

If you drink tank water... get a filter!

Bottled Water

This presents with its own problems since many plastic bottles contain xeno-estrogens which mess with our hormones. If possible use your own filter and purchase safe reusable bottles in glass or stainless steel.

Flavoured Water

If you are not a fan of plain water (please make sure it's fluoride and chloride free water) try flavouring it with pieces of fruit or slices of citrus. I keep ice cube trays of lemon juice in my freezer and either add hot or cold water to a cube depending on the weather.

Another favourite of mine is cucumber and orange - sounds really odd but the taste is sensational!!

Water Chestnuts

If you have not tried water chestnuts you may not have eaten much Asian food. They are a light crisp bulb that grows in waterways or paddy fields and are great in stir-fries.

They are an aquatic vegetable, not a nut as the name suggests, and is the bulb of a type of grass that grows in marshy areas.

100g of water chestnuts gives us:

- 7% of DV in Vitamin C (thyroid pathway, adrenals)
- 6% of DV in Vitamin E (thyroid pathway)
- 9% of DV in Vitamin B1 (thyroid, hair, hyperthyroidism)
- 12% of DV in Vitamin B2 (thyroid pathway)
- 5% of DV in Vitamin B3 (mental health)
- 5% of DV in Vitamin B5 (food conversion, energy production)
- 16% of DV in Vitamin B6 (mental health)
- 4% of DV in Folate (MTHFR, liver health)
- 5% of DV in Magnesium (stress, sugar)
- 6% of DV in Phosphorus (bones, liver)
- 17% of DV in Potassium (thyroid, fatigue, fluid)
- 3% of DV in Zinc (thyroid, immune, mental health)
- 16% of DV in Copper (skin, nerves, bones)
- 17% of DV in Manganese (thyroid pathway)
- 1% of DV in Selenium (thyroid pathway)
- 12% of DV in Dietary Fibre (hormone clearance, gut health)
- 3% of DV in Protein (thyroid pathway)
- 74% water content
- Glycemic Load of 9

This means that these amazing little balls are:

- High in antioxidants (disease reducing)
- Helps lower Blood Pressure
- Reduce the risk of heart disease
- Encourage weight loss
- Supports healthy digestion

If you are interested in Ayurveda, these calm the pitta dosha and are a natural diuretic.

Watercress

Watercress is a cruciferous vegetable which contains goitrogens. This chemical can produce goiters and may interfere with thyroid hormone production by blocking iodine. If you choose to eat these foods for all of the other health giving benefits, be sure you are eating an iodine rich diet also. During my research, all articles stated that watercress was high in iodine itself, however I could not find any definitive amounts recorded.

Recent research suggests, that once cooked, goitrogen chemicals are no longer present in food. While this may be true, it is always wise to test foods over a period of time with blood tests before and after to see if they have had any detrimental or positive effects on thyroid function.

That said, watercress has an amazing lineup of nutrients, so it is worth trying. I make it (occasionally) into soup with potatoes and chicken stock and it is so good!

Studies done on watercress has shown:

- ☐ It has anti-cancer properties
- ☐ Can reduce blood triglyceride levels by 10%
- ☐ Can lower incidence of cataracts and macular degeneration
- ☐ May suppress breast cancer cell development
- ☐ May reduce the risk of colon cancer
- ☐ Is anti-inflammatory
- ☐ Lowers blood pressure
- ☐ Strengthens bones and teeth
- ☐ Improves skin, hair and nail health
- ☐ Reduces DNA damage

1 cup (34g) chopped watercress contains:

- ☐ 22% of DV in Vitamin A (thyroid pathway)
- ☐ 24% of DV in Vitamin C (thyroid pathway, adrenal health, antioxidant, immunity)
- ☐ 2% of DV in Vitamin D (bones, hormones)
- ☐ 106% of DV in Vitamin K (blood, bones)
- ☐ 2% of DV in Vitamin B1 (thyroid health, hair health, hyperthyroidism)
- ☐ 2% of DV in Vitamin B2 (thyroid pathway)
- ☐ 1% of DV in Vitamin B5 (food conversion, energy)
- ☐ 2% of DV in Vitamin B6 (mental health)
- ☐ 1% of DV in Folate (MTHFR, liver health)
- ☐ 4% of DV in Calcium (bone health)
- ☐ 2% of DV in Magnesium (stress, sugar)
- ☐ 2% of DV in Phosphorus (liver health, bone health)
- ☐ 3% of DV in Potassium (thyroid health, fluid retention, fatigue)
- ☐ 4% of DV in Manganese (thyroid pathway)

- ☐ 1% of DV in Dietary Fibre (hormone clearance, gut health)
- ☐ 2% of DV in Protein (thyroid pathway)
- ☐ 93% Water

Watercress, although full of nutrients should not be consumed long term in huge amounts, and should always be washed thoroughly as it is grown in waterways. If you have kidney disease or are pregnant, discuss it with your practitioner before adding it to your diet regularly.

Watermelon

Richer in lycopene than tomatoes and more bioavailable, the lovely watermelon is anti-inflammatory a great source of antioxidants and phytonutrients.

1 cup (150g) of diced fresh watermelon contains:

- ☐ 3% of DV in Vitamin B1 (Thyroid health)
- ☐ 2% of DV in Vitamin B2 (thyroid pathway)
- ☐ 2% of DV in Vitamin B3 (mental health)
- ☐ 3% of DV in Vitamin B6 (mental health)
- ☐ 5% of DV in Biotin (hair, skin, nails, sugar)
- ☐ 7% of DV in Folate (liver health, MTHFR)
- ☐ 3% of DV in Pantothenic Acid (hormones, stress, food conversion)
- ☐ 18% of DV in Vitamin A (thyroid pathway)
- ☐ 21% of DV in Vitamin C (thyroid pathway, adrenal health, Immune health)
- ☐ 7% of DV in Copper (skin, nerves)
- ☐ 2% of DV in Iron (thyroid pathway, fatigue)
- ☐ 4% of DV in Magnesium (stress, sugar)
- ☐ 3% of DV in Manganese (thyroid pathway)
- ☐ 3% of DV in Molybdenum (thyroid health, Wilson's disease)
- ☐ 2% of DV in Phosphorus (bone health, liver health)
- ☐ 5% of DV in Potassium (thyroid health, fluid retention, fatigue)
- ☐ 1% of DV in Selenium (thyroid pathway)
- ☐ 1% of DV in Zinc (thyroid health, mental health, immune, wound healing)
- ☐ 7% of DV in Protein (thyroid pathway)
- ☐ Glycemic Load of 3

This information adds up to some amazing benefits of eating watermelon which include:

- Hydrates the body
- Healthy digestive tract
- Promotes collagen growth
- Cancer prevention
- Soothes sore muscles
- Improves heart health
- The juice of watermelon flushes out the kidneys

And they are so easy to grow if you have space!

Weight Lifting

The act of resistance training or lifting weights builds muscle. More muscle means a higher metabolism which is why men seem to lose weight easier than women, they have a higher muscle ratio in their bodies.

When we want to lose weight we have a tendency to feel like we have to jog, ride, zumba or other cardio efforts to make it happen. Lifting weights will actually help the process much quicker. We still need cardio for our heart health, but weights will help our bodies change.

Add to the physical benefits, the psychological benefits of feeling strong and empowered, it has a carry over effect that helps us to improve other areas of our lives.

Weight Loss

For those with hypothyroidism (and a few with hyperthyroidism although not as common) weight loss is only second to fatigue as the symptom that is most wanted to be reversed.

Because it is incredibly hard for the impaired thyroid metabolism to speed up and lose weight, often protocols that promise quick weight loss are tried instead of a sensible longer term diet.

The thing about quick weight loss is the danger it poses. You see our fat cells are also our guardians. They hold onto and protect us from toxins, chemicals, hormones, heavy metals and other pathogens.

When we start losing weight, those pathogens and toxins are dumped into the bloodstream, which is why when we go on a detox diet we feel crappy for the first week or so.

If we lose a lot of weight quickly, we are dumping a HUGE amount of toxic rubbish into our bloodstream quicker than our compromised livers can deal with.

Here's where it gets scary.

There are many instances where women have discovered they have breast cancer after massive weight loss and have declared how grateful they were that they had lost the weight or they may never have found the lump.

Is it possible that the massive toxic dump caused the lump? Many health authorities believe so.

It is extremely important to put in place detox methods when losing large amounts of weight to help remove the lost toxins safely.

Wentz, Izabella

Known as the Thyroid Pharmacist, Izabella is an author, speaker and has made a film called The Thyroid Secret.

Her passion comes from her own battles with Hashimoto's Disease and that is the focus of her wisdom.

You can find her at https://thyroidpharmacist.com/

White Potato

People struggle with potato, and think it contributes to weight gain, but it is actually what we put on the potato or how we cook it that causes the issues.

In fact there are many cases now of people going on "potato only diets" for weight loss. Recently a guy in Australia ate nothing but spud's for a whole year and lost 50kg. No I don't recommend this, just a fun fact to illustrate that it is possibly what we put on the potato that is the problem.

Why do I love it for thyroid issues?

1 cup (173g or 1 medium) of baked potato gives us:

- 32% of DRI in Vitamin B6 (mental health)
- 26% of DRI in Potassium (thyroid health)
- 22% of DRI in Copper (be careful allergy people)

- ☐ 22% of DRI in Vitamin C (Adrenals)
- ☐ 19% of DRI in Manganese (thyroid health)
- ☐ 17% of DRI in Phosphorus (liver health)
- ☐ 15% of DRI in Vitamin B3 (mental health)
- ☐ 15% of DRI in Fibre (hormone clearance)
- ☐ 10% of DRI in Iron (thyroid pathway)
- ☐ 6% of DRI in Vitamin B2 (thyroid pathway)
- ☐ 12% of DRI in Folate (liver & MTHFR)
- ☐ 4% of DRI in Vitamin K (blood and bones)
- ☐ 3% of DRI in Calcium (bones)
- ☐ 12% of DRI in Magnesium (sugar & Stress)
- ☐ 6% of DRI in Zinc (healing & Hormones)
- ☐ 1% of DRI in Selenium (thyroid pathway)
- ☐ 1% of DRI in Omega 3s (mental health & so much more)
- ☐ Contains a small amount of ALL amino acids
- ☐ 9% of DRI in Protein
- ☐ They are astringent which means they dry up fluid in the body.

So this adds up to the experts saying this about potatoes:

- ☐ Lowers Blood pressure
- ☐ Builds cells
- ☐ Helps regulate the nervous system
- ☐ Helps make serotonin
- ☐ Helps make melatonin
- ☐ Cardiovascular protection
- ☐ Helps prevent strokes
- ☐ Contains cancer protease inhibitors (Potatoes are a main component of The Gerson Therapy which is often used for cancer)

So all of these wonderful benefits though are assuming we are not eating the potato dripping in butter or cheese, or fried to within an inch of its life.

Wilson's Disease

A rare disorder that causes an accumulation of copper in the liver and other organs.

It is generally diagnosed under the age of 35 and can be life threatening due to the copper not being eliminated as it should be.

Wilson's Disease is inherited and can cause liver cirrhosis, liver failure, neurological issues, kidney problems, blood problems and psychological problems such as depression, and bipolar.

Often confused with liver disease, Wilson's Disease is diagnosed via genetic testing and a liver biopsy.

If diagnosed, treatment includes zinc which prevents copper absorption, and chelating agents.

Wilson's Thyroid Syndrome

Also called Wilson's Temperature Syndrome, this issue is defined by a constant low body temperature and the inability or lowered ability to convert T4 (inactive hormone) into T3 (active hormone).

It is considered a mild form of hypothyroidism and is generally corrected by prescribing T3.

If this is an issue for you then correcting the thyroid pathway, particularly the conversion components is important.

Withania

Also known as Ashwagandha, this herb appears in almost every thyroid supplement. Although I think it's brilliant for thyroid people who don't take any medication, I would urge careful monitoring when using this herb if you are on medication as it can swing you into both hyper and hypo states which can make you feel awful.

I tend to use Rhodiola instead if taking thyroid medication of any kind.

Withania is used for anaemia, immune deficiency, fatigue, physical stress, convalescence, insomnia, osteoarthritis, fibromyalgia.

It is an adaptogen, a mild sedative, anti-inflammatory, immune modulating and anti-anaemic.

Wound Healing

The speed of which we heal from a cut or wound is affected by the nutrients we eat.

Thyroid patients often are low in zinc, which is one of our main wound healing micronutrients.

If you find you are an extremely slow healer, it may be worth talking to your practitioner about supplementing with zinc.

X

Xerox

Are you an exact copy of someone else on this planet?

Even if you are an identical twin, you will still have different bacteria in your gut, react differently, feel stress differently, have different likes and dislikes and often have different points of view.

Because we are not exact thyroid copies of other thyroid people, we should never assume that what others have done to heal themselves will work for us. We cannot follow a cookie cutter program and expect the same results as someone else.

First we must understand our own body, learn the thyroid language, be familiar with the Thyroid Pathway and only then can we choose a program that best suits us individually and tweak it as we go along.

It is pure madness to think if we follow somebody else's assembly instructions for their body that we can put back together our own body.

Do all of those programs work? Of course! They have worked for at the very least one person.... the person who designed it. Remember that when you are beating yourself up for not getting better on a cookie cutter program.

Xeno-estrogens

Xeno-estrogens are not hormones however they behave like they are. Also called estrogen mimics, there are many natural and artificial substances that fall into this category.

Considered the primary cause of estrogen dominance, consuming or using too many of these items will cause the body to think it has excess estrogen and it will act accordingly by interrupting hormone balance. Anything that causes hormone imbalance will cause thyroid imbalance.

I remember watching Gray's Anatomy years ago and hearing Izzy (yes that long ago) say that some shampoos were like a placenta in a bottle. That was the moment I really understood how bad some commercial hair and skin products really were.

Xeno-estrogens include:

- Commercially raised animal protein and dairy products
- Oral contraceptive Pill
- Hormone replacement therapy
- Disposable menstrual products
- Tap water (distilled water removes everything)
- Insecticides and pesticides
- Dryer Sheets
- Phthalates (soft plastics, takeaway coffee containers, plastic wraps)
- Parabens (shampoos, toothpastes, lotions, soaps)
- Soy protein and soy protein isolate
- Artificial additives (MSG, colours, flavours)
- Bisphenol-A BPA (plastics, plastic lining in some tinned foods)
- Don't store food in plastic containers
- Avoid perfumes - we even spray them directly onto our thyroid!

Effects of xeno-estrogens:

- Early puberty (girls getting their period at six, little boys developing man boobs)
- Early Menopause
- Man boobs (sorry, there is no other obvious way of saying that, but they occur from excess estrogens
- Infertility
- Erectile dysfunction and low testosterone
- Promote hormonal derived breast cancer

X-Rays

Most people are aware these days that X-rays can cause damage due to the radiation it provides, but repeated X-rays also increase the risk of thyroid cancer.

While we can't avoid them all the time, we can certainly mitigate some of them.

The dentist is a great example. Unless you have really damaged teeth, or there is another oral problem, you don't need mouth X-rays as often as they suggest.

I always put mine off every year until they really nag me, because I have good teeth with only 3 fillings from when I was really young. So unless something changes I will continue avoiding the X-ray (by the way, I don't have the fluoride treatment either).

If you must have the X-ray (be sensible and do it if you need to) then ask for a lead lined cover or blanket to place over your neck and thyroid so that it doesn't get zapped.

The same goes if you have had a broken bone or any other reason you need an xray, ask for the lead blanket to cover your thyroid. It takes only a minute to ask and them to get it, so don't feel bad about asking.

Xylitol

This sugar substitute is actually a naturally occurring alcohol found in plants.

It can be used the same as sugar 1:1 in all recipes and beverages.

What's great about xylitol?

- It tastes sweet like sugar
- It does not cause decay in the mouth
- Can reduce bacteria that causes ear infections
- Can be used in a neti pot to rinse out sinus passages (reduces symptoms more than saline)
- Reduces dry mouth issues
- Animal studies have shown improved fat metabolism when consuming xylitol
- Completely safe up to 50g a day for adults and 20g a day for children

The downsides are:

- Excessive amounts over long periods (a few years) may cause tumours
- May cause diarrhoea, gas and bloating
- Can be expensive

Y

Youthful

I felt like I lost the best part of my "adult youth" because all of my 20s and 30s were sucked into a thyroid world I didn't understand and made me feel less than.

It is only now that I am about to hit 50 I feel like I have the energy to be a 20 something.

At first I struggled with this, because I was wanting to do things and experience things that were not exactly for my age group. But now I have other thoughts about that and since many of you fall into my age bracket I thought I would share them.

I am really happy to be reliving my younger days. I have more money now so can do many of the things I wouldn't have been able to then. Our son is an adult, so I can try a few riskier things. I don't care as much now about what people think of me, so am happy to try things that may go against the norm.

Many people around us right now are thinking hubby and I are going through a mid-life crisis. But really, all we are doing is all the things we have ever wanted to do because now we have the money, don't have school fees to pay and don't need to find a babysitter.

If you feel like you have missed the "fun years" I beg you to take control of your health, learn the thyroid language through this Thyroid Encyclopedia, enrol in my Thyroid Pathway Course to understand your thyroid world, and let's get to having those fun years again shall we?

I'll be waiting for you.

Yeast Infection

An uncomfortable issue that causes the genital areas to become flooded with yeast organisms.

It causes itchiness, discomfort, irritation, and an odour and is also called vaginal candidiasis.

This often occurs when the body and gut are extremely out of balance, for example too much sugar has been consumed, or after a course of antibiotics but can also happen when removing sugar as the bad bacteria migrate to somewhere it can flourish. In the latter case it only lasts a day or two.

There are over the counter products to treat this if things get really intense, otherwise here are some natural options that may take a day or two longer but may be better for the body:

- Probiotics that contain GR-1 (Lactobacillus rhamnosus) and RC-14 (Lactobacillus reuteri) and SB (saccharomyces boulardii)
- 2 drops of tea tree oil (as long as you are not allergic) in 1 ounce of coconut oil, then soak in a tampon and insert. Change regularly
- Inserting plain yogurt vaginally
- Wear loose clothes of natural fibres
- Use plain soap such as Castile soap for cleaning
- Avoid perfumed products vaginally including soaking in bubble baths.

Yellow Dock

An herb used for dermatitis, psoriasis, chronic skin disorders, constipation, rheumatism, osteoarthritis, rheumatoid arthritis.

It is considered a mild laxative, cholagogue (discharge of bile) and depurative (purify & detoxifying).

Yellow Skin

Yellowing of the skin is common with thyroid disease. It may not be as obvious in many cases like malaria induced type yellow, but it is noticeable when compared to someone else with similar skin tone.

I first noticed it on myself in a photo with a friend of mine who had similar fair complexion. I thought it was the camera at first but realised my friend didn't look yellow. Looking at the palms of my hands showed that I had a distinct yellowing at the time.

After studying I discovered there were a few reasons this could be happening in thyroid disease:

- Hashimoto's people struggle to convert beta-carotene into Vitamin A
- Liver health is responsible for 70% of conversion of thyroid hormone
- Jaundice is common in hyperthyroidism

I no longer have the yellowing, so for me it was connected to liver health which I have cleaned up and continue to work on.

Yin Yoga

This was the first kind of yoga I ever tried a few years ago and it is a slow, stretching form of Yoga which is perfect for beginners and people who don't feel all that flexible.

Yin Yoga is a specific type of yoga which helps the lymphatic system, flexibility, the overstimulated mind and helps the connective tissues, tendons and ligaments because it holds stretches for long periods of time. Some even use it as a form of meditation.

Regular practice of this form of yoga is said to:

- Improve circulation
- Improve flexibility
- Reduce stress
- Reduce anxiety
- Improve joint health
- Calm the mind and body
- Regulates energy levels
- Reduce frequency of migraines
- Reduce TMJ pain

All these areas which are often weaknesses for thyroid people we can then feel better which in turn will help us want to do more.

Having excess weight, there are always yoga positions I cannot get into, but Yin Yoga is not a problem. It is non confronting and has a huge impact on the body. I was sore for days after trying it which completely surprised me.

Yogurt

While yogurt is considered a healthy food for gut flora it is also a dairy food, which means often people are intolerant or sensitive to it.

Particularly thyroid people who are trying to reduce antibody levels, dairy along with gluten and soy needs to be removed.

The other surprising thing about yogurt is that some of the low fat yogurts on offer can contain up to 11 teaspoons of sugar. This is because they trade the fat for sugar so it tastes good.

I guess the moral of the story here is, if you need to improve your gut flora, then perhaps a probiotic may be better for your overall health than a pot of yogurt.

Z

Zigzag

Healing never comes in a straight line. Ever.

There will be days you feel brilliant and days you feel like you're dying from nothing more that detox symptoms. On those days I keep in mind this quote by the late Charlotte Gerson:

Nobody ever died from healing.

Often when we are in the throws of detoxing because we are doing something different and scary it is easy to give up because of fear. But just remember, your body had to endure a lot to get where it is today and it has carefully hidden away all of the toxins and pathogens that it thought was unsafe. It is going to be rough letting go of them, there is no question about that.

That is where your bravery, courage and determination come in.

Zig when you need to zig and zag when you need to zag. Listen to your body and remember the most beautiful of scenic roads are the windiest.

Zinc

Zinc is an extremely important micronutrient for thyroid people and it is estimated nearly 50% of the population are deficient as it is no longer in our soils.

Zinc is required for:

- ☐ Production of T3
- ☐ Reducing thyroid antibodies
- ☐ Wound Healing

- ☐ Absorption of B-Vitamins
- ☐ Cellular immunity
- ☐ Improves insulin activity
- ☐ Cadmium excretion

Deficiency Symptoms of Zinc include:

- ☐ Stretch marks
- ☐ White spots on nails
- ☐ Picky eating
- ☐ Translucent fingernails
- ☐ Acne
- ☐ Alopecia
- ☐ Brittle nails
- ☐ Poor immunity
- ☐ Depression
- ☐ Dermatitis
- ☐ Slow wound healing
- ☐ Poor concentration and memory
- ☐ Poor vision
- ☐ Sleep issues
- ☐ Hair loss and early greying
- ☐ Low progesterone levels

Factors that contribute to Zinc deficiency:

- ☐ Mercury blocks Zinc
- ☐ Cadmium blocks Zinc
- ☐ High copper levels block Zinc
- ☐ Excess sweating loses zinc
- ☐ Pregnancy & breastfeeding consumes zinc
- ☐ Stress consumes zinc
- ☐ Diuretics & ACE inhibitors flushes out zinc
- ☐ Oral contraceptive Pill flushes out zinc
- ☐ HRT - hormone replacement therapy flushes zinc

Food sources of Zinc include:

- Oysters (highest source), seafood, beef, egg yolks
- Sunflower seeds, Pumpkin seeds
- Ginger, wholegrains, capscium

Daily Requirements of Zinc:

- Adult - 15mg or 0.2 mg/kg
- Lactation - 19mg

Zoodles

Noodles made out of zucchini (courgettes) made a life-changing appearance in carb free kitchens over a decade ago.

Now you can find zoodle makers in just about any kitchen store and the term zoodles are a blanket term for any kind of vegetable based noodle.

Zoodles made from carrots, sweet potatoes, zucchini, and many other vegetables have exploded into our kitchens and you don't need to buy a fancy zoodle maker if you don't want to - you can simply make pappardelle noodles by using your vegetable peeler and peeling off long thin pieces of the vegetable.

For a gluten free and dairy free pasta alternative try combining courgette Zoodles with bacon, onion, basil and raw sour cream for a creamy blissful treat.

Zizyphus

An herb used for anxiety, insomnia, emotional stress, night sweats, irritability, palpitations and hypertension.

It is considered a hypnotic, mild sedative, hypotensive and anxiolytic.

Use cautiously when severe diarrhoea is present.

Zucchini

We call them zucchini in Australia but in other places they are known as courgettes.

They are a forgotten vegetable, but they are great for many people because they don't have a really distinct flavour which means they can be hidden easily in lots of meals.

The reason I love them for thyroid disease is that 1 medium zucchini contains:

- ☐ 8% of DV in Vitamin A (thyroid pathway)
- ☐ 56% of DV in Vitamin C (adrenal health)
- ☐ 1% of DV in Vitamin E (thyroid pathway)
- ☐ 11% of DV in Vitamin K (blood and bones)
- ☐ 6% of DV in Vitamin B1 (thyroid health)
- ☐ 16% of DV in Vitamin B2 (thyroid pathway)
- ☐ 5% of DV in Vitamin B3 (mental health)
- ☐ 21% of DV in Vitamin B6 (mental health)
- ☐ 14% of DV in Folate (MTHFR)
- ☐ 3% of DV in calcium (bone health)
- ☐ 4% of DV in Iron (thyroid pathway, fatigue)
- ☐ 8% of DV in Magnesium (stress, sugar)
- ☐ 7% of DV in Phosphorus (liver health)
- ☐ 15% of DV in Potassium (thyroid health, fatigue)
- ☐ 1% of DV in Sodium (adrenals)
- ☐ 4% of DV in Zinc (immune system)
- ☐ 5% of DV in copper (skin, nerves)
- ☐ 17% of Manganese (thyroid pathway)
- ☐ 1% of DV in Selenium (thyroid pathway)
- ☐ 5% of DV in Protein (thyroid pathway)
- ☐ Glycemic Load of 3

You can turn zucchini into zoodles and replace spaghetti or fettuccine. I often make zucchini boats where I stuff them with a mix of other veg. And don't forget grating them into fritters or just steamed. So versatile and so full of many of the micronutrients thyroid people need.

About the Author

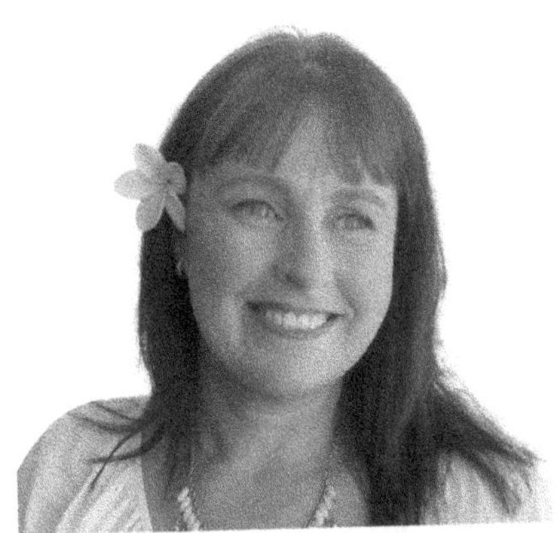

Kylie Wolfig is a qualified practicing Naturopath, Nutritionist, Herbalist, and author of four books about thyroid disease. She is the founder of Thyroid School, an online educational platform created to empower people with thyroid disease by demystifying the illness and inspiring them to take on the challenges by providing an extensive array of resources that ignites them to not just get well, but to knock thyroid disease out of the park!

Drawing from her personal 28-year journey living with thyroid disease and her professional experience, Kylie has helped over 12,000 people enjoy a better quality of life while dealing with the everyday challenges of the illness. She holds an Advanced Diploma in Naturopathy, Nutrition, and Western Herbal Medicine and is a member of the Australian Natural Therapists Association.

Kylie has been featured in Conscious Living magazine, Elephant Journal, Thrive Global, Everyday Health, and has also spoken at the Conscious Living Expo and Every Woman Expo.

Kylie lives in Perth, Australia, with her husband and beloved shoe collection.

www.ingramcontent.com/pod-product-compliance
Lightning Source LLC
Chambersburg PA
CBHW080555030426
42336CB00019B/3201